P9-BZH-345

Quality Management in Health Care
Principles and Methods

Second Edition

Donald E. Lighter, MD, MBA, FAAP
Director of The Institute for Healthcare Quality Research and Education
Clinical Associate Professor, University of Tennessee Medical Center
Professor, College of Business Administration,
University of Tennessee, Knoxville
Knoxville, Tennessee

Douglas C. Fair
Director of Statistical Applications
InfinityQS International, Inc., an SPC Software company
Manassas, Virginia

JONES AND BARTLETT PUBLISHERS
Sudbury, Massachusetts
BOSTON   TORONTO   LONDON   SINGAPORE

World Headquarters

Jones and Bartlett Publishers
40 Tall Pine Drive
Sudbury, MA 01776
978-443-5000
info@jbpub.com
www.jbpub.com

Jones and Bartlett Publishers
Canada
2406 Nikanna Road
Mississauga, ON L5C 2W6
CANADA

Jones and Bartlett Publishers
International
Barb House, Barb Mews
London W6 7PA
UK

Copyright © 2004 by Jones and Bartlett Publishers, Inc.

Library of Congress Cataloging-in-Publication Data

Lighter, Donald E.
    Quality management in health care : principles and methods /
Donald E. Lighter and Douglas C. Fair. — 2nd ed.
        p. cm.
    Rev. ed. of: Principles and methods of quality management in
health care / Donald E. Lighter, Douglas C. Fair. 2000.
    Includes bibliographical references and index.
    ISBN 0-7637-3218-4
    1. Medical care—Quality control. 2. Medical care—Quality
control—Statistical methods. 3. Medical care—United States
—Quality control.   I. Fair, Douglas C., 1964- . II. Lighter,
Donald E. Principles and methods of quality management in
health care. III. Title.
    [DNLM: 1. Quality Assurance, Health Care—organization &
administration. 2. Statistics—methods. 3. Total Quality
Management—methods.   W 84.1 L723q 2004]
RA399.A1L54 2004
362.1'0973—dc22

                                    2003023651

All rights reserved. No part of the material protected by this copyright notice may be reproduced or
utilized in any form, electronic or mechanical, including photocopying, recording, or any information
storage or retrieval system, without written permission from the copyright owner.

Production Credits:
Publisher: Michael Brown
Associate Editor: Chambers Moore
Production Manager: Amy Rose
Associate Production Editor: Renée Sekerak
Marketing Manager: Joy Stark-Vancs
Manufacturing and Inventory Coordinator: Amy Bacus
Composition: Bookwrights Inc.
Art Creation: Smolinski Studios
Cover Design: Kristin E. Ohlin
Printing and Binding: Malloy, Inc.
Cover Printing: Malloy, Inc.

Printed in the United States of America
08 07 06 05 04   10 9 8 7 6 5 4 3 2 1

Table of Contents

Contributors

Donald E. Lighter, MD, MBA, FAAP

Director of The Institute for Healthcare Quality Research and Education
Clinical Associate Professor University of Tennessee Medical Center
Professor College of Business Administration
University of Tennessee, Knoxville
Knoxville, Tennessee

Douglas C. Fair

Director of Statistical Applications at
InfinityQS International, Inc.
Manassas, VA

Neda Lewis, RN, CCM

Nashville, Tennessee

Sally A. Lighter, JD

Executive Director of The Institute for Healthcare Quality Research
and Education
Knoxville, Tennessee

Curtis P. McLaughlin, DBA

Professor Emeritus of Business Administration and Health Policy
and Administration
University of North Carolina
Chapel Hill, North Carolina

Foreword to the First Edition

Dr. Donald Lighter and Mr. Douglas Fair have written a very valuable book for the health care industry. They have argued persuasively that quality improvement (QI) is part of the solution to the crisis gripping the health care industry, and it is a solution that should be embraced by providers. The alternative to providers embracing the quality of delivered health care is that insurance companies will embrace quality as a strategy.

Other industries in the United States have undergone similar crises in the last few decades. Their costs have grown and their quality has suffered. In many of those manufacturing industries, the driving force has been international competition. Drs. Deming and Juran have repeatedly shown how delivered costs have declined due to systemic application of quality improvement principles in industry after industry. Now it is time for the health care industry to lower costs and improve delivered quality through systemic quality improvement.

Escalating costs and declining quality have been serious issues in the health care industry. However, the driving force has not been international competition. The driving forces have been much closer to home. Those forces have included a growing role for the government due to increased health care expenditures by the government, a growing role for insurance companies trying to control costs, and Internet-empowered patients who can benchmark the quality of care. Although the forces are different from the international competition driving quality improvement in manufacturing, the results are the same: quality improvement is needed to meet demands for quality while simultaneously reducing the cost of delivered health care. This is the solution the authors convincingly advocate in this book.

As we enter the new millennium, the term "managed care" has become synonymous with the pejorative term "managed cost." Many insurance companies and health maintenance organization (HMO) insurance plans have focused on controlling costs by denying care. Such firms are missing an historic opportunity to compete on the basis of quality. Who has ever said that they will accept lower quality health care if it is offered at a lower price? What hospital has been recognized for lowering the cost of delivered care by denying treatment? What physician has been recognized for denying or skimping on care and thereby lowering costs? Indeed, such health care strategies often deliver those physicians into litigation in a defenseless position. If insurance companies are missing an historic opportunity to compete on the basis of quality, then others should pick up the mantle of quality and compete on that basis. Quality in health care should be a natural fit for physicians and hospitals because quality is consistent with the Hippocratic oath and the reason why many entered the practice of medicine.

Consistent with the Hippocratic oath, this book shows physicians and other health care providers how to improve the quality of delivered care and simultaneously lower costs. Then, health care providers can rightly claim the high ground in the controversy surrounding the health care industry.

—Michael J. Stahl, PhD Program Director, Physician Executive MBA
Distinguished Professor of Management
College of Business The University of Tennessee, Knoxville
Knoxville, Tennessee

Foreword to the Second Edition

The last thirty years have witnessed a remarkable array of medical advances with equally impressive clinical outcomes. Chemotherapy has cured many with cancer; hip and knee replacements have brought mobility to the lame; in-vitro fertilization has made childless couples parents; and organ transplantation has realized a functional life for those who otherwise would have died. And yet, both the patients and their physicians are increasingly dissatisfied. Some suggest that this is a result of disparate expectations. Patients have health goals that may not be achievable. After all, certain diseases and death are not curable. Doctors know they can deliver far more than they are currently delivering. Lack of time and lack of insurance are just two of the many roadblocks. I would argue that for both patients and physicians, the major source of dissatisfaction is the obvious need for the entire health care system to improve its quality.

A precise definition of quality remains nebulous—indeed, all participants in the system view quality from their own perspectives. Nevertheless, the specifications of a quality health care system are being defined. Are therapies safe? Are they effective? Is their availability timely? Are clinical decisions based on the best available scientifically sound evidence with consideration of the physician's skills, the surgeon's skills, and the patient's values?

At first glance, such quality domains may not seem to be measurable. In realty, they are. Although information technology is lagging behind, the major obstacle to implementing quality improvement methodology and its associated statistical processes is psychological, not technological. Physicians have found it difficult to accept the tenets of process improvement for health care. Many health care providers recoil at the idea that all work is a process, whether it be in an industrial setting or in a hospital system and that, therefore, the principles of quality improvement can be successfully applied to the provision of health care. As with evidence-based medicine (another concept of interest but not of acceptance into clinical practice), physicians argue that the delivery of quality clinical care depends solely on experience and expertise. Thus, physicians and other health care providers come to believe that they are performing well. And yet, too many reports documenting a lack of access and the prevalence of medical errors suggest otherwise. Furthermore, the very thought of quality oversight of performance or of public reporting of results is, at best, met with opposition and, at worst, summarily rejected by the physician community.

The consequences of physician unwillingness to participate in data collection for either quality improvement or accountability are numerous. The government, the managed care industry, and large employers have come to agree that non-doctors should monitor physician performance and non-doctors should stimulate change in physician behavior—that it is non-doctors who are the only reliable advocates for quality. Managed care companies treat all physicians as essentially identical, whether a physician has been in practice for one year or two dozen, their care is considered the same. There is no premium awarded for better outcomes or for expertise.

The authors of this text not only successfully argue that statistical methods can be applied to improving the quality of our current health care system, but they also provide the tools necessary to do so. Kept in the forefront is the essential concept that providers, patients, payers, and policy makers are part of a single interacting system. No one part acts without affecting all the others. Doctors can certainly be the leaders and even set the agenda for restoring medicine's pre-eminent place in our society; but they cannot do it alone, nor can they believe that simply restoring physicians' autonomy and authority will solve the quality problem.

Health care providers can participate in quality improvement. They need not abandon the dual realities that, while such processes as length-of-stay can be shortened, they cannot shorten the time necessary for compassion, for healing, and for counseling. Furthermore, these two realities are not at odds. The public has come to recognize that their health care system is not performing as well as it could. They have embraced the idea of quality improvement and demanded its implementation.

What is Bastille Day? To many, it was the start of the French Revolution. Actually, it was the *end* of the French Revolution. The people of France had already changed their concept of government. The years that followed were simply the implementation of that change in thinking. American health care has reached its Bastille Day. Our society has changed its concept of health care. Quality is demanded. Now, it is all about implementation.

—Michael J. Goldberg, MD
Tufts-New England Medical Center
Boston, Massachusetts
February 2004

Preface

Efforts to improve health care performance are replete in health care today. Unfortunately, these efforts often mimic those of past generations of quality assurance committees and fail to encompass the true nature of the new paradigm. Quality improvement has been well accepted in American industry—indeed, in similar settings throughout the world—for over five decades, and the slow adoption of these principles and practices by the health care industry has led to cumbersome inefficiencies and intrusions by regulatory agencies, payers, and government. Fortunately, the trend has reversed, and many segments of the industry now are using newer methods of improving the quality of care and services while attenuating cost containment pressures from society.

The purpose of this book is to provide a foundation for the implementation of quality improvement activities for both providers and payers in the health care industry. Topics cover the breadth of quality improvement in the industry, concentrating on quantitative methods that can prove helpful in ensuring that quality improvement efforts are documented effectively. Topic areas include

- overview of the health care system and the need for quality improvement
- group processes for quality improvement
- process orientation: evaluation and management of work flow processes
- statistical process control: basic to advanced
- advanced statistical techniques for quality improvement
- clinical practice guidelines
- care management
- techniques for implementing quality improvement changes
- the legal and regulatory environment of health care
- the future of performance improvement in health care

Emphasis on the group process, including organizing people and corporate resources for quality improvement efforts, weaves through several chapters of the book because these efforts will usually be rewarded with great success. An attempt has also been made to provide readers with an overview of the health care industry that substantiates the need for quality improvement efforts. With the astronomical rises in health care costs in the United States in the 1970s and 1980s, numerous regulatory agencies arose to "control" costs. In the wake of those efforts, traditional quality assurance efforts have summarily failed to maintain an adequate level of care to suit American society, necessitating a shift to the quality improvement model. The first chapter details changes in society and the health care delivery system that have mandated the quality improvement movement in health care. Additionally, Chapter 11 describes the plethora of regulatory and accreditation organizations that have permanently changed the health care system.

Health care in the United States has been lauded for decades as the most sophisticated and effective in the world. In recent years, however, performance measures for the health care industry have indicated that the measured performance lags behind many other developed countries. Some measures, such as infant mortality rates, now are seriously below those of other major industrial countries that spend far less per capita on health care. It seems propitious that now it is time for us to adapt Deming's "new philosophy" of quality to the health care system by placing the customer first and demonstrating quality to our peers, payers, and the public. It is no longer sufficient to say that we are the best; we must also demonstrate our preeminence using the principles outlined in this book. Many health care organizations are fragmented, and workers are demoralized by developments in the industry over the past decade, making the need for adopting the quality framework even more acute. The most successful health care organizations in the world, just as in other industries, have incorporated the quality improvement philosophy into the culture of the organization. The tools in this book should help any organization achieve the goal of transforming its culture into one that provides value for all stakeholders.

The quality revolution has been fairly quiet so far, but it is growing in volume and pitch. Organizations such as the Foundation for Accountability, the Institute for Healthcare Improvement, the Institute for Healthcare Quality Research and Education, and many others around the United States are helping health care leaders move their organizations into the new paradigm. These efforts must stress the incorporation of the quality philosophy into organizational cultures; simply creating quality management departments that conduct annual projects will no longer suffice to achieve the goal of elevating the quality of health care services to the levels necessary in the new millennium. Rather, health care leaders must foster the adoption of quality improvement principles throughout their organizations in order to instill in all workers the drive to continually improve their work and the service that they provide the company's customers. Creating the environment in which this goal can be achieved is the prime task of every manager.

This book, then, is designed for students of health care quality, health care managers, and health professionals such as physicians and nurses who want to create environments in which quality can be measured and improved and where workers achieve self-actualization through job satisfaction. From the most elementary to the most sophisticated approaches to quality measurement and intervention, the book details the uses of quality improvement science to deal with the issues facing the health care delivery system today. Our hope is that, using these tools and collaborating in a true quality improvement environment created by health care industry leaders, the health care industry can increasingly demonstrate value for consumers and health care workers.

Acknowledgments

A project such as this could never have been accomplished without team-work. Just as we discuss in several of the chapters in the book, teams help produce some of the best quality results in nearly any endeavor. In particular, the authors would like to thank the people who have provided material for chapters in the book: Curtis McLaughlin, DBA, for his immeasurable help with the first chapter of the book and insight into the publishing process; Neda Lewis, RN, who contributed a great deal of information to Chapter 8 on clinical practice guidelines, based on her extensive experience in the health care quality improvement field; and Michael Stahl, PhD, who directs the Physician Executive MBA program at the University of Tennessee, for serving as a valuable mentor throughout the production process. Thanks also to the wonderful people at Lyle-Kearsley Systems, the makers of InfinityQS SPC software, which made development of the charts in this text a snap.

But one of the people who provided the greatest amount of help is Amy Lighter-Steill, a budding law student with a strong literary background, who painstakingly reviewed the entire manuscript for syntactic and rhetorical precision. Without her help, the book you have before you could never have been finished.

Mr. Stephen Wise, a good friend, has provided insightful counsel on statistical methods in the creation of this work and in so many years past. Two other good friends, David Sylwester, PhD, and Ray Phillippi, PhD, provided substantial insight into advanced statistical methods for quality improvement based on their collective expertise. They methodically reviewed the information on statistical approaches in quality improvement, adding significantly to the value of that information. Anyone knowing the rigorous approach taken by statisticians will quickly realize what an effort they made to ensure that the information presented in that chapter reflected current knowledge in the field.

The people who deserve our most heartfelt gratitude, however, are our wonderful families—Jody, Douglas, and Connor Fair and Sally, Marc, Megan, and Caitlin Lighter—who, through all of the travel, research, and late nights, have supported, encouraged, and uplifted us. Thank you for being our inspiration, our love, and our dearest friends.

Chapter 1

The Rationale for Quality Improvement in Health Care

DONALD E. LIGHTER
CURTIS P. McLAUGHLIN

◈ Introduction

During the last decade of the 20th century, the health care delivery system changed more than it had in the previous 30 years. Just the threat of increased incursion of the federal government into health care created conditions that have changed forever the way that physicians and institutions practice medicine. A strong consumer movement has created demands on the system at unprecedented levels at the same time that financial constraints from payers have peaked. Although the influence of managed care has waned in the first few years of the new millennium, pressure on health care revenues has reached a critical phase in both public and private sectors. In a reflection of the declining business cycle, employee benefit programs have shifted more of the cost of care to employees at a time when health care costs have resumed double-digit inflationary increases. Even with increased sophistication and technological advancement, the cost of care still far outstrips the perceived societal benefit. Cost containment in any economic system can lead to deterioration in the quality of a product or service, but payers and consumers have insisted that providers maintain quality while reducing costs; i.e., stakeholders are insisting on increased value in the health care delivery system.

The purpose of this book is to equip health care professionals with the understanding and tools necessary to evaluate and improve the quality of care. Starting with a review of the issues that presage the need for quality improvement and measurement, the book outlines a methodical path to improving performance in the health care environment. Chapters 2 through 7 address the group procedures, process analyses, and statistical techniques that form the foundation of quality management in medicine. Specific applications of these quality improvement methods are described in Chapters 8 through 10, where interventions like clinical practice guidelines and care management are described in depth. Finally, the legal implications of continuous quality improvement, as well as industry-tested methods of organizational improvement, are enumerated to provide an overview of issues that must be addressed during quality management activities to ensure compliance with applicable laws.

◆ Changing Health Care Environment

One of the major drivers of the quality improvement (QI) movement in the United States and in many other industrial economies throughout the world is the escalating cost of care seen over the past two or three decades. The most significant economic figures about the cost of health care in the United States relate to the growing share of our national wealth allocated to the health care industry. Health care expenditures rose 40-fold between 1960 and 1997. Even adjusted for the growth in the population and for price infla- tion, the actual or "real" per capita amount of goods and services produced in the health sector rose fourfold during that same period (Iglehart, 1999; Levit, et al., 1996). The share of the US gross domestic product devoted to health has risen from approximately 5% in 1960 to 14.1% in 2001 (Department of Health and Human Services, 1998). Until the late 1990s, when increases at- tenuated due to cost containment initiatives on the part of payers, price increases in the health sector were much greater than for the economy as a whole. Figure 1.1 illustrates the growth in health care expenditures as a per- centage of gross domestic product (GDP), and Figure 1.2 shows growth in health care expenditures in constant dollars and on a per capita basis. The figures indicate that national expenditures for health care have increased nearly fivefold in constant dollars from 1980 to 2001, and health care costs as a percentage of GDP have increased over 60% during that same time period. Although the rate of increase showed signs of attenuating in the 1990s, the long-term trend has resumed in the new millennium, i.e., health care costs have started to grow again relative to the national economy.

Some of this real growth has come from the aging of the population. The percentage of the population over 65 years of age grew from about 8% in 1950 to about 13% in 1995, and that percentage promises to grow in the new millennium (US Census Bureau, 1996). The elderly tend to be high con- sumers of health care, but much of the growth in expenditures is related to the increasing supply of providers and the sophistication of medical technol- ogy. There has been an explosion of medical science and clinical capabilities since the end of World War II, and funding these developments has been one of the greatest strains on the health care financing system.

At the same time that health care expenditures were rising at an alarm- ing rate, American industry was besieged by increasing international compe- tition from Japan, Europe, and growing economies in Latin America and the Far East. Formerly secure industries that produced automobiles and steel were enduring fierce waves of competition from these aggressive contenders, and the philosophy of "lean and mean" manufacturing became dominant in

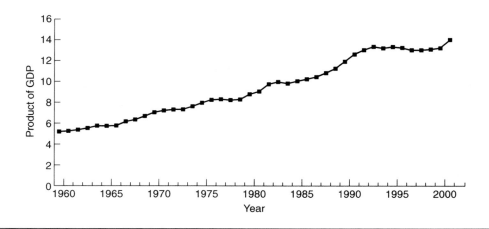

Figure 1.1 Growth of Health Care Expenditures as a Percentage of GDP

the 1960s and 1970s. American industry embarked on a massive effort to improve efficiency, with focus on just-in-time manufacturing, lean manufacturing, and (TQM) management. Because of expansive domestic demand for services, the health care industry did not face such pressures, so the techniques applied by American industry to reduce waste and improve productivity were not immediately recognized as applicable to the medical industry.

In the 1980s and 1990s, society also began to question the efficiency and effectiveness of the health care delivery system, highlighted by the fact that many other countries of the world spend significantly less per capita without any apparent differences in health outcomes such as infant mortality or male life expectancy and sometimes with even better performance in these areas. Studies of health care expenditures clarified the point that among developed nations there is little, if any, correlation between health care expenditure per capita and measures like male life expectancy or perinatal mortality (Phelps, 1997).

The use of insurance to pay for health care is a relatively recent phenomenon, and as the health insurance industry has matured, the cost of health care has become increasingly uncontrollable. The advent of Medicare and Medicaid in the 1960s heightened demand for medical services and exacerbated the upward pressure on costs, leading to a period of nearly unrestrained inflation in the health care sector (Keightley, 1993). Health insurers became reluctant middlemen in the system—society demanded curbs on costs that the health care delivery system was unable or unwilling to effect, so health insurers were thrust into the position of policing abuses and inappropriate utilization in the system. In such an imperfect system, consumers began to question the utility of the entire system, from the services they received in hospitals and doctors' offices to the decisions made by the insurance companies regarding the services deemed appropriate or inappropriate for funding.

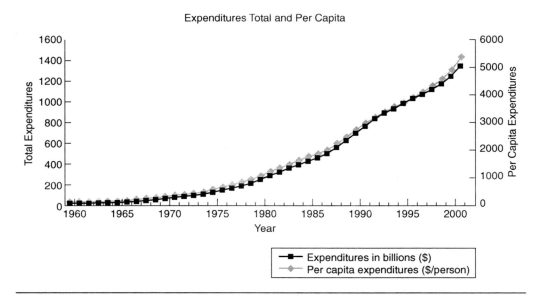

Figure 1.2 Health Costs in Total Expenditures and Expenditures Per Capita (Constant Dollars)

In response to these societal demands, the health care industry has begun to adapt the tenets of TQM to nearly every aspect of health services. Although techniques such as statistical process control and change management were readily adaptable to the business aspects of health care, these same methods have been more slowly accepted as being applicable to clinical medicine.

◆ Growth of QI in Health Care

In the 1980s American products such as automobiles began to lose out in world and domestic markets on the bases of both price and quality. American industry had become less competitive, especially with the Japanese, whose standard of living was rapidly improving at the same time. The success of the Japanese, using the concepts of American quality engineers such as Deming and Juran that were not yet popular in the United States, demonstrated the benefit of these approaches, and Japanese companies flooded US markets with goods that gradually encroached on the market share of American products. Belatedly, American manufacturers began to adopt this TQM or "Kaizen" approach. Not only did the Japanese adopt these American concepts, they began to develop their own embellishments and modifications following the work of Ishikawa, Taguchi, and others. In response, American industry embarked on a massive effort to improve efficiency, focusing on just-in-time manufacturing, lean manufacturing, and TQM (Bounds, et al., 1994). Much of this effort involved "discovering" the techniques of Japanese management—techniques that the Japanese had learned from leading American thinkers and consultants. These approaches involved a strategic commitment to QI and driving out waste by reducing variation (using a series of techniques that will be discussed later in this book) and employee empowerment to encourage the process to move ahead rapidly. By the mid-1990s, American manufacturers had regained their presence as formidable competitors, and the growth in the US trade deficit had slowed somewhat (Figure 1.3). However, one of the areas where they felt at a competitive disadvantage was in the relative cost of health care for their employees. Industry leaders began pointing to the cost of employee health benefits as a major competitive disadvantage in global markets. In response to aggressive efforts at cost containment, industry became concerned with the quality of care, leading to demands for quality measurement throughout the system. Health care administrators adopted TQM rather quickly, but clinicians have been slower to recognize the value of the approach for medical practice.

The pendulum of public perception swings frequently from demands for access to assurances of quality of care, furthering the acceptance of TQM in clinical health care. On one hand, the public desires unfettered access to providers of all types, but on the other hand, they seek guarantees that the quality of care that they receive is exceptional at every encounter. Consumerism in health care climaxed at the end of the 20th century, and the demands of the new paradigm are rapidly forcing the health care delivery system to implement QI methods to promote preventive care and improve access to appropriate services. For example, insurers can no longer simply serve as an intermediary that pays claims. The exigencies of the marketplace demand that insurers screen their networks of doctors and monitor hospitals for quality and access to care and then initiate efforts to improve any deficiencies that they find. QI projects have proliferated in the marketplace as inappropriate variation is identified and efforts are made to eliminate it throughout the system. These activities sometimes become the most important determinants of the resources and services available in a community, and providers have lost the influence that they once enjoyed in directing resource allocation. In fact, consumers and payers have become instrumental in shaping the health care environment based on QI activities that identify effective diagnosis and treatment modalities.

In addition to the rise of consumers and payers in determining resource allocation, other workers in the health care delivery system have become more influential in matching resources to customer needs. The idea that organizations should systematically and continuously improve their internal and external processes by involving workers as participants became popular in the United States in the 1970s and 1980s and, in health care, even later. The earlier model, often called Taylorism or "the one best way," called for management to design the process and then instruct the work force to use it without deviation (Taylor, 1911). It was a paternalistic approach in which the bulk of the workers were expected to check their brains in their lockers

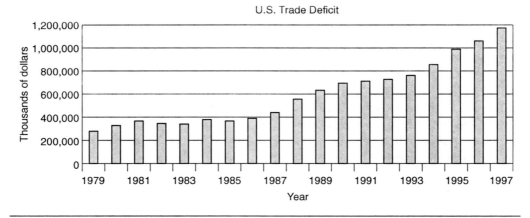

Figure 1.3 Historical Pattern of the U.S. Trade Deficit.

before coming to work. In the true spirit of continuous QI, many health care organizations in the United States have adopted methods and procedures that are beginning to tap the wealth of experience and information in the work force to promote new methods of solving age-old problems.

Health care did not quickly follow the precepts of TQM that had been adopted by American industry. Analysis of health records with statistical process control and QI methods languished until the introduction of diagnosis-related groups (DRGs) in the 1980s. Prior to the use of DRGs, coding of medical diagnostic and therapeutic interventions relied on the complex international classification of diseases (ICD), current procedural terminology (CPT), and health care procedure code systems (HCPCS) that often lacked the level of detail necessary for thorough analyses. Systems such as DRGs, designed by a group from Yale, and the ambulatory care groups designed by Starfield and associates (Johns Hopkins University School of Hygiene and Public Health, 1998), provided clustering of diagnoses and/or procedures that made statistical analyses more useful. Prior to these innovative methods of defining services, interorganizational or intraorganizational comparisons of cost or quality were fraught with inequities and discrepancies. The introduction of coding systems for product definition was one of the key factors that signaled the beginning of the end of health care as a cottage industry.

Once these measurements became more ubiquitous and acceptable, the primary payers in the American health care system, employers and their insurance intermediaries, began to question the efficiency of health care and to demand cost cutting as well as proof that value was being delivered. Just as they began to expect quality from their employees and suppliers, they increased the pressure on health care providers for changes in their ways of doing business. As the largest purchaser of health care in the United States, the federal government also sought optimum value in the care that they subsidized. Additionally, Medicare and Medicaid agencies insisted on lowered costs and more efficient utilization of services, cutting deeply into health industry revenues. The bargaining power of the federal government created discounts that not only exceeded those of other payers but also established lower payment levels that drove down revenues throughout the industry.

◆ ## Transition to Integrated Health Care Delivery Systems

The transition from cottage industry to integration has not been smooth for the health care industry. Boynton, Victor, and Pine (1993) have suggested that any industry moving out of the craft (or cottage industry) mode goes through a series of stages in which it successively refines and stabilizes its products and processes, moving first from craft (individual creator) toward mass production of the dominant product type. This stage is followed by process performance enhancement, then by efficient customization of that product or service through mass customization techniques. However, this sequence of stages was aborted in health care by the unwillingness of both providers and patients to accept mass-produced health care (McLaughlin and Kaluzny, 1997). Industrialization took place technically in the development of the large capital-intensive hospitals and integrated health care systems, but these alone did not necessarily bring about improvements in quality of care or costs. However, as these organizations matured, many observers realized the potential of continuous process improvement techniques in health care.

In spite of the cottage industry nature of the health care delivery system, medical technology advanced in giant leaps. Some examples:

◆ Plain x-rays were replaced by exceedingly more detailed imaging studies that could detect metabolic anomalies in addition to revealing underlying anatomic features.

◆ Surgeons adopted endoscopic surgical techniques that produced incredible improvements in the morbidity and mortality of surgical procedures.

◆ The pharmaceutical industry produced new drugs to improve the quality of life and reduce the cost of care, literally changing how medicine is practiced.

◆ Computer technology enhanced information transfer between providers, making consultation and team approaches to care easier to implement.

With each advance came new pressures to provide ever more sophisticated services to the public, and the costs of these new care modalities soared. In most other industries, improvements in technology decrease costs of production, but in health care, these improvements have only led to escalating demand and higher prices. Health care organizations were faced with large capital expenditures just to keep up with these technological "miracles." With societal pressures to reduce costs, physicians and hospitals were caught in a difficult bind that forced them to find ways of providing new technologies and services in more cost-effective ways. Other industries in the United States had already pioneered the means to achieve this capital efficiency, namely, mergers and acquisitions. Thus were born the ever-growing integrated medical delivery systems.

Insurers faced similar pressures. Employers insisted on cost containment but in most cases did not want to stand in the way of employees obtaining appropriate, necessary care. In response to their customers, health insurance plans devised managed care. Moving from traditional indemnity plans, insurers created preferred provider organizations (PPOs), which usually involved simple brokering arrangements between employers and providers for reduced rates. However, because PPOs provided little oversight or analysis of the health care that the system reimbursed, the limitations of PPOs in ensuring the quality of care soon became evident and led to the development of health maintenance organizations (HMOs) that not only negotiated better rates and shifted financial risk to providers, but also monitored the quality of care as provider incentives changed. At the end of the 20th century, HMOs and PPOs had become the predominant forms of insurance in the marketplace, and the demands for quality management burgeoned beyond anyone's expectations. In the new millennium, the marketplace backlash that fostered a decline in the popularity of managed care has led to increasing health care costs, with a subsequent search for effective methods of improving quality of care while attenuating costs.

◆ Delicate Balance Between Quality and Access

A number of forces have arisen to counterbalance the cost-cutting efforts of managed care organizations, including

- ◆ medical-legal pressures in response to increasing restrictions on access to care
- ◆ federal QI regulations promulgated by the Centers for Medicare and Medicaid Services (CMS; formerly the Health Care Financing Administration or HCFA)
- ◆ pressure from state and federal governments for managed care organizations to assist in funding medical education programs that languished as traditional governmental sources of funding disappeared

In spite of these influences, patient access to care and satisfaction sometimes suffered. Fragmented health care processes, the target of managed care organizations, persisted in handing patients off from department to department and specialist to specialist, with little thought given to the experience of the patient. Waiting times were long, patients had little say in their treatments, and no one seemed to own a process from beginning to end (Lathrop, 1993). Many processes of care had grown almost serendipitously, burdened with steps that had been introduced idiosyncratically or for reasons involving legal defensiveness or financial gain. Meanwhile, payers and board members of health care organizations began to demand the same attention to process improvement from health care providers that they expected from other suppliers. Federal and state program administrators, seeing very wide variation in the costs and outcomes of the care they were purchasing, began to insist on prospective reimbursement (case-based payment), putting hospitals at financial risk for excessive costs. Capitation and discounted fee-for-service contracts also brought the need for efficiency home to physicians, who found themselves implementing cost reduction by omitting or denying care. However, the acceptability of cost-cutting efforts and reduced access to care soon began to rest on the condition that quality was not markedly reduced.

As this process of industrializing health care has progressed, the concern for the QI aspects of this transition has become institutionalized. The Joint Commission for Accreditation of Healthcare Organizations has required that certified institutions have a QI process in place that goes beyond traditional quality assurance, introducing such QI tools as root cause analysis and failure mode and effects analysis. Congress has mandated that the CMS publish rudimentary report cards on selected costs and outcomes for physicians and hospitals. The accrediting agency for HMOs, the National Committee for Quality Assurance, evaluates quality of services and outcomes of care for managed care organizations and their associated service companies. PPOs have a similar organization, the Utilization Review Accreditation Commission, which has aggressively developed programs for a number of other health care-related service companies such as workmen's compensation. However, organizations satisfying accreditation requirements do not necessarily implement successful QI programs, and sometimes compliance with accrediting bodies is perfunctory at best (Linder, 1991).

Observing the effects of cost containment on patient utilization patterns, providers often express concern that payers sacrifice quality for reduced cost. The premise that more is better, i.e., the philosophy that higher health care expenditures connote higher quality of care, is slowly being replaced with a new paradigm that evaluates access to care in terms of quality of care. Numerous papers and studies have suggested that more care is not always conducive to better outcomes (Navarro, 1999; Rawlins, 1999; Craig, et al., 1978; Sullivan, 1998; Hamburger and Kaplan, 1989). As physicians and other providers have become familiar with the tenets of QI, the standard for measuring quality has changed from simply providing unlimited access to actually measuring outcomes of specific interventions in specific disease processes. Although access to care can be unduly limited and affect the quality of care, a fine balance exists between access and quality, and the line is being redrawn regularly as more QI studies and innovations are being applied in the health care delivery system. Providers, like payers, are slowly coming to the realization that measurement of quality and outcomes must become an integral part of the system if scarce resources are to be properly allocated.

◆ Next Level: Systemwide QI

Perhaps the most significant innovation of 20th century health care was the recognition that quality health care is a measurable entity that can be scientifically studied. With this new awareness came a mandate to design systems to measure and improve processes of care, based on the needs of the consumers of these services, rather than on profits or provider convenience. Society has come to demand such efforts, and although the definition of quality remains nebulous, the features of quality health care are becoming better focused through the efforts of organizations like the CMS, the National Committee for Quality Assurance, the Joint Commission, the Utilization Review Accreditation Commission, and others. Through these associations, society is increasing pressure on the health care industry to instill value into health care services and to demonstrate continuous QI scientifically.

The Institute of Medicine published a landmark work, *Crossing the Quality Chasm*, in 2001 (Institute of Medicine, 2001) that pointed out the serious problems in the US health care system and made concrete recommendations for improvement, including measuring health care effectiveness and applying QI techniques that have been perfected in other segments of the economy, such as the airline industry. The recommendations called the US health care system to task for not adopting these measures earlier and for tolerating error rates that compared with the worst industrial performance. Since then, a number of efforts have been mounted, including those of the Leapfrog Group (*http://www.leapfroggroup.org*), a consortium of major businesses in the United States that have set standards for health care organizations to reduce errors and improve the quality of care.

System wide accountability becomes a natural consequence of this new approach because providers are rewarded for quality outcomes, and interventions are designed to improve systems of care. Designing QI methods into the entire health care system will be the only viable option for achieving this new level of value. The end result will be cost-effective, high-quality health care that is affordable for all Americans.

◆ Discussion Points

1. What major trends changed the health care system in the latter decades of the 20th century? How have different providers within the health care delivery system responded to these trends?

2. How has quality improvement become important in health care? Have providers and health care institutions adopted quality improvement concepts easily?

3. What barriers to the adoption of quality improvement in health care must be overcome for the quality improvement interventions to succeed in a hospital? A clinic? A home health care company?

4. Describe the relationship between quality improvement and access to care. How can providers work to improve quality at the same time that payers are reducing access to services?

5. How have accreditation organizations, such as the Joint Commission on Accreditation of Healthcare Organizations, the National Commission for Quality Assurance, and the Utilization Review Accreditation Commission, contributed to the growth of quality improvement in health care? Can standards be counterproductive?

6. How has cost containment affected the US health care system? What has been the effect on quality of care?

7. What industry groups outside of health care have been active in promoting quality health care in the United States? What initiatives have they undertaken to improve the quality of care?

◆ **Notes**

Bounds G., Yorks L., Adams M., Ranney G. (1994). *Beyond total quality management: Toward the emerging paradigm*. New York: McGraw–Hill.

Boynton A. C., Victor B., Pine J. (1993). New competitive strategies: Challenges to organizations and information technology. *IBM Systems Journal, 32*(1), 40–64.

Bureau of Economic Analysis. (1998). *GDP and other major NIDP series*. Retrieved June 2003, from *http://www.bea.doc.gov/bea/dn/0898nip3/tab2a.htm*

Bureau of Economic Analysis. (1999). *International accounts data*. Retrieved June 2003, from *http://www.bea.doc.gov/bea/ai/0798bpr/tab1-2.htm*

Craig W., Uman S., Shaw W., Ramgopal V., Eagan L., Leopold E. (1978). Hospital use of antimicrobial drugs: Survey at 19 hospitals and results of antimicrobial control program. *Annals of Internal Medicine, 89*(5), 793–795.

Department of Health and Human Services. (1998). *1998 Green book: Background material and data on programs within the jurisdiction of the committee*. Retrieved June 2003, from *http://aspe.os.dhhs.gov/98gb/apenc.htm*

Hamburger J. I., and Kaplan M. M. (1989). Hypothyroidism: Don't treat patients who don't have it. *Postgraduate Medicine, 86*(1), 67–74.

Iglehart J. (1999). The American health care system—Expenditures [Electronic version]. *The New England Journal of Medicine, 340*(1). Retrieved June 2003, from *http://www.nejm.org/content/1999/0340/0001/0070.asp*

Institute of Medicine. (2001). *Crossing the quality chasm: A new health system for the 21st century*. Washington, DC: National Academy Press.

Johns Hopkins University School of Hygiene and Public Health. (1998). *The Johns Hopkins ACG case-mix system*. Retrieved June 2003, from *http://acg.jhsph.edu/what/what.html*

Keightley S. Y. (1993). Sessions focus on health care crisis and reform [Electronic version]. *The Tech, 113*(42). Retrieved June 1999, from *http://www.tech.mit.edu/V113/N42/health.42n.txt.html*

Lathrop J. P. (1993). *Restructuring health care: The patient-focused paradigm*. San Francisco: Jossey–Bass.

Levit K., Lazenby H., Braden B., Cowan C., McDonnell P., Sivarajan L., et al. (1996). National health expenditures—1995. *Health Care Financing Review, 18*(1), 175–214.

Linder J. (1991). Outcomes measurement: Compliance tool or strategic initiative? *Health Care Management Review, 16*(4), 21–33.

McLaughlin C. P., and Kaluzny A. D. (1997). Total quality management issues in managed care. *Journal of Health Care Finance, 24*(1), 10–16.

Navarro R. P. (1999). Cost and quality implications of inappropriate anti-infective use. *Managed Care Interface, 12*(1), 67–68.

Phelps C. E. (1997). *Health economics* (2nd ed.). Reading, MA: Addison–Wesley.

Rawlins M. (1999). In pursuit of quality: The National Institute for Clinical Excellence. *Lancet, 353*(9158), 1079–1082.

Sullivan J. A. (1998). Hypertension in the elderly: Don't treat too quickly! *Journal of Emergency Nursing, 24*(1), 20–23.

Taylor F. (1911). *The principles of scientific management.* New York: Harper.

US Census Bureau. (1996). *Current population reports: P25-1130 population projections of the United States by age, sex, race and Hispanic origin: 1995 to 2050.* Retrieved June 2003, from *http://www.census.gov/prod/1/pop/p25-1130*

Chapter 2

Group Processes in Health Care Quality Improvement

DONALD E. LIGHTER

◈ Introduction

Teamwork is the cornerstone of quality improvement efforts. As health care has become more complex over the past 50 years, no single entity has had resources sufficient to deliver the breadth of health care services to a population. Unfortunately, the diversity and complexity of services has led to fragmentation in the health care delivery system, and the consequent inefficiencies have increased the cost of health care without adding to quality. One of the major thrusts of quality improvement efforts is to capitalize on the group process to solve problems collaboratively. Health care has long been aware of the value of the group process because teams have treated complex patients for many years. However, the rule that the physician is the captain of the team changes when the subject matter waxes managerial rather than clinical. Physicians and other health professionals make good team members when they are aware of the rules of the game and their opinions are respected. In their 1982 best-seller, *In Search of Excellence,* Peters and Waterman noted that America's best-run companies "treat the rank and file as the root source of quality and productivity gain" (Peters and Waterman, 1982). A recent survey of business managers demonstrated that one of the important causes of failure of quality improvement programs is that employees are not adequately trained in communications and group discussion (Tamimi and Sebastianelli, 1998).

The health care delivery system can implement the team approach effectively. The Geisinger Clinic has demonstrated excellent results using collaborative decision-making through teams (Ziegenfuss, et al., 1998). Throughout the 1990s, Geisinger created a number of functional teams, which they termed "boards," organized around clinical conditions or functional areas such as general medicine, cardiothoracic surgery, etc. During the 5-year period that was studied in the report, these teams undertook nearly 50 projects, and 60% of the projects had positive outcomes. Only three projects had negative outcomes, and the remainder had mixed or inconclusive outcomes.

The Geisinger staff learned a number of important lessons through these teams, not the least of which was of the benefits of the team approach to problem solving and organizational communications. Board members demonstrated greater sensitivity to the problems of other staff members, leading to a greater level of teamwork.

The Blue Cross network of southeast Michigan demonstrated a similar success using quality improvement teams. During the first year, the health plan successfully applied the team concept to continuous quality improvement (CQI) projects in a number of clinical and administrative situations, with one team's efforts resulting in a 50% reduction in credentialing turn-around time. Their endorsement of the use of teams in CQI projects is based on their success in these service areas.

The 2002 Malcolm Baldrige National Quality Award recipient in the health care category, SSM Health Care of St. Louis, also took the team approach to new levels (SSM, 2003). Through the use of clinical collaboratives, SSM Health Care teams have demonstrated favorable results in management of patients with congestive heart failure and ischemic heart disease and those requiring anticoagulation therapy. The multi-institutional organization supported 85 teams in 2002 and implemented clinical pathways for several clinical conditions; over the past 5 years, these efforts have proven successful in improving performance measures in numerous clinical areas.

The value of teams has been demonstrated throughout the business world. As health care moves into an era of continuous quality improvement, the team approach will gain even more importance, not just for providing innovation, but also for improving the work environment (Macy and Izumi, 1993). Clinical and work site outcomes have been effectively improved through team techniques in nursing units (Wood, Farrow, and Elliott, 1994). Specific group interventions using health care teams have shown great promise in improving patient compliance with treatment regimens and enhancing patient satisfaction in a number of clinical situations (Adorian, et al., 1990; Collighan, et al., 1993; Noffsinger, 1999). This chapter describes some of the team enhancement and operational techniques that can improve the success of teams in the organization.

◆ Teamwork Concepts

A basic understanding of group dynamics provides an appreciation of the fundamentals of organizing and promoting teams within an organization. Studies of groups over the years have lead to some observations of group behavior that are very helpful in organizing and motivating teams.

- ◆ Teams can be used as a medium for change, but those who are to change must be involved in the group.
- ◆ Team member motivation will be highest when the team member is invested in the results.

◆ Changes recommended by teams should relate to the purpose of the team.
◆ Prestigious team members exert greater influence on the team.
◆ Teams function best when all members are exhibiting similar behavior; i.e., some members of the group are not demonstrating deviant behavior relative to the norm of the group.
◆ The best method of change is to create a shared perception of the need for change and allow the group to exert influence over deviant members.
◆ Information must be equally available to all members of the group.
◆ Change must be uniform throughout the group to avoid loss of group effectiveness.

Interestingly, these principles of group dynamics were published by a number of authors over 25 years ago (Cartwright, 1978) but continue to have relevance in considering team interactions. Team effectiveness depends on successful group interactions, and these criteria should be continually reevaluated during the creation and ongoing operation of organizational teams.

Many organizations now use multidisciplinary or cross-functional teams to deal with almost all organizational functions, with the goal of ensuring that everyone who might be affected by a team's proposed changes will have the opportunity to influence the recommendations. Efforts at making changes benefit significantly when everyone affected by a change feels some ownership in the new process. Thus, health care organizations that are trying to change physician practice patterns now include physicians in development teams to incorporate the unique perspective brought by these professionals, as well as to have "champions" who will assist in implementing suggested changes. A number of factors can lead to the success of teams (Guzzo and Shea, 1992).

First, the team must have a meaningful, clearly defined task, and its objectives should be clear and well articulated. Members should have unique and meaningful tasks, and the performance of individual members should be assessed and feedback provided. In addition, there should be regular feedback on the team's success in considering its objectives.

Teams are usually formed around a specific task, and accomplishment of the task should be the primary goal of the team. For progress to be measured, however, the task must be well delineated and often divided into more manageable subtasks. The techniques described later in this chapter can assist teams with the job of clarifying the task at hand. Once the task has been defined, objectives must be listed so that the team has a clear path to success. Often, a timeline is attached to the objectives to provide milestones against which the team can measure progress toward the goal.

Team members should have responsibilities reflecting their abilities and interests. Frequently, team members are selected because of their position in the organization, but efforts should be made to ensure that members are also invested in the team's work. Team members with many other responsibilities may not have the time to commit to the project, so their participation and later endorsement of the results will most likely be suboptimal. As a team is being selected, new members should be screened for their interest in the team's activities; then each team member should participate in a conditioning process to improve commitment to the team. Conditioning members for a team may simply involve a personal discussion with the team leader, but if the team's activities are complex, then a formal training process, including background education regarding the technical aspects of the project, may prove useful. In either event, the team leader should quickly become familiar with the interests, organizational responsibilities, and capabilities of each member so that as specific tasks arise during the team's work, appropriate assignments can be made. Once the group is functioning, team leaders should continually monitor members for waning interest and intervene to maintain high levels of commitment. As members complete projects, the team leader must ensure that the work is recognized both at the team level and at the organizational level. As part of this process, the leader can periodically summarize and update the team and management staff about the team's progress.

Cross-functional teams can sometimes drift from their original purpose as members from different sections of the organization use the team to solve problems in their sections. Maintaining focus presents a challenge to the team leader because deviating from the team's purpose can prove fractious. For example, a team that is convened for improving waiting times in the operating theater should not end up with recommendations on new instrument sterilization techniques unless the recommendation relates somehow to the original problem. Team members become disaffected and are unlikely to support changes that do not relate to the original reason that they joined the team. On the other hand, a leader should always seek ways to relate issues brought by team members to the team's central function. One reason for having diverse membership is to bring all possible issues to the team's attention. New issues should not be discounted without deliberation.

Other considerations for team management deal with promoting productive interactions between team members, as well as communicating the team's efforts and results internally and externally (Firth-Cozens, 1998). Team leaders must be sensitive to interpersonal issues, especially those that could lead to conflict between members of the group. Conflict is a natural part of the work of any group, and well-managed conflict can lead to constructive change. In general, promotion of good communication between team members, as well as with organizational management, will prove effective in converting conflict into change. Depending on the nature of the group's work and organizational communication mechanisms, the team can use any number of modalities to publicize its accomplishments. Many organizations are turning to the corporate intranet and extranet to disseminate group information, as well as facilitate interaction between team members. Lacking these electronic alternatives, a simple newsletter often proves effective for disseminating the group's reports to internal and external customers.

◆ Use of Teams in Organizations

A successful team project must address several issues. Quality improvement (QI) efforts require substantial planning and project design in order to succeed, and preliminary planning efforts are nearly always rewarded with a successful QI intervention. W. Edwards Deming (1986) was a pioneer in QI in Japanese and American industry, and he articulated 14 principles that guide QI efforts around the world. They can be adapted to health care as follows.

1. Create constancy of organizational purpose to become more competitive and excel in the business and clinical aspects of the organization's endeavors.
2. Adapt to the new economic age. Issues like managed care, capitation, and reduced reimbursement will not disappear, and the old economic order is past.
3. Abandon the quality assurance approach. Inspection, artificial targets, and punitive measures are valueless in the new health care environment.
4. Value business relationships on total quality management. Evaluate each supplier's costs based on a proper economic evaluation that includes all the costs and benefits related to the product.
5. Adopt a QI approach to continuously evaluate and enhance the organization's services and products. Successfully applied, this approach can minimize total costs and maximize economic returns.
6. Include continuing education in every worker's job profile.
7. Improve management techniques and styles to incorporate leadership principles that empower workers and place managers in charge of improving processes to create a better environment for achievement of goals.
8. Drive out fear. Make every worker unafraid to speak out and suggest innovation. Change the environment so that error reporting is encouraged and mistakes are handled to improve quality.
9. Eliminate functional silos in the organization. Encourage communications throughout the enterprise to promote teamwork and learning.
10. Abolish slogans, exhortations, and targets for the work force. Involve professional and support workers in activities designed to improve the quality of outputs and not just to lower costs.
11. Eradicate the barriers in the system that does not allow workers to feel pride in their work. Empower workers to feel ownership of their work. Make workers accountable, but also grant authority to improve processes and themselves.
12. Eliminate any impediment that keeps professionals from feeling pride in their work. Ensure that resources are adequate to support professional activity.

13. Implement continuing education and self-improvement throughout the organization. Capitalize on newer forms of just-in-time training, as well as the need for humans to continually improve themselves and their performance.
14. Transformation to a QI organization requires a sea change in philosophy. Everyone in the organization must be committed to the change for success.

Although some of these principles seem relatively foreign in the health care industry, their validity has been proven repeatedly in the industrial sector.

In accordance with these basic tenets, an approach to team projects can be outlined that will optimize the possibility of success: (1) select projects that have a high probability of successful completion, (2) choose team members who will contribute to the project, (3) gather all appropriate data for analysis and review by the team, (4) prepare the team for the task, (5) coordinate meetings and team activities to maximize productivity, and (6) finalize recommendations and ensure that team members are credited with the success.

Team-building efforts frequently help promote group identification and team effectiveness. Techniques that have been highly successful in the industrial sector can prove useful for health care as well.

Project Selection

The general principles listed in Table 2.1 are often helpful when considering a process for intervention. Internal customers actually implement any project designed by the team, so their commitment to these interventions is paramount. Cost and staff resources constitute important issues in most organizations, and the team must be cognizant of staffing and budget resources in each work area affected by the intervention. The "What's in it for me?" principle cannot be ignored. The duration of the project and the rapidity with which results can be obtained present special problems in health care because some disease interventions take months or years to demonstrate improvement. Long-cycle continuous quality improvement (CQI) projects are more difficult to implement in American health care because most managers are burdened with a relatively short financial time horizon. Rapid cycle improvement projects that identify an issue, measure current performance, create an intervention with short-term effects, then measure results and disseminate the change can produce measurable results in days or weeks and make more sense in today's environment.

Another important issue for most internal customers involves the guinea pig factor. Most organizational divisions cannot afford the disruptions caused by a poorly functioning project, which may disable an entire operational area for long periods of time. Claims management in a health insurance company

Table 2.1 Project Selection Criteria

STAKEHOLDER	CRITERIA
Internal Customers	Project is achievable using existing resources and budgets
	Project will improve some area that involves the individual's work or compensation
	Cycle time is short so that results can be produced quickly
	Process to be improved is not already being transformed
	Interventions require minimal re-education or re-engineering
	Interventions have been piloted on smaller systems prior to implementation system wide
	Addresses business goals of the organization
Executive Management	Project addresses issues that have been identified as key by executive management
	Cost-benefit ratio is favorable
	Disruption to existing operations is minimized
	Project has no known adverse collateral effects
	Improvement will benefit profitability and/or customer satisfaction
External Customers	Project will improve the quality of the products or services bought from the organization
	Project will improve the process of acquiring the products or services
	Cost will fall
Regulators	Project will not violate any regulations or contractual obligation
	Reports of effects on any regulated organizational functions are readily available
Accreditation Agencies	Project will improve the quality of products or services, allowing better performance on accreditation reviews

provides a good example. If a change causes the process to stop for several hours or days, then the company will be besieged by angry calls from providers and members and could even be in violation of the law. Thus, any project that could disrupt operations should be piloted first to eliminate any potentially devastating problems.

One criterion that is shared by internal customers and executive management mandates that the project must relate to the business goals of the organization. Executive managers are more likely to identify business goals as an important issue because they have the responsibility of thinking strategically about the system that they oversee; however, contemporary managers are increasingly involving line staff in strategic planning and goal setting, disseminating the accountability for meeting goals throughout the organization. Executive managers are also concerned about cost, but they must also evaluate improvement projects for benefits accrued as well as cost. Analysis of possible side effects provides useful information to executive managers because they must anticipate problems that could occur in order to make strategic decisions regarding resource allocation.

Improvements must demonstrate value for external customers to be viable. If the project cannot address the concerns or perceived needs of the organization's customers, then it probably is not a productive use of resources. In most cases, external customers are most concerned with cost and access, but if there is any doubt about customers' needs, a survey can provide very useful information. Customer opinions can be garnered in a number of ways at various points of contact with the health care delivery system, and managers should avail themselves of as much of this information as possible in deciding which projects to select. External customers also include employers, who often have strong opinions about the direction the health care system should be taking. These very important clients should be allowed input into decisions regarding projects.

Finally, in today's health care system, with myriad regulatory and accrediting bodies to which organizations are accountable, any project must conform to rules and regulations. For example, if a managed care organization is working toward certification by the National Committee for Quality Assurance (NCQA), projects will probably be directed at improving performance of measures that will enhance the NCQA review. Hospitals will select projects that enhance their status with the Joint Commission for Accreditation of Healthcare Organizations, trying to squeeze twice the benefit out of the study.

Selecting the Team

The process of team selection depends heavily on organizational structure. Some organizations will appoint people to teams through a relatively straightforward top-down procedure. Others promote the formation of cross-functional task forces, usually through the initial appointment of an oversight team that helps guide the project team's activities. The oversight team consists of five or six manager-level staff members who can convene the project team using staff from any operational area of the company. Figure 2.1 illustrates reporting relationships of these teams and management. Each oversight team can manage from one to three project teams, depending on the nature and complexity of the projects. The project teams must have a team leader and staff members who are expert in areas that are important to the success of the project. Thus, the oversight teams have an important responsibility to create project teams that have the necessary expertise for the pro-

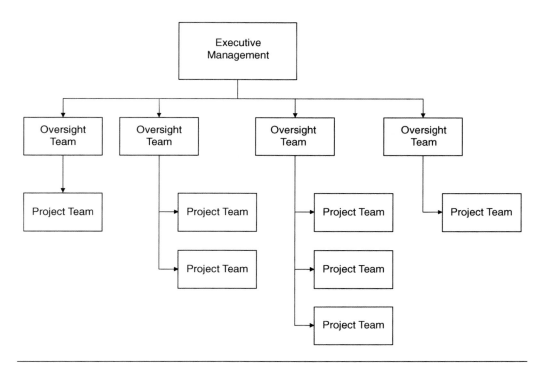

Figure 2.1 Reporting Relationships of Project Teams

ject. In some organizations, the oversight teams will also have the task of establishing parameters for the project, including goals and objectives, needed resources, and baseline information. Smaller organizations may eliminate the oversight teams and have executive managers provide these functions for the project teams. Whoever provides this oversight, however, must have regular meetings with the project team leader(s) to ensure that project goals are being met in a timely manner. Additionally, the oversight team members should be at a level in the organization that allows the team to cut through bureaucratic red tape and expedite the work of the project teams. As the project team nears completion of the design and testing phase of the project, the oversight team also needs to prepare the results for presentation to executive management and ensure that the project can be implemented.

The team leader facilitates meetings, manages administrative details of the meetings, and interacts with the oversight team. The leader should have good people skills and a demonstrated ability to lead through example and encouragement. An effective leader also easily shares responsibility with other team members and ensures that everyone on the team has an opportunity to provide input into the process. Finally, the team leader should be conversant in QI science or have access to a professional during the team's deliberations.

Project team members are selected for their expertise and commitment to the team's goals. Part of the charge by management for project teams should include management assurance that the work of the project team is part of each member's job, not just an extra responsibility. Team members will each be responsible for some of the work of the group, and that time must come out of the members' regular work time to avoid burnout. Executive managers must ensure that the team members have adequate time available to accomplish their goals.

Preparing for Team Meetings

The oversight team usually prepares the materials for the first meeting of the project team. These materials should include

◆   an overview of the project and its ramifications for the organization
◆   the rationale for the project (based on the criteria in Table 2.1)
◆   the boundaries of the project
◆   the criteria for improvement, including possible performance measures
◆   the timeline for the project team's work
◆   oversight of team membership
◆   meeting parameters—e.g., how often, where, and when to meet; selection of team leader
◆   baseline data from company records, customer surveys, etc.

Any other information that is felt pertinent to the work of the project team should be included, e.g., a market analysis of competitors' activities in the target area or any specific directions from executive management. The packet should be provided to the team prior to the first meeting so that all members can be prepared for discussion. Table 2.2 provides the framework in greater detail. For companies that have corporate intranet resources, dissemination of these materials can be performed electronically.

Team Meetings

Effective meetings require planning and skill. The team leader needs to prepare an agenda for each meeting and supply team members with needed materials at least a week in advance of the meeting, and the minutes of the last meeting should be included in the packet. A sample format for meeting minutes is provided in Figure 2.2. Team members can be encouraged to prepare for the meeting using techniques such as "finding Waldo" in the packet—the team leader places some marker in the meeting materials and provides a reward for the person finding "Waldo." The tenets of QI necessitate an evaluation of the meeting, often most effectively collected on a standard questionnaire at the end of the meeting. An example questionnaire is included as Figure 2.3. At the end of each meeting, team members can complete the survey, providing the team leader with immediate feedback and direction for future meetings. The results of the survey should be included in the minutes of the meeting.

Table 2.2 Framework for Project Team

PARAMETER	DESCRIPTION
Process or system to be improved	Description of process, with flowchart as appropriate
	Description of boundaries of project, e.g., what parts of process should not be included
Rationale for project	Customer or corporate data supporting decision to work on process
	Executive management decision rationale for project
	Need for more data to further study the process
Goals for project	Changes in outcome measures that are expected from the project
	Should be limited to two or three changes at the most
Time line for the team's work	Duration of team activities
	Timing for implementation of project
	Cycles for measurement and revision of the intervention
Team logistics	Oversight team or management staff involved in the project
	Team leader
	Organizational positions and members of team
	Reporting intervals
Resources available	Financial
	Computer and information
	Clerical support
	Executive management
	Training
	Supplies

Team leaders must have meeting leadership skills that facilitate the group's discussions. The team leader should not allow anyone to dominate the discussion, and all points of view should be allowed. Periodic restatement of the discussion keeps team members focused on the issue and allows for an estimate of consensus. When the discussion seems to be drifting from the central topic, intervention by the team leader can change a lost meeting into a productive one. Each agenda item can be assigned a time limit so that the team leader can enforce the limit if the dialogue seems to be counter-productive.

The team leader should maintain meeting records with appropriate clerical support, and the example format for minutes in Figure 2.2 can facilitate the process. Storyboards provide an effective method for presenting team efforts to the rest of the organization. The leader and one or two other team members can assemble the storyboard from the minutes of each meeting, and

Project Meeting Minutes

Team Name: _____ Project Name: _____

Team Leader: _____ Meeting Date: _____ Time: _____

Members Present: Members Absent:

Agenda Item	Discussion	Resolution	Action	Person Responsible

Figure 2.2 Sample Format for Meeting Minutes

Meeting Evaluation					
Team Name: _____			*Date:* _____		

1. Was the meeting of sufficient duration to complete the tasks assigned?   Yes   No

2. Did the team accomplish all of its objectives for the meeting?   Yes   No

3. Did you have an opportunity to present your views and ideas?   Yes   No

		Poor				*Excellent*
4.	How would you rate the quality of the discussion?	1	2	3	4	5
5.	How would you rate the time allotted for discussion?	1	2	3	4	5
6.	How would you rate the quality of team interactions?	1	2	3	4	5

7. What would you suggest to improve the team's meetings?

_____

_____

_____

_____

_____

_____

_____

_____

Figure 2.3 Sample Meeting Evaluation Questionnaire

by the time the project team's work is completed, the entire process will be represented in a pictorial format. Storyboards simply take the work of the team and put it into a graphic and pictorial format. The storyboard may contain photographs, data tables, graphs, and brief textual descriptions that describe (1) the problem with the existing process, (2) the team assembled to solve the problem, (3) possible interventions considered for solution, (4) the intervention finally chosen, along with the rationale for this decision, (5) an implementation schedule, and (6) results of implementation.

Phone Center Project Team

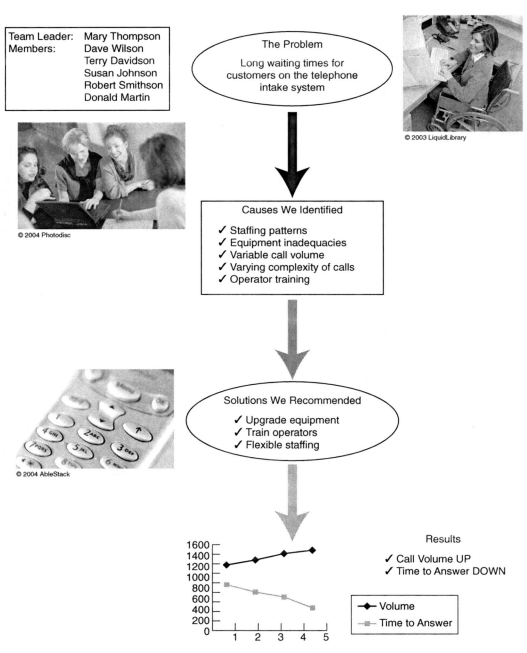

Team Leader: Mary Thompson
Members: Dave Wilson
Terry Davidson
Susan Johnson
Robert Smithson
Donald Martin

© 2004 Photodisc

© 2003 LiquidLibrary

The Problem

Long waiting times for customers on the telephone intake system

Causes We Identified

✓ Staffing patterns
✓ Equipment inadequacies
✓ Variable call volume
✓ Varying complexity of calls
✓ Operator training

© 2004 AbleStack

Solutions We Recommended

✓ Upgrade equipment
✓ Train operators
✓ Flexible staffing

Results

✓ Call Volume UP
✓ Time to Answer DOWN

◆ Volume
▪ Time to Answer

Figure 2.4 Example Storyboard for Project Team

Computer graphics tools make creation of a storyboard much less difficult than it was previously. The example storyboard in Figure 2.4 was created using the program Visio. Although this example is relatively uncomplicated, some complex projects can stretch nearly around a room! Typically, the storyboard will consist of each of the sections of the chart (shown in Figure 2.4 as an individual page, enlarged and placed in a conspicuous location for staff viewing.

◆ Group Process Techniques

Storyboarding is one example of a number of group process tools that can be used to improve the way that teams function. Several other QI approaches prove helpful in moving teams into a proactive position to solve the target problem, including

- ◆ brainstorming
- ◆ brainwriting
- ◆ nominal group technique
- ◆ benefits and barriers exercise
- ◆ list reduction
- ◆ multivoting

These approaches have specific applications in the group process, and their value has been proven in numerous environments.

Brainstorming

Perhaps the most widely recognized technique, brainstorming provides many new ideas very quickly. Brainstorming yields a broad range of ideas and can sometimes cut through stalemates in deliberations. The spontaneity of the brainstorming procedure generates a rich spectrum of creative proposals, as well as some untenable ideas. However, no idea is off limits when a team brainstorms possible solutions. The best brainstorming sessions are open, avoid disparagement of team members, and include the entire team equally.

Brainstorming is a simple process, but several important principles must be followed. The procedure involves the following steps.

1. Definition of the problem in a single statement phrased as a "who, what, or how" statement, such as "How can we improve patient compliance with antihypertensive medications?"
2. Allowing a few minutes for the team to consider the issue. During this time, no discussion should be allowed.
3. Having someone record ideas on a flip chart while the team present their ideas. The recorder should log the ideas verbatim, with little or no editorializing. Other team members should not provide any editorial comment either.

The process of presenting and recording ideas should continue until no new ideas occur for several minutes. For teams in which all members contribute equally, the open brainstorming process works well; however, when one or two members tend to dominate the group, the team leader may wish to have team members take turns presenting a single idea until all ideas have been introduced. The two most important principles of brainstorming provide that (1) all team members participate equally, and (2) no commentary can be made on ideas as they are presented.

The list should be exhaustive, and ideas are often duplicative as team members build on other ideas, but each suggestion should be left on the list until the brainstorming exercise is completed. Another technique, called list reduction, is used to pare the list to a more manageable size. List reduction will be discussed later in this chapter. Team members should be encouraged to produce suggestions that may seem outrageous, because those ideas often spur others to even greater creativity. Participants can use proposals on the list as a basis for other ideas.

No limit should be placed on the number of ideas considered by the group during brainstorming. If ideas are generated too quickly, more than one recorder may be needed to capture all of the team's contributions. If more than one recorder is used, then all of the charts must remain visible to the entire group so that team members can build on other ideas.

One of the best traits of brainstorming is the wealth of ideas generated in a very short time. If team members are sufficiently empowered and feel equal in the effort, brainstorming can prove to be a most effective method of generating creative concepts that can prove valuable in QI efforts.

Brainwriting

In some instances, a team must generate ideas through a brainwriting effort. The team may have problems communicating, the subject may be too controversial, or one or two members may dominate the team, thus thwarting brainstorming efforts. Brainwriting, a nonverbal form of brainstorming, then becomes a suitable alternative. In brainwriting, all ideas are written on sheets of paper by the individual team members, rather than verbalized. The process is usually conducted as follows.

1. Team members are each given several sheets of paper.
2. As in brainstorming, the problem is presented as a "what, where, how" question.
3. Each team member then puts up to five ideas on each sheet and places the completed sheets in the center of the table.
4. The cycle continues until no new ideas are generated or 10 minutes have passed.
5. The sheets are consolidated, and a final list is created.

The group can further refine the ideas using the list reduction technique described later in the chapter. Properly applied, brainwriting can be as effective as brainstorming in producing innovative ideas.

Nominal Group Technique

Another method for brainstorming in groups that have dominant members or when the group is unusually reticent to deal with an issue is the nominal group technique (NGT). Some teams have problems generating new ideas due to difficult relationships that exist or have developed over time. The NGT provides the means by which all group members can participate in a modified brainstorming exercise. The procedure is similar to the brainwriting process and can be outlined as follows.

1. The problem is presented, as in the other techniques, in a "where, what, or how" format.
2. Each group member writes down as many ideas as possible in a 10-minute period.
3. The team is polled, with each member presenting one idea at a time, until all ideas are recorded on a flip chart. During this time, no discussion is allowed, and team members can present ideas that are not on their lists; however, each member has a turn in the process.
4. If team members pass on one turn, they may add another idea during the next time around the group.
5. The process continues until all team members pass or a time limit is reached.
6. The ideas are then combined or clarified through group discussion. If an idea is to be changed, anyone contributing to the idea must agree to the change.

List reduction can be used to help organize the ideas into a more manageable form. NGT is often an excellent alternative to brainstorming in situations where team interactions are more reserved and creativity needs encouragement. Team members who have difficulty expressing opinions in regular team meetings are often empowered to contribute to the NGT process. Sometimes, team-building techniques may be useful before the group begins work so that all team members can feel empowered to participate.

Benefits and Barriers Exercise

Occasionally, a team may not recognize the benefits of proposed changes. The team may also find organizational biases against the change, dooming their efforts to failure before a potential change can be implemented. The benefits and barriers exercise (BBE) can help overcome these problems and encourage acceptance of proposed changes throughout the organization. Just by performing the exercise and including individuals who are perceived as being unreceptive to the group's ideas, the group can help overcome some of the barriers that exist within the organization.

In most cases, the BBE proceeds after a concept has been developed by brainstorming or one of the other idea-creation techniques. However, some teams may find the exercise helpful as a preliminary task to determine the extent and locus of organizational resistance to the change that has been conceived by the group. In general, the more substantial the change, the greater the need for the BBE. For example, if a major QI initiative is being proposed that crosses several departmental boundaries, the BBE becomes essential to avoid resistance and duplication of effort.

The exercise is similar to the other idea-generating techniques described previously. The BBE, however, relies on smaller groups to enhance individual contributions.

1. The large group is divided into smaller teams of four to seven individuals. These groups should each have a leader who provides direction and keeps the group on task. The groups should include a cross-section of the organization to encourage sharing of concepts between departments.
2. While one person in the group records ideas on a flipchart or white board, the leader should begin to solicit input on the benefits of the proposed change for each individual and department. Any of the previously described methods may be used, but NGT is most frequently employed.
3. Each subgroup should evaluate benefits for three distinct stakeholders: individuals, work groups, and the organization. Most experts recommend that the group deal with individual and work group benefits before contending with the organization.
4. Using the techniques of multivoting or list reduction (described later in the chapter), each subgroup should prioritize the top three benefits for each stakeholder group.
5. At this point, the entire team should reassemble for presentation of the lists by each subgroup. The leader or designated presenter from each subgroup should enumerate the results, and all ideas should be listed within the view of the entire team. Additionally, the subgroup leader should provide an assessment of the effectiveness of the process for that subgroup.
6. After the benefits are shared with the entire team, the subgroups should next convene to evaluate possible organizational barriers. The individual and work group barriers are not assessed at this time, because such discussions could lead to unnecessary controversy that would inhibit the group process. In most cases, as organizational barriers are identified by the subgroups, the nidus for the barrier becomes readily apparent.

7. Again, the subgroups reduce the number of barriers to three using multivoting and list reduction.
8. The subgroups then report to the full team with the prioritized lists. The team may discuss the lists or simply accept them for use in planning interventions.
9. The team leader organizes the lists after the meeting and assembles the information into a report. In most cases, the list should be disseminated to team members for input prior to finalizing the issues and submitting the information to senior management.

A typical exercise identifies benefits and barriers but does not address approaches to eliminating barriers. Because team members may have vested interests as they reveal barriers, they could become defensive and fail to provide appropriate suggestions for interventions. These problems are usually handled in separate meetings involving implementation planning.

As should be evident, the BBE can tread into some very sensitive and emotional areas. Exploring benefits before barriers sets the tone of the exercise, defusing some of the emotions that may arise. A facilitator from outside the organization may help keep the team on track by effectively managing interpersonal conflicts in the group and reducing disruptive behaviors such as pulling rank or unproductive digression. Professional meeting managers can serve as neutral discussion leaders and continually direct the team toward a goal.

One important prerequisite for success is the distribution of details of the proposed change prior to the meeting so that team members are completely informed before the exercise. If the plan is elaborate, then the team should have the information at least a week in advance to ensure adequate preparation for the exercise. Additionally, the team must seriously evaluate all barriers identified by the subgroups. Even if the barrier does not seem to be of significance on first inspection, it may prove to be critical during implementation. Thus, even though the team may pare a list down to a few important issues, all of the barriers defined by the subgroups should be included in the final report.

Ideally, a BBE team should have enough members to create effective subgroups. In most cases, at least three to six subgroups of five people each should be formed, meaning a team size of 15 to 30 people. The team should include members from all departments that will be affected by or be involved in implementation of the planned change, and the team leader must ensure that participants are chosen carefully to improve chances for success. Smaller organizations may have too few people to assemble such a large team, and in those cases, the entire team may be involved in the exercise, rather than subgroups. The subgroups should have at least five people and no more than eight people to optimize group interactions.

Other important considerations include the need for everyone in the room to see the list of suggestions as it is presented to the team. If available, a computer projection system can often assist in this effort. If flipcharts are used, the recorder must write large enough for everyone in the room to see, and as a page is filled, it is torn off the palette and taped to the wall. The facilitator or BBE team leader then uses the information on the computer or on the flipchart sheets to create the final report.

The BBE can prove to be crucial when change is difficult for an organization to achieve. Properly deployed, a BBE cannot only help senior management inform the organization's staff of the potential benefits of a new course, but it can also help uncover other barriers that had previously been unrecognized.

List Reduction

As mentioned in previous sections, list reduction is a useful approach to consolidating groups of brainstorming ideas, and the technique is usually applied at the end of or shortly after the brainstorming process. The goal of list reduction and its companion procedure, multivoting, is to take a large disaggregated list of ideas and make the list more usable. After a brainstorming session, the list of ideas typically is long and duplicative, and sometimes the list will contain ideas that are only marginally relevant. The process of list reduction provides the group with an opportunity to work together to determine which ideas should be pursued, combined with others, or eliminated. The procedure for list reduction mimics that of brainstorming or the NGT.

1. Present the entire list of ideas to the team, preferably using flipcharts or computer projection equipment.
2. Have the group consider each item with a "yes" or "no" vote. If the majority of the team votes "no," then indicate that the idea will be eliminated.
3. After all ideas have been considered, return to each of the eliminated ideas and ask the group if each one should be added back. Even if only one person feels that the idea should be returned to the list, it should be added back.
4. Combine ideas on the list using an iterative process where each idea is compared with the others to determine if they are similar enough to be merged. Gain consensus for each combination.
5. Rank the remaining ideas according to criteria that the team suggests. Some common ranking schemes include economic importance, probability of successful implementation, cost of implementation, and acceptability to senior management. Frequently, senior management will provide the criteria for the team to consider, but the team should provide the final ranking.
6. Have the team reevaluate the ideas according to the listed criteria to make certain that each idea conforms to all of the criteria. (An example evaluation matrix is included as Table 2.3.)

Table 2.3 List Reduction Matrix

	COST	EASE	PROFIT	MALPRACTICE RISK
Hire personnel	−	−	−	+
Upgrade equipment	+	+	−	+
Train personnel	+	−	−	+
Improve collections	+	−	+	+
Reduce paperwork	+	+	+	+

As can be seen in Table 2.3, some of the ideas have positive effects on the criteria, and others have adverse effects. The most appealing ideas are those that satisfy the most criteria, and convincing senior management of the worth of a plan is much easier if pertinent criteria are affirmed.

As the team is reducing and combining ideas, several important principles should be observed. First, the rationale for putting an idea back on the list after it has been voted off should be explained to the group. In a sense, each team member has a "reverse veto" power to put ideas that have been eliminated by a vote back onto the list. Under these circumstances, the team member must explain the rationale for placing the idea back on the list. Additionally, the team must reach consensus on the final ranking of the ideas on the list. Occasionally, however, the team is left with several comparable choices after several iterations of list reduction. At this point, multivoting can prove to be a useful technique to finalize the list.

Multivoting

This approach can narrow a list to a final selection, and it can be used, like list reduction, after a session that produces a multitude of unorganized ideas. The concept of multivoting allows an idea that has a simple majority to gain popularity, even if it is not one of the top choices. The procedure is as follows.

1. Using a list of ideas from one of the idea-creation techniques, number each item in sequence.
2. Allow each member of the team to vote for one third of the items.
3. Tally the votes, either by secret ballot or a show of hands, and reduce the list by eliminating the items receiving the fewest votes.
4. Repeat the process until a single item emerges as the clear winner. If a single concept is not chosen, then have the team reach consensus on the remaining items.

The procedure is quite straightforward unless there is a tie among three or more alternatives at the end of the multivoting process. In that case, the team must reach consensus on which of the remaining choices would be optimal, and if the group cannot agree, then the NGT can be applied to settle the stalemate.

If the issues are controversial or if some team members are reluctant to contribute in an open forum, then a modified NGT approach could prove useful. In this scenario, the team develops a list of choices that is used as the basis for the multivoting process. Team members then are allowed to vote for a number of choices on each round of voting, using the rule of thumb in Table 2.4 to determine the number of votes. With the NGT, the voting proceeds as previously described but by secret ballot. After each round of voting, a scorekeeper records the scores and reduces the list. Voting continues until the list becomes manageable. If the list is particularly long, the voting process may also include ranking so that the choices are also prioritized. After each round of voting, each choice is then ranked by the number of first-, second-, and third-place votes it received, as well as the total number of votes of any kind. Although these procedures and scoring methods tend to be more complicated, they provide the group with more information about the priorities of the team members.

Although the goal of any of these exercises is to achieve consensus, multivoting does not always lead to agreement. Instead, the procedure often leads to the best compromise for the team. Each remaining choice should be discussed after each round so that team members can express changing perceptions of remaining items. For example, as choices are narrowed, a team member may develop opposition to one of the remaining items. The team leader must encourage expression of these opinions during discussion so that team members understand fully the nature of the issues before the group. Finally, multivoting is not a process that should supplant the adequate collection and analysis of data. The group should not be asked to form a consensus around an idea that has no evidentiary foundation. Multivoting is particularly useful in larger groups that have too many people for effective discussion of every issue. By reducing the number of issues for consideration, the group can spend more time evaluating those issues that show the greatest promise.

Table 2.4 Votes per Team Member in Multivoting Procedure

NUMBER OF ITEMS	NUMBER OF VOTES
<10	2
10–15	3
15–25	4
26–35	6
>35	8

◆ # Special Situations: Team-Building Approaches

In most organizations, team members will know each other well enough to work together on the project. However, the team leader should assess the interaction between group members to determine the need for measures to improve the effectiveness of the team. A number of these interventions are listed and described in Table 2.5. These techniques are particularly effective if the group is newly formed and when members are somewhat reticent to interact in the group.

Introduction Techniques

The first few entries in Table 2.5 involve introduction of members to each other within the group. These techniques may involve individuals introducing themselves or introducing each other after getting some information about another team member. One of the most useful methods of gaining team cooperation is to help members feel comfortable with each other, and it is incumbent upon the team leader to ensure that the introductions are kept very positive and upbeat.

Some of the more innovative introduction techniques involve goal setting and work mapping. In goal setting, each team member includes two goals for the team in the introduction, with a brief explanation of why the goals are important both individually and for the organization. The team leader can often emphasize these goals by recording them for the group's use on a

Table 2.5 Approaches to Building Teams

TECHNIQUE	TIMING	DESCRIPTION
Mutual introductions	Initial, when members do not know each other	Assign team members to pairs who do not know each other
		Have each person ask the other a defined list of questions about family, job, background
		Have each person introduce the other in the pair to the group
Individual introductions	Initial	Have each team member introduce himself and include one unusual characteristic, e.g., a special hobby, famous relative, etc.
PowerPoint introductions	Initial	Have each team member prepare a short PowerPoint presentation on her life, including any pictures

continues

Table 2.5 *continued*

Technique	Timing	Description
Goal setting introductions	Initial	Each team member introduces himself and then provides two goals that he hopes that the group will achieve
Work map	Anytime	Make a map of the building in which people work and have each person put their work area on the map
		Use the map to discuss work interactions and networking possibilities
Case solutions	Anytime	Divide the team into smaller groups of three or four people per group
		Present a business case similar to the present problem
		Have each subgroup find solutions and report to the entire team
Obstacles to quality	Anytime, especially when team seems stalemated	Divide the team into subgroups of 3–4 persons
		Provide each subgroup with an equal number of Deming's Fourteen Principles
		Have each subgroup identify obstacles to quality for their principles
		Each subgroup then presents their list to the team for review and discussion
		Alternatively, have the subgroups trade lists and have the second subgroup suggest solutions to the problems
Group consultant	Periodically throughout team work cycle	Each team member is asked to be the group consultant for one meeting
		The group consultant observes the meeting and critiques interactions
		The group consultant reports back to the team leader, who then shares observations with the group periodically
WIIFM (What's In It For Me)	Initially for introductions or periodically for stalemate resolution	Brainstorm with team members the personal goals that can be served through the success of the team
Meeting debriefing	Anytime	Have the team critique the meeting, either verbally or by using a form, after each meeting

flipchart or computer projection system. At the end of the introductions, the team leader may wish to amplify any of the goals, but none should be discarded so that every team member feels empowered. Work mapping produces a diagram of each team member's physical location in the organization. Each team member proceeds with an introduction and then indicates his or her work location on a master chart in the front of the room. At the end of the introductions, the team leader may want to comment on the distribution of team members, e.g., that members come from diverse locations within the institution or that team members are relatively close to one another in the facility in spite of their different functions. The team can gain a greater level of cohesiveness through such techniques. The work mapping exercise can also point out opportunities for team members to network on other issues in addition to those that concern the team effort.

Stalemate-Breaking Techniques

At times, even the best teams reach a stalemate in their deliberations. The team leader has a number of options to alleviate the impasse that can also restore some of the team confidence lost when it seems that the group is not functioning effectively. Teams that cannot move ahead with a project often become disillusioned with the team process and can become increasingly ineffective at completing the project because they lack the collective confidence to succeed. Several exercises can be of help.

The *case solutions* technique can be applied at any time, and for some teams, it can provide a good warm-up exercise prior to initiating work on the project. Business case studies abound in the literature, in textbooks, and on the Internet. A few Internet sites that have case studies are included in Table 2.6. The team leader should select a business case that is similar to the team's project or to the cause of the team's deadlock and then direct the team to solve the problem. If the team is large, it may be divided into smaller units that then share their solutions with the larger group. By moving the problem outside the organization, the group can often achieve a degree of objectivity that provides better solutions without disrupting team unity. Once the solution has been effected, the team should then be ready to move ahead with the organization's project.

The *obstacles to quality* exercise helps team members define the issues that are causing the team's stalemate. In this exercise, the team is divided into smaller groups, and each group is given a roughly equal number of Deming's 14 principles. Each group determines how the current impasse creates barriers to fulfilling the quality principles and then presents the results to the team. The groups can then reconvene to propose possible solutions to the barriers using the principles of QI. Sometimes the team leader may want to have the entire team work on solutions if there are just a few barriers. In either case, the team should clearly identify the barriers to QI and suggest methods of moving beyond the gridlock.

Table 2.6 Case Studies Available on the Internet

SITE NAME OR SPONSOR	URL	DESCRIPTION
Monash University	http://www.monash.edu.au/casestudies/	Case studies in a variety of industries on business and health care topics
Businesscases.org	http://www.businesscases.org	Commercial site with business cases for purchase (provided for information only, not an endorsement)
Times100	http://www.thetimes100.co.uk/	Free business case studies written by business school faculty on leading international businesses
Biz/ed (UK)	http://www.bized.ac.uk/virtual/economy/studies/	Case studies on people, business, and government, with a British flavor
Department of Public Enterprise, Ireland	http://www.ecommercegov.ie/ebcip/index.html	Short case studies on e-commerce applications in a number of industries
The Financial Times	http://www.longman.co.uk/tt_secbus/resources/bus_arch.htm	Business case studies from The Financial Times, a leading business periodical
University of Virginia	http://www.darden.virginia.edu/collection/index.htm	Well-known resource for case studies from the University of Virginia
Department of Innovation and Information Economy, Sport and Recreation Queensland	http://www.iib.qld.gov.au/using/Case%20Studies/BC_Case_Studies.htm	Use of information technology to solve small business challenges

Even if the team is functioning well, the use of a team consultant can often maintain the team's effectiveness unobtrusively. The team consultant concept is designed to provide team members with insight into the team's functional status as well as to provide the team leader with useful feedback on the team's operations. A different member of the team is chosen as consultant for each meeting, and that member observes the work of the team without participating in the group. At the end of the meeting, the team consultant reports to the team leader. Frequently, a team consultant will bring insights to the team's operations that have eluded the team leader, so the team leader can benefit from the exercise as well. The report of the team consultant can remain confidential or be conveyed to the team at the next meeting at the discretion of the team leader.

The "What's in it for me?" (WIIFM) exercise is a useful tool at the beginning of a project or when a project seems to be at a stalemate. WIIFM is essentially a brainstorming session in which team members list the benefits of the project to themselves and their work. Conducted in the same manner as any other idea-creation exercise, the WIIFM question is always "How will this project benefit me personally as well as my work?" The answers to the question can help others in the group discern new ways of understanding how the project can benefit them personally, thus renewing or creating commitment to the project. The WIIFM procedure can be used at the beginning of the project to gain early dedication of the team, at the end of the project as a sort of BBE, or at times when the team seems bogged down and cannot reach a consensus on a course of action. Additionally, when team members recognize that they will benefit from the project as much as other team members, greater solidarity can be achieved.

Finally, debriefing the team after each meeting, as suggested earlier in the chapter, can provide a means for team members to express problems with meetings or the progress of the project. Many times, the process of debriefing is informal and simply provides time at the end of the meeting for each team member to express opinions about the meeting and the project. Some teams, however, require a more formal process of completing a form with an appraisal of the meeting, using a form such as the one in Figure 2.3. As a team-building tool, the meeting appraisal can serve as a springboard for team members to openly discuss progress and thus build relationships between team members.

◆ Teamwork: The Key to Higher Quality

Perhaps the cornerstone of QI, teamwork has assumed an increasingly important role in American industry. Teams handle subjects from the mundane to the complex, and the ability to participate in and manage teams has become the most crucial skill that a manager can have. As health care organizations and providers move into an increasingly consumer-driven marketplace, the use of teams to design and implement creative solutions to marketplace challenges could be the defining trait for successful organizations.

◆ Discussion Points

1. How are teams useful to modern organizations? How do teams enhance the decision-making process?
2. What motivates team members? How can a team leader structure a team to ensure equal input from each member?
3. What are the important issues to remember when selecting a project for a team? Include the issues that are specific to the health care industry.
4. What steps should be taken to prepare for a team meeting? Who should assume responsibility for organizing meetings? How does this work in your organization?
5. List the techniques for developing ideas in a group. Briefly describe each and give examples of how the techniques could be used.
6. Discuss the techniques used for narrowing a list of ideas into a few useful concepts. Give examples of how these techniques can be used.
7. Describe methods of improving team function and describe the circumstances in which they should be applied.

◆ Notes

Adorian D., Silverberg D., Tomer D., Wamosher Z. (1990). Group discussions with the healthcare team: A method of improving care of hypertension in general practice. *Journal of Human Hypertension, 4*, 265–268.

Cartwright D. (1978). Achieving change in people: Some applications of group dynamics theory. In W. L. French, C. H. Bell, and R. A. Zawacki (Eds.). *Organization development: Theory, practice, and research*. Dallas, TX: Business Publications.

Collighan G., et al. (1993). An evaluation of the multidisciplinary approach to psychiatric diagnosis in elderly people. *British Medical Journal, 306*, 821–824.

Deming W. E. (1986). *Out of the crisis*. Cambridge, MA: MIT Press.

Firth-Cozens J. (1998). Celebrating teamwork [Electronic version]. *British Medical Journal* Dec;7 Suppl:S3–7. Retrieved March 1999, from *http://www.bmj.com/misc/qhc*

Guzzo R. A., and Shea G. P. (1992). Group performance and intergroup relations in organizations. In M. D. Dunnette and L. M. Hough (Eds.). *Handbook of industrial and organizational psychology*. Palo Alto, CA: Consulting Psychologists' Press.

Macy B. A. and Izumi H. (1993). Organizational change, design and work innovation: A meta-analysis of 131 North American field studies: 1961–91. In W. A. Pasmore and R. W. Woodman (Eds.). *Research in organizational change and development, 7*, 235–313. Greenwich, CT: JAI Press.

Noffsinger E. B. (1999). Answering physician concerns about drop-in group medical appointments. *Group Practice Journal, 48*(2), 14–21.

Peters T. J., and Waterman R. H. (1982). *In search of excellence: Lessons from America's best-run companies*. New York: Warner Books.

SSM (2003). *First health care winner. National Baldrige Award*. Retrieved June 2003, from *http://www.ssmhc.com*

Tamimi N., and Sebastianelli R. (1998). The barriers to total quality management. *Quality Progress, 31*(6), 57–60.

Wood N., et al. (1994). A review of primary health care organization. *Journal of Clinical Nursing, 3,* 243–250.

Ziegenfuss J.T. Jr., Munzenrider R. F., Fisher K., Noll S., Poss L. K., Lartin-Drake J. (1998). Engineering quality through organization change: A study of patient care initiatives by teams. *American Journal of Medical Quality, 13*(1), 44–51.

Chapter 3

Process Orientation in Health Care Quality

DONALD E. LIGHTER

◆ Introduction

Although the doctor–patient relationship has achieved something of a sanctified position in society, the interaction between physicians and their "customers" can be correctly characterized in quality improvement terms as a process. One of the basic tenets of quality improvement is that "all work is a process," and provision of health care services is no exception. Because every health care service can be characterized in this manner, the principles of quality improvement can be applied successfully.

In spite of the highly personal and sometimes lifesaving nature of health care services, the precepts of continuous quality improvement are important in evaluating the quality of care. Viewing these services as processes is the first step in applying techniques to improve care at each step along the clinical path. Products and services in the health care industry can be divided into a number of categories.

◆ Administrative services: insurance claims, financial management and reporting, human resources, regulatory compliance, materials management, facilities management, patient record-keeping
◆ Clinical services: provider services, imaging and laboratory, therapeutic services, patient education, surgical services
◆ Durable medical equipment: delivery, setup, and training for medical equipment used by patients in a variety of settings
◆ Hospital services: nonclinical inpatient and outpatient services
◆ Pharmaceutical and therapeutic services: drugs (oral and injectable), therapies requiring human intervention (e.g., physical and occupational therapy)

Each of these categories requires somewhat different interventions for improving quality, but the principles that underlie the identification of quality issues and the creation of solutions are the same.

For example, health care insurers deal with most of the administrative issues involved with payment for services, but providers such as physicians and hospitals also influence the system by the quality of the insurance forms that they send to the insurance companies. Quality issues for insurers include concerns for several processes, such as receiving and entering claims into the insurer's computer system, ensuring the completeness and accuracy of claim information, determining if the claim contains covered services for the member and plan, determining if the person listed on the claim is an eligible member, checking the eligibility of the provider to perform the listed services, and evaluating the appropriateness of the service for the diagnosis. These are just a few of the myriad processes applied to claims submitted to insurance companies. Fortunately, most of the work is done electronically, but the computer programs must be continually tested for errors and changed as new members and benefit structures are added.

From the perspective of providers, other processes must be established to collect and submit billing data. These include capturing billing information at the time of the provider–patient encounter, coding information in a format appropriate for the insurer, ensuring eligibility of the patient for the insurance company to be billed, placing the billing information on the appropriate form for the insurer, submitting the bill within the time limits set by the insurer, tracking the status of the bill until it is paid, and properly crediting payments to the correct accounts.

Although most insurance companies are highly automated, many of the processes in physicians' offices are performed manually. Thus, different quality issues must be addressed, not only because the processes are different, but also because of differences in the business environment.

Clinical processes present a completely different set of quality challenges. At the bridge between the 20th and 21st centuries, physicians have a long history of evaluating clinical problems using the scientific method, insisting on appropriate experimental designs and proper statistical analysis. These investigations often require substantial resources and long time periods for success, and such studies are often ambivalent in their results. The scientific method has led to the advanced understanding of diseases and interventions that exists in modern health care; however, the current state of knowledge is inadequate for completely understanding many of the most common diseases encountered by the average provider. Most interventions are still relatively clumsy attempts to mimic the reparative or preventive capacity of the body, so these imperfect therapies can cause problems as well as produce cures. Every disease can be considered a process or series of processes; thus, the same quality improvement measures applied in other processes can be applied to disease processes as well. In fact, the disease management programs noted in later chapters describe these applications. Unfortunately, disease processes have a number of important features that differentiate them from administrative processes, including

◆   longer term for the process to evolve
◆   a substantial number of controlled and uncontrolled variables

◆ incomplete understanding of disease pathophysiology
◆ therapies directed at symptoms, rather than underlying cause
◆ human factors relating to response and adherence to treatment recommendations
◆ human factors relating to diagnosis and treatment

These factors complicate the quality improvement approach to diseases, but the complexity involved in analyzing disease states in quality improvement terms can be approached in several ways, which will be discussed in later chapters.

In short, virtually all of health care can be described using the process-analysis tools of quality improvement. Complexity aside, breaking down health care services into component processes can help identify opportunities for improving the care that people receive. Whether the analysis is performed on a defined population in a state or region or on individuals, quality improvement process-analysis tools can prove useful in defining possible areas for intervention.

◆ Process-Analysis Tools

Understanding the process that is to be improved often presents a major challenge. Without the organizing influence of quality improvement (QI), some processes can appear chaotic; thus, the initial phase of a QI intervention involves gaining in-depth knowledge of the process with the use of the tools listed in Table 3.1. Each of these tools will be discussed in greater detail throughout the remainder of the chapter.

Flowcharts

Basic Flowcharts

Gaining an overview of a process serves to provide an impression of the complexity of intervention targets. Flowcharts have the advantage of providing such an overview while also including the details necessary to determine potential areas for intervention. Most flowcharts in QI have a fairly well-defined structure, but they allow enough variation to describe nearly any process. In their most elemental form, flowcharts simply outline the path that an input takes through a process to produce an output. A sample flowchart for accessing an automated teller machine (ATM) is included in Figure 3.1.

The flowchart starts with an input—in this case, the customer inserting the ATM card—and then each step in the process is detailed with a symbol that represents the nature of the event. Figure 3.2 lists the various shapes, along with the interpretation of each. Although there are a number of other shapes that are used in flowchart diagrams, those listed in Figure 3.2 are the most common.

Table 3.1 Process-Analysis Tools

Type	Name	Application
Flowcharts	Basic flowchart	Characterization of process; steps from input to output
	PERT (arrow) diagram	Identification of critical path in process
	Cost of quality analysis	Determination of costs of QI interventions
	Critical to quality analysis	Identification of steps in process that are critical to QI intervention
	Deployment flowchart	Steps in the process that are required for appropriate implementation of the process
	Requirements and measures tree	Relates customers, process requirements, and performance measures
	Top-down flowchart	Orders process by layers of steps; allows prioritization of steps
Relationships diagrams	Relations diagram	Diagrams cause and effect relationships in box and arrow format
	Tree diagram	Identification of actions required to solve a problem; allows specific identification of solutions
	Root cause diagram	Find a root cause by becoming more specific at each level of specification
	Work flow diagram	Characterize the flow of resources and inputs into a process
Matrices	Basic matrix	Tabular representation of data; helps define relationships between variables
	L-shaped matrix	Commonly used for defining relationship between 2 variables or in data collection
	T-shaped matrix	Used for determining relationship between 2 variables and a 3rd
	Y-shaped matrix	Used to determine interactions among 3 variables
	X-shaped matrix	Relates 4 groups of variables, with each group relating to 2 other groups
	Decision matrix	Weighs and scores alternative courses of action, problems, or solutions for optimization
	Performance–importance matrix	Assessment of customer perceptions of importance and performance for products and services

Table 3.1 *continued*

TYPE	NAME	APPLICATION
Matrices	Kepner–Tregoe matrix (is–is not matrix)	Identification of causes of problems in processes by asking common questions: who, what, when, where, how?
	Plan–results matrix	Compare plans with results to determine interventions necessary for improvement
	Requirements matrix	Identifies and characterizes outputs necessary for internal and external customers
	Effective–achievable matrix	Prioritization of choices in process design and evaluation

QI, quality improvement; PERT, program evaluation and review technique.

Flowchart construction is relatively straightforward and usually leads to a better understanding of the process being examined. For clinical processes, a flowchart can outline the critical pathway that must be followed for a process to be completed successfully. The following approach will lead to creation of a successful chart.

1. List the steps involved in the process.
2. Determine the order in which the steps occur.
3. Separate the steps into operations and procedures. In general, an operation is performed on an input, whereas a procedure is often a subprocess.
4. Decide where decision points occur and place the decision diamond shapes accordingly.
5. Connect the shapes with the appropriate connectors (see Figure 3.2).

Software programs make the task of creating flowcharts much easier, and such tools allow moving and renaming the nodes of the flowchart. Additionally, using modern computer networking and groupware tools, the flowchart can be created collaboratively.

Program Evaluation and Review Technique Diagram

The critical path method was created in the early 1950s. It was rapidly adapted by the US Navy to manage the Polaris missile project in the late 1950s, for which it was renamed the program evaluation and review technique (PERT). Other terms used for this technique include arrow diagram and critical path scheduling. The focus of the PERT diagram is the critical path, the path between the inputs and outputs that involves all required steps. Although alternative and subsidiary pathways are included in the PERT diagram, the critical pathway is used to determine the time required

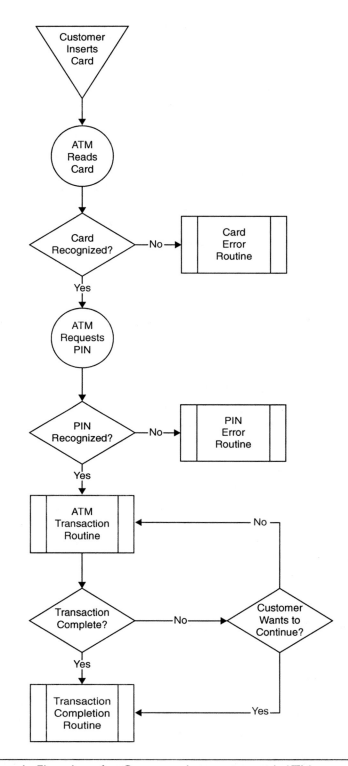

Figure 3.1 Sample Flowchart for Customer Interaction with ATM

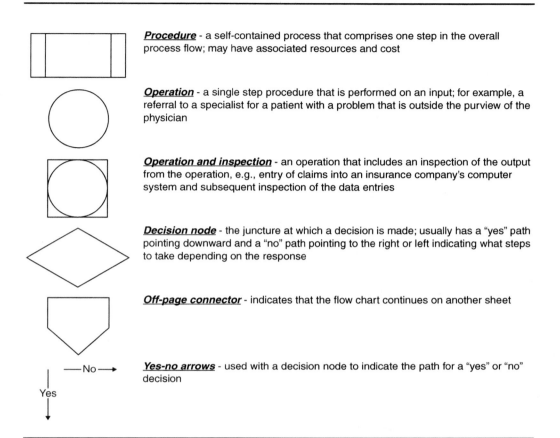

Procedure - a self-contained process that comprises one step in the overall process flow; may have associated resources and cost

Operation - a single step procedure that is performed on an input; for example, a referral to a specialist for a patient with a problem that is outside the purview of the physician

Operation and inspection - an operation that includes an inspection of the output from the operation, e.g., entry of claims into an insurance company's computer system and subsequent inspection of the data entries

Decision node - the juncture at which a decision is made; usually has a "yes" path pointing downward and a "no" path pointing to the right or left indicating what steps to take depending on the response

Off-page connector - indicates that the flow chart continues on another sheet

Yes-no arrows - used with a decision node to indicate the path for a "yes" or "no" decision

Figure 3.2 Flowchart Symbols

for completion of the process. PERT analysis can be performed manually, but a number of very effective computerized tools exist for the creation of PERT diagrams. The program Microsoft Project was used to create the model in Figure 3.3, and such simple diagrams can readily be made much more complex using these types of computerized tools. Figure 3.3 depicts a generic team project, primarily to illustrate the features of a PERT diagram. PERT diagrams have several important features that are discussed below.

PERT boxes can contain a number of parameters, and they are placed in the large box as shown in Figure 3.3. Other parameters can also be used, including the following:

◆ earliest start: the earliest time in the process that this particular step can start
◆ duration: the duration of this step in the process
◆ earliest finish: the earliest time in the duration of the process that this step can end
  ◆ earliest finish: earliest start + duration of task
◆ latest start: the latest time in the process that this step can start

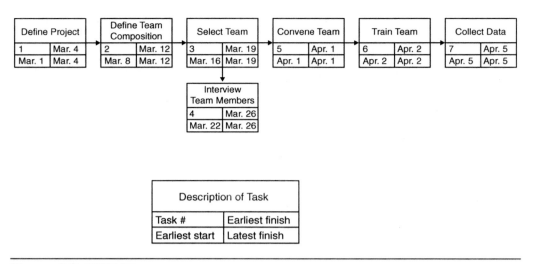

Figure 3.3 PERT Diagram

◆ slack: any extra time that must be added for interruptions or delays
  ◆ slack: latest start—earliest finish
◆ latest finish: the latest time in the process that the step can end; also, the smallest of the latest starts for all the tasks leading out of the current task

These numbers are important for determining the efficiency of a process and whether the process can meet capability estimates.

The steps involved in creating a PERT diagram are straightforward but require in-depth understanding of the process.

1. Define the steps in the process. Place them in order on a flowchart.
2. Determine the duration of each of the steps, including the shortest time and the longest time necessary to complete the step.
3. Construct the PERT statistics based on the duration data, including earliest start, latest start, earliest finish, latest finish, and slack for each step.
4. Complete the boxes in the PERT diagram with the numbers from the analysis in the previous step (step 3).
5. Calculate total time for the process (the sum of the durations plus the slack times for each step) and compare them to standards or benchmarks.
6. Evaluate possible interventions for improvement, such as those steps with the longest durations and largest slack times.

PERT analysis augments basic flowcharts by adding a dimension of resource utilization and time. Using the data from the PERT diagram, a QI team focuses on specific areas for intervention, with better targets and more objective measures of improvement.

Cost of Quality Analysis

An important variant of the basic flowchart is termed a cost of quality analysis. Poor quality produces costs; e.g., from rework, products that are unusable, or liability associated with poor quality. For example, radiologists reject poor quality x-rays as unreadable, leading to a repeat procedure. The cost of repeating the x-ray will be included in the overall cost to the institution, leading to higher prices and lowering of the organization's competitiveness. The cost of quality analysis provides insight into the steps in the process that could be revised or eliminated in order to reduce the cost of quality lapses.

The analysis begins with a flowchart. Steps that are related to inspection or rework are identified in the flowchart, and the process is re-evaluated for changes in preceding or subsequent procedures that will reduce the need for inspection and rework. The process is then redesigned and piloted, and the changes are adopted if they successfully eliminate the quality problem.

Figure 3.4 demonstrates an example of a cost of quality analysis for an outpatient laboratory. Outpatient testing centers often receive orders from physicians for tests that involve some preparation on the part of the patient: overnight fasting, consumption of some test material prior to the procedure, etc. This scenario posits that a physician has ordered such a test and the patient appears at the outpatient diagnostic center for completion of the procedure. The registration process for the patient involves several steps, some of which could be deemed "inspection steps" because they involve evaluation of the registration process and potential rework. The steps that lead to rework are circled in dotted lines, and they involve problems with communication, either between the diagnostic center and the patient or between the physician's office and the outpatient center. Solid circles indicate conditions in which rework will not be required but that could lead to quality problems.

The *Patient Presents at Facility* circle could describe a situation in which a patient appears at the center unprepared for a test. In such cases, the patient may have misunderstood the instructions for preparation or simply failed to prepare adequately (for example, forgot to abstain from food or drink overnight to prepare for a fasting blood sugar test). Elimination of this cost of quality entails working with the physician's office to ensure education of the patient on proper preparation for the test and verification by the physician's office that the patient is prepared prior to appearing at the center. The *Order Received from Doctor* decision point diamond that is encircled involves failure of the physician's office to contact the center with orders. The delays caused by this quality problem can disrupt operations as well as increase patient anxiety over the procedure. Improved communication between the physician's office and the center, perhaps by using an online ordering system, can ameliorate this type of problem. The step labeled *Register*

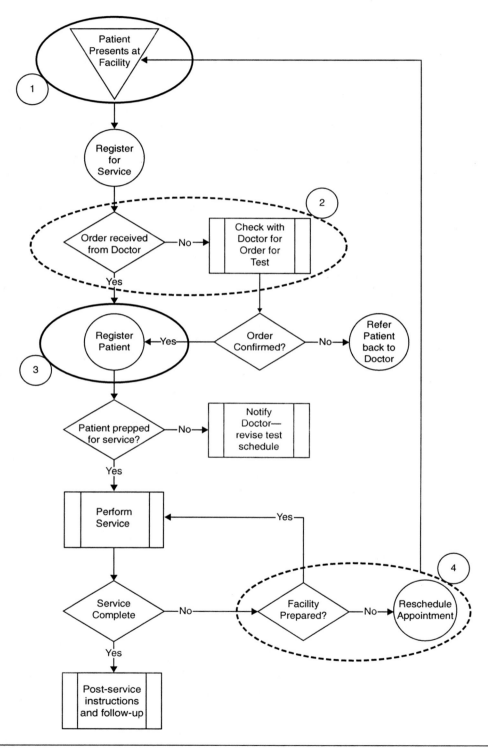

Figure 3.4 Cost of Quality Analysis

Patient that has a cost of quality concerns problems with patient registration, e.g., lack of insurance information or perhaps appropriate permissions for a procedure if the patient is a minor. Proper notification of the patient prior to the visit and preregistration over the telephone may help reduce the disruption caused by this type of error. Finally, the *Reschedule Appointment* quality circle indicates that the problem will again cause rework. In this case, the center is not prepared for the patient's test and must either delay the test or reschedule, causing downtime and undue pressure on the schedule on another day. The improvement team may determine that better internal communication may alleviate this problem and allow the center to prepare for each day's tests the night before.

The cost of quality analysis is particularly useful when processes are complex because it can identify significant areas of rework and inspection that add to process costs. Elimination of inspection and rework often improves customer and employee satisfaction by reducing waiting times and the feeling of needless repetition of work. One of Deming's 14 Principles (discussed in Chapter 2) mandates elimination of rework and inspection by designing QI into each process; the cost of quality analysis is an effective tool for achieving this goal.

Critical to Quality Analysis

Similar to the cost of quality analysis, the critical to quality analysis evaluates inputs and outputs for potential improvements. Typically, a critical to quality analysis is performed to ensure that all the steps required to produce high-quality output are included in a flowchart, so it can be viewed as an obligatory step in the creation of a flowchart. Once the flowchart has been constructed, the information (shown in Table 3.2) is collected and analyzed for those inputs that are critical to producing quality output. The steps in the flowchart that involve the critical inputs should be highlighted for the attention of the QI team. In most cases, the team will develop performance measures that monitor these inputs for lapses in quality that can affect the value of the service to clients.

An example of an application of critical to quality analysis is in the cycle for producing clinical practice guidelines (CPGs) (discussed in detail in Chapter 8, "Clinical Processes: Clinical Practice Guidelines"). After a CPG is created, expert panels of providers usually review the guideline for those elements that are of greatest importance in ensuring quality care. For example, in a CPG for diabetes mellitus, a critical step may be a biannual foot exam by the primary care physician. The result of that examination would be considered a critical input in the process of care for the diabetic patient because a missed skin ulcer could lead to secondary infection and subsequent amputation. Thus, a performance measure can be designed to evaluate the efficacy with which the system provides regular foot exams for diabetic patients through the primary care physicians in a care network. Frequently, however, a critical to quality analysis is not performed before performance measures

Table 3.2 Critical to Quality Analysis Table

ITEM TYPE	PROVIDER NEEDS	CLIENT NEEDS
Inputs	Source of input	Quality of input
	Timing of input in process	Importance of input
	Importance of input	
	Quality of input	
	Specifications of input required by process	
Outputs	Quality of output	Quality of output
	Which clients receive the output	Importance of output
		Timing of output
	Importance of timing of output for process success	Specifications of output required by client
		Specifications of output desired by client

are identified and interventions designed, which usually leads to inappropriate interventions for improvement and, in some cases, diminished quality of care due to pushback from providers.

Deployment Flowchart

After appropriately identifying those inputs and outputs of critical value to the process, the next procedure for a QI team involves deployment of the process. The thrust of this flowchart variant is to identify who in the organization is required to implement a process. Although usually reserved for implementation planning, a deployment flowchart can also be useful in identifying individuals or departments in the organization that are responsible for particular procedures.

An example of a deployment flowchart, created in the computer program Visio (a graphical program designed for organization charts), is presented in Figure 3.5. The flowchart is arranged so that responsibilities are clearly outlined for each person or department involved in accomplishing the task. The flowchart in Figure 3.5 represents a computerized laboratory system. The four participants in the process are placed at the top of the chart, and the tasks for each are placed in order below them. The sequence of events can then be determined by connecting the tasks in the order that they should occur. In some cases, conflicts in sequencing can be discovered as the process is being charted, adding to the value of the deployment flowchart.

To create the deployment flowchart using a computer graphics program:

1. Define the major steps in the process. Create labeled boxes for each step.

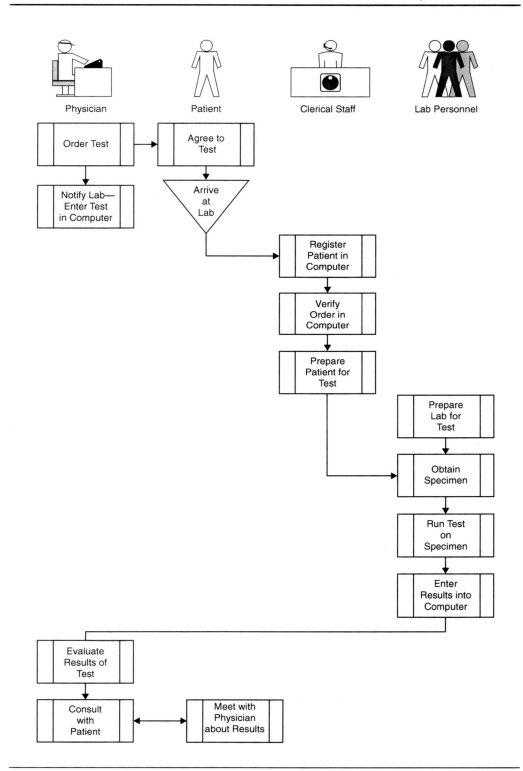

Figure 3.5 Deployment Flowchart

2. Determine all individuals and departments involved in the process.
3. Place the individuals and/or departments across the top of the flow-chart design page.
4. Place the tasks in order below the individual/department responsible for the task.
5. Connect the tasks in sequence.

The deployment flowchart can also be created using paper and pencil, but the computerized method provides greater flexibility and a printable product for distribution.

Requirements and Measures Tree

As planning for a process progresses, the improvement team needs to remain focused on customer needs. In order to maintain that focus, the team can construct a modified flowchart called a requirements and measures tree (RMT). The RMT relates the elements of a product or service that customers value to the process. QI teams frequently refer to the RMT to order priorities in a process to ensure that customer needs are being met as the process is designed or re-engineered. Teams often find the technique most helpful not only during the development process but also when trying to organize complex sets of requirements or measures or when a visual representation of these relationships is useful for improving understanding.

The RMT in Figure 3.6 demonstrates the technique applied to producing Health Plan Employer Data and Information Set (HEDIS) measures for a health plan. Increasingly, health plans are being called upon to produce performance measures perceived to be of value to the public. The National Committee for Quality Assurance (NCQA) has published a set of measures known as HEDIS, which includes descriptive measures of health plan activities, from clinical and patient satisfaction measures to administrative effectiveness metrics. Producing these measures requires a complex internal process in most health plans, but the information is used by a number of internal and external customers. The RMT in Figure 3.6 defines these relationships.

The procedure for producing a RMT is as follows:

1. Select a product or service output from the process.
2. Define all potential internal and external customers for the product or service.
3. List all requirements for each of the customers. Look for duplication or overlap in requirements so that the list may be consolidated.
4. Determine measures for each of the requirements, but pare the list to a reasonable number.
5. Define the measure in terms of data required to produce the measure, who will be responsible for producing the measure, and how it will be distributed.

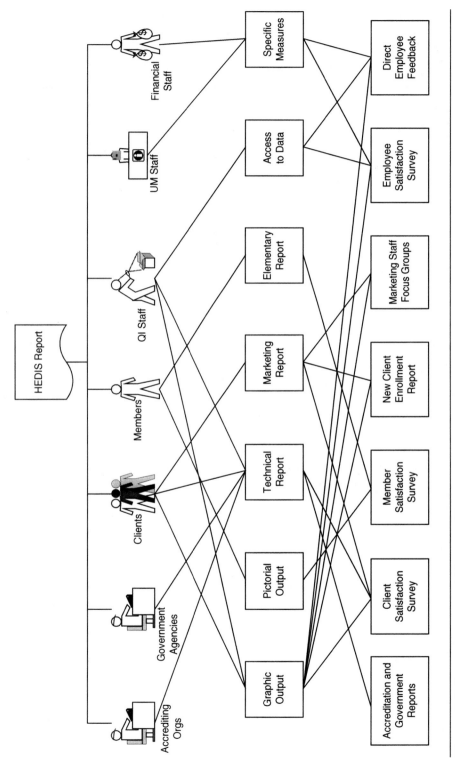

Figure 3.6 Requirements and Measures Tree

Based on information in Table 3.3.

Table 3.3 Customers and Requirements for HEDIS Measures

CUSTOMERS FOR HEDIS REPORT	REPORT REQUIREMENTS	PROCESS REQUIREMENTS	QUALITY MEASURE
Accrediting organizations	Specific format Submission deadline Audited	Validated data base Audited report Data collection and analysis by deadline	Accreditation status Score on accreditation relating to HEDIS
Government agencies	Graphic format Submission deadline Supporting report	Graphic presentation software Report meeting government standards	QI recommendations from CMS and state Medicaid bureau
Clients (employers)	Graphic format Marketing presentation Explanation of measures	Graphic presentation software Detailed explanation Marketing input Details for client	Employer satisfaction survey
Members	Pictorial format 8th-grade reading level Nontechnical explanation	Easily understood pictures Simple explanation of importance Reading level check	Member satisfaction survey Disenrollment data
Potential clients	Graphic format Other marketing materials Comparison with competitors	Graphic presentation software Marketing input Competitor data	New client enrollment Marketing staff focus groups regarding use of information in sales
Plan QI staff	Supporting data Report deadline Year-to-year comparison	Access to database Data collection and analysis by planning deadline Data from previous years	Employee satisfaction survey Direct feedback on report
Plan UM staff	Graphic format Subset of measures relating to utilization and member satisfaction	Graphic presentation software Subset of measures for their needs	Employee satisfaction survey Direct feedback on report

Table 3.3 *continued*

CUSTOMERS FOR HEDIS REPORT	REPORT REQUIREMENTS	PROCESS REQUIREMENTS	QUALITY MEASURE
Plan financial staff	Graphic format Subset of measures relating to financial performance	Graphic presentation software Financial subset of measures	Employee satisfaction survey Direct feedback on report

HEDIS, health plan employer data and information set; CMS, Centers for Medicare and Medicaid Services; UM, utilization management.

The RMT provides a quick overview of customer requirements and the methods used to measure the requirements. Additionally, however, this tool reveals relationships between measures that can reduce the chance that a particular output may escape measurement. For example, in Figure 3.6, the graphic output of the report needs to be measured in nearly all of the organization's surveys of members, clients, and employees; however, satisfaction with the pictorial output will only require measurement in the member survey. Thus, the RMT helps ensure that all pertinent customers will evaluate a particular output.

Top-Down Flowchart

Just as a deployment flowchart identifies responsible individuals and departments for a process, the top-down flowchart orders the steps of a process by importance. The top-down flowchart provides an overview of the process steps ranked by the improvement team or by those responsible for implementing the process, providing helpful information for allocating scarce resources to a project and ensuring that adequate resources are available for critical steps before the process is initialized. Additionally, the hierarchy established by the top-down flowchart can direct QI efforts by focusing on crucial stages and ensuring that all subprocedures are included in process planning.

Creating a top-down flowchart follows many of the same procedures used for other flowcharts, and computer tools make the task much easier.

1. Define the process and put the major steps of the process in boxes at the top of a page.
2. Determine subprocedures for each of the major steps and list them in order below each major step.
3. Connect the procedures and subprocedures using arrows as in a typical flowchart.
4. Seek input regarding the hierarchy of steps from those who will implement the process.

An example of a top-down flowchart is included in Figure 3.7, detailing the process of delivering a patient to the operating room from the surgical floor. The figure illustrates the sequencing that takes place in creating the top-down flowchart, although in this case, the procedures were sequential and not arranged in order of importance. For example, the verification of the patient's identification is no less important than any other step in the process; however, a top-down flowchart was chosen to demonstrate how a process could be analyzed by procedures and subprocedures.

In addition to its use in process planning, the top-down flowchart can be used as a quick way to flowchart an existing process that has seemingly grown to unexpected proportions because it prioritizes steps and simplifies the task of re-engineering the process. As a process is evaluated, the top-down flowchart provides information that can identify sources of waste and rework.

Relationship Diagrams

As processes become more complex, interrelationships begin to grow among various inputs and outputs; as these interactions increase, the probability of problems increases as well. For example, in the patient preparation for surgery scenario represented in Figure 3.7, the patient cannot be prepped for the operating room prior to being transported there. Thus, there is a relationship between transportation to the pre-op preparation area and the efficiency with which the patient may be prepared for a timely surgical start. Relationship diagrams, the topic of this section, can characterize these types of interactions.

Relations Diagram

A simple relations diagram indicates cause-and-effect relationships that may be affecting the efficiency of the process. As the least sophisticated of the relationship diagrams, this tool can often be completed quickly by a QI team, defining interactions between variables or concepts that can lead to improvement in the process. Prior to implementation of the process, a relations diagram can establish which inputs and outputs will require monitoring to optimize efficiency. Another common application of the relations diagram is in matrix format, where it is used for comparing ideas or process components in pairs.

A relations diagram and a matrix are found in Figure 3.8. The project is the installation of an electronic medical records system in a clinic, and the relations diagram represents a small proportion of the interactions involved in the implementation plan. The mix of concepts and actions is one of the most useful aspects in the relations diagram, but as the number of these items increases, many QI teams will eliminate the concepts in favor of simplifying the diagram. The matrix presents the same information in tabular format, which is more readable for some team members (see Figure 3.8, *bottom*).

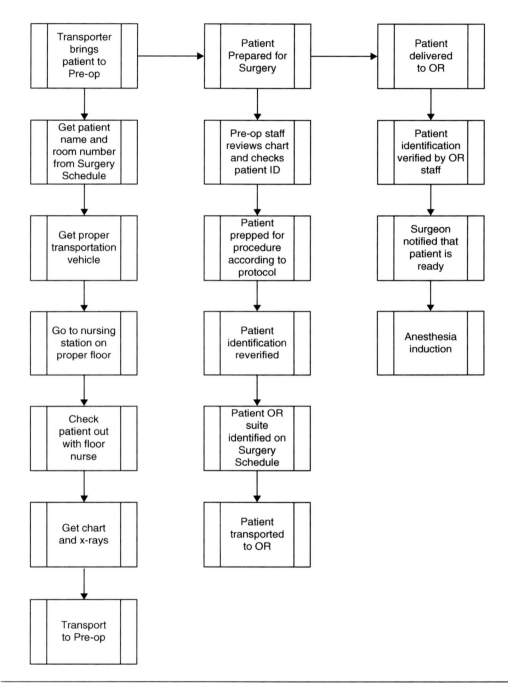

Figure 3.7 Top-Down Flowchart

OR, operating room; ID, identification

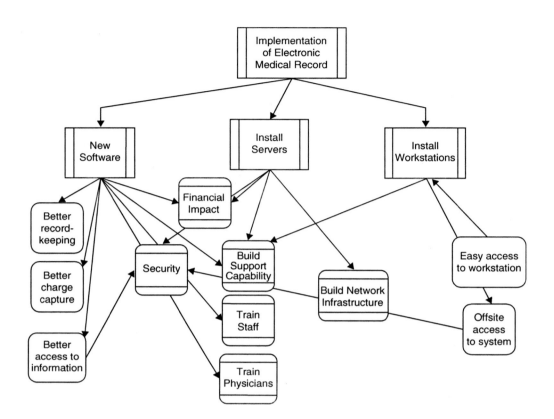

	New Software	Install Servers	Install Workstations
Financial impact	X	X	X
Build support capability			X
Security	X	X	X
Easy access to workstations			X
Offsite access to system	X		X
Train staff	X	X	X
Train physicians	X		X

Figure 3.8 Relations Diagram and Matrix

Construction of a relations diagram follows a system similar to the design of flowcharts.

1. List all possible concepts and issues for a project; if the list is too long, then combine some concepts or divide the list into subprojects of related ideas.
2. Place the components on sticky notes or note cards and connect the cards that are related. Some computer programs (e.g., Visio) can simplify the process by automating this step.

3. Work with the QI team and those responsible for implementing the project to refine the relationships between the concepts and issues.

If the list of ideas is too long, e.g., more than 50 concepts, then the relations diagram will not work well. In such cases, the project can be divided into smaller parts for analysis, with the caveat that a single concept may be placed in more than one subproject. Each concept should be evaluated using the query "What other ideas does this concept affect?" Each relationship should be only one way; i.e., there should be no double-headed arrows. These two-way relationships cloud interpretation of the diagram because prioritizing concepts and deployment issues becomes difficult without knowing which issues are of greater importance.

Tree Diagram

Most people are familiar with the concept of the tree diagram because it provides a logical framework for organizing complex systems or illustrating the branching logic of a decision support system. In a QI system, the tree diagram is often used to move from a general concept or goal to specific actions. It is particularly useful when there are many possible ways to achieve a goal or the objective is very complex. Tree diagrams present complex decision paths in relatively straightforward graphical diagrams and can be used to provide an overview of complex processes.

The approach to creating a tree diagram focuses on organizing a decision sequence into a logical order and then using brainstorming techniques to determine the means for accomplishing each action. Computer programs are very useful for creating tree diagrams; the diagram in Figure 3.9 was created with Visio. The procedure for constructing a tree diagram is as follows.

1. Define the goal of the diagram. This step is usually performed by the organization during strategic planning sessions or by mandate from senior management.
2. Determine what steps need to occur to achieve the goal. In most circumstances, this stage of the process will generate several possibilities, but if the number of possibilities exceeds five or six, then the project should be redefined to keep the number of branches on the tree manageable.
3. After these possibilities are defined, each is further dissected into more branches until the team feels that the tree is complete, i.e., the ends of the branches represent specific actions to be accomplished.
4. After all of the branches have been defined, the team re-evaluates the tree to ensure that each task shows all the actions necessary to complete the task. Additionally, the team should evaluate all actions to confirm that each is necessary to accomplish the goal.
5. Include implementation teams in the planning process to determine if each action is achievable.

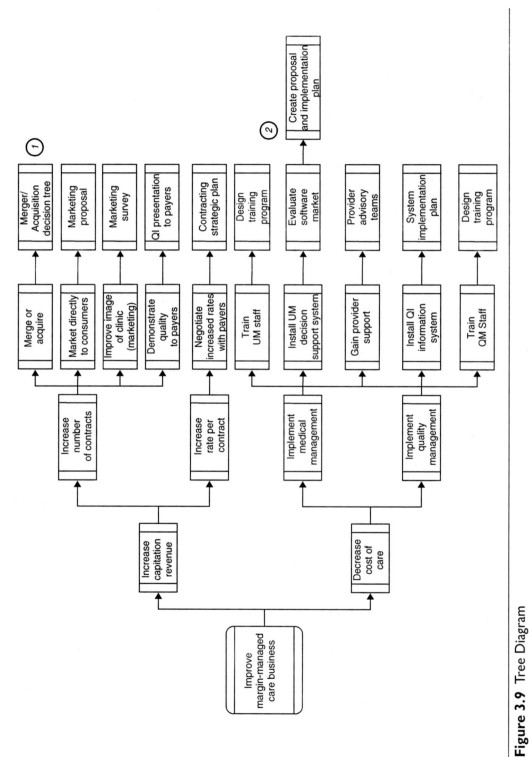

Figure 3.9 Tree Diagram

QM, quality management

Figure 3.9 exemplifies a preliminary tree diagram for improving the return on capitated contracts for a provider organization. Although this diagram is certainly not exhaustive for the problem of improving the financial performance in a capitated system, it illustrates several features of a tree diagram. For example, the branches of the tree lead inexorably to actions for each division. In some cases, as with the area marked with the *circled 1*, the branch may end in a reference to another decision tree that evaluates issues beyond the scope of the current tree. Notably, the tree branches do not necessarily end in the same place. The area indicated by the *circled 2* on the diagram indicates a branch that ended beyond the level of the others. Careful examination of the diagram will also reveal that the tree is not symmetrical; there are no rules that indicate the need for symmetry.

As the tree is created, the improvement team may complete one branch at a time or several branches at once. There are advantages to each approach, and the team will usually indicate a preference. Completing all branches at the same time may make the team more cognizant of similarities among the paths and lead to consolidation of the tree into fewer branches. On the other hand, evaluating one branch at a time allows the team to concentrate on one issue and formulate the best approach to each process.

The usefulness of tree diagrams should not be underestimated because they can be applied to several types of problems, such as determining a list of potential approaches to solving a problem, determining the cause of a problem, and characterizing the path for decision making.

Root Cause Diagram

One specific application of the tree diagram is the root cause diagram, often called the why–why diagram, which addresses the determination of the cause of a problem. Figure 3.10 presents a root cause diagram for a problem with waiting time in a radiology department. This variation of the tree diagram demonstrates the versatility of the concept, as well as the ability of tree diagrams to visually present the logic behind decisions. The radiology scheduling diagram also illustrates a method of indicating related concepts on the diagram at the connection designated by the *circled 1*. The transportation problem noted in the diagram relates two different concepts, i.e., that transporters are not available at a specific time and that transporters are not scheduled according to the needs of the radiology department. This relationship can be indicated by a connection between the boxes.

Ishikawa (Fish Bone) Diagram

Root cause diagrams provide insight into reasons and solutions for process problems. Kaoru Ishikawa introduced another method of evaluating root causes in the 1960s, often nicknamed the fish bone diagram because of its appearance. An example of an Ishikawa diagram, concerning low immunization

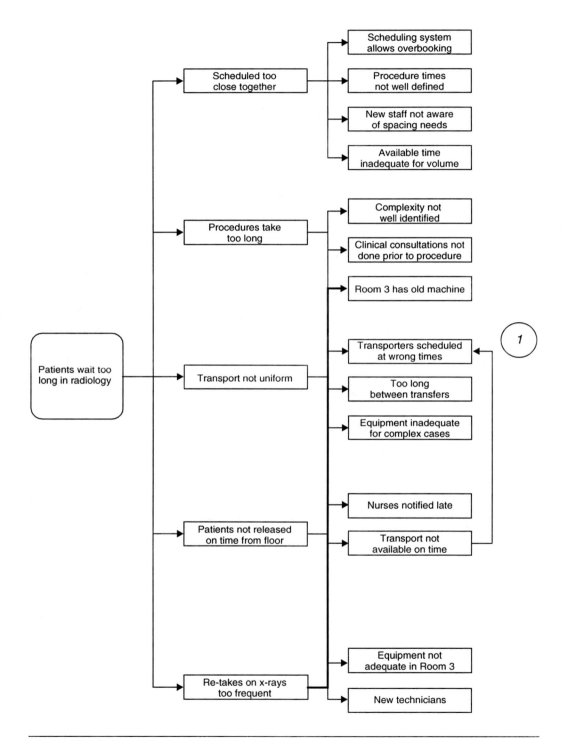

Figure 3.10 Root Cause (Why–Why) Diagram

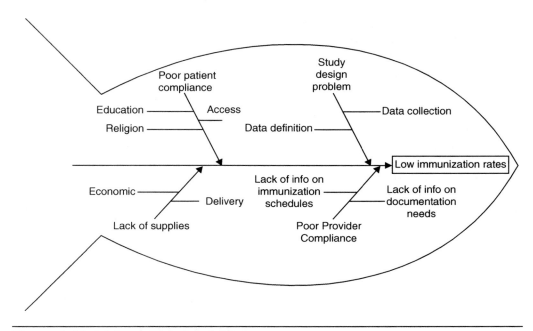

Figure 3.11 Ishikawa (Fish Bone) Diagram

rates, is presented in Figure 3.11. The main stem of the fish bone leads to the defined problem, in this case, low immunization rates. The branches leading to the main stem represent major areas of concern and often fall into categories such as people, materials, equipment, measurement, or environment.

The procedure for constructing an Ishikawa diagram relies on brainstorming, stimulating the QI team to think of reasons for the problem.

1. Determine the major problem for analysis.
2. Assemble a team of improvement professionals as well as operations staff concerned with the problem.
3. Construct the main stem of the diagram with the problem described at the end.
4. Brainstorm the major concerns as branches off the main stem.
5. Once the major concern branches are complete, combine any that are redundant or that should be subbranches.
6. After the group has agreed on the major branches, brainstorm each branch for root causes.
7. After the root causes are identified, combine any that are redundant.
8. Brainstorm root causes for any other factors that should be included as causes on the chart under the root cause branches.

The process is finished when no more branches are added.

The fishbone format is well established in QI, primarily because it can visually present a large number of root causes and issues in a relatively compact format. Some QI professionals prioritize the placement of major branches, with the branches deemed by the group to be more important placed nearer the "head" of the fish.

Work Flow Diagram

The work flow diagram shows movement within a process by people, materials, paperwork, or information. A floor plan of the work site is overlaid with the movement of the item of interest upon the floor plan, with the goal of identifying redundant motion and inefficiency. The most frequent use of these diagrams in health care is for examining traffic flow patterns in clinics and hospital systems. Figure 3.12 presents a work flow diagram for a clinic visit, demonstrating the redundancy in the patient's movement within the clinic. The method of developing a work flow diagram is straightforward.

1. Determine the item of interest that moves, e.g., people, paper, data, supplies, and materials.
2. Identify the realm within which the object moves.
3. Draw a floor plan of the realm. Computer software is very helpful for this task.
4. Develop a flowchart of the process for the object of interest that lists process steps in sequence.
5. Draw lines on the floor plan indicating every step that the object of interest takes in order to produce an output.
6. Analyze the workflow for overlap and inefficiency, e.g., excessive or unnecessary movement or motions that are repetitive.
7. Examine the floor plan or process flow for opportunities to improve the efficiency of the process.

If the object of interest is electronic information, the process is the same, but the diagram is different. The same principles apply if the information is not visible, as with paperwork, but the diagram will include features such as the person or site for information delivery and distribution. Implementation of a groupware installation in an organization can be analyzed using these techniques, with the goal of expediting movement of information throughout the company.

Matrices

Just as flowcharts form the backbone of process analysis, matrices have similar utility in helping understand and characterize issues for improvement. Matrices compare a number of entities with each other, and the flexibility of these tools makes them particularly useful in QI as well as in other areas of the company. For example, by using a matrix to compare product

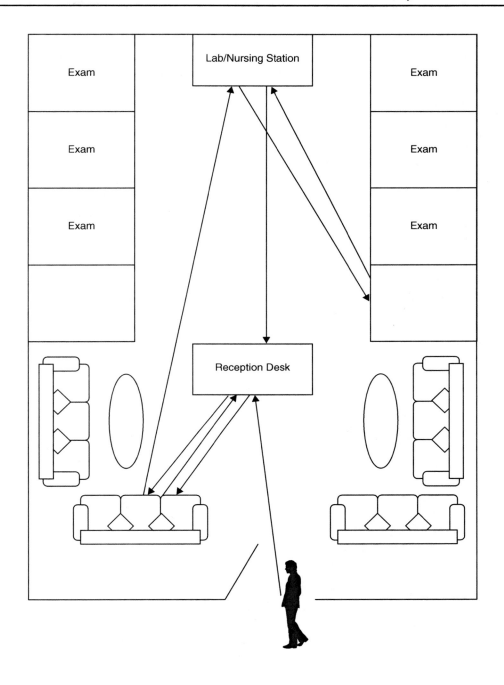

Figure 3.12 Work Flow Diagram

characteristics with customer needs, a marketing department can tailor sales materials to specific customer groups. Matrices have applications across the organization, and an understanding of the use of matrices can prove useful in a variety of business analyses.

Basic Matrices

Comparing two or more attributes using a matrix provides insight into relationships that are of importance to a QI effort. Most QI teams are familiar with the 1 × 1 matrix, sometimes called the L-shaped matrix, because spreadsheet programs are designed to easily create comparisons with rows and columns. Matrices have several other forms and can compare three or four variables in a manner similar to the two-variable comparisons. This section will explore the use of matrices for QI applications.

L-Shaped Matrix Perhaps the most ubiquitous of the matrices, the L-shaped matrix relates two variables in a row and column format. Although these matrices can be created manually, computer spreadsheet programs produce this format quickly and easily, as shown in Table 3.4. The data in Table 3.4 represent the total number of visits in each department of a multispecialty clinic. Data in a matrix must be related for the matrix to be useful.

Computer spreadsheet programs are powerful tools that facilitate organization of data in a matrix (sometimes called relational) format and then provide functions to perform mathematical operations on the data. Most spreadsheet programs now have graphing tools as well; these expedite the task of changing tabular data into many different types of graphical output. The functions that can be applied to data in spreadsheet programs now range from engineering to statistics, making these computerized tools particularly versatile.

The assignment of parameters to columns and rows is usually inconsequential to the creation of an L-shaped matrix. However, in some applications, the matrix will be more understandable to intended users if certain

Table 3.4 L-Shaped Matrix—Office Visits by Department

	January	February	March	April	May	June	Total
Pediatrics	563	872	743	498	459	401	3536
Family Practice	493	784	792	509	632	384	3894
Internal Medicine	287	345	408	392	410	273	2115
Obstetrics	308	297	310	283	312	294	1804
Gynecology	194	234	219	229	175	215	1266

conventions are observed. In most cases, the decision is one of personal preference, but if the data are to be graphically presented, then rows are generally used for an identifying attribute (company or department name), and the columns are used for measurement parameters (revenues, months of the year, output). Most spreadsheet software programs assume this type of row and column orientation in creating graphs from tabular data, so observing this simple rule can facilitate the process of creating the graph from a data table.

T-Shaped Matrix Another version of the matrix that compares two variables with a third is deemed the 1 × 2 or T-shaped matrix. Named for its structure, the T-shaped matrix places the comparison variable as a column and the other two variables as rows. An example is found in Table 3.5. Following the previous example (Table 3.4), the multispecialty clinic compared revenues between the clinics and added the revenue variable to the matrix, making it T-shaped.

The T-shaped matrix provides a concise view of several parameters and variables simultaneously. This matrix is most commonly used to compare multiple parameters within several categories in an easily understandable format.

Y-Shaped Matrix Yet another variation on the matrix theme is the Y-shaped matrix, which, like the T-shaped matrix, is used to demonstrate relationships between three groups of variables. The Y-shaped matrix, however, compares each group to the other two groups, i.e., a 2 × 1 comparison. Although more complex in design, the Y-shaped matrix imparts substantial insight into relationships among three variables as shown in Figure 3.13, which relates physician and operational variables to performance measures in an operating room. The entries in each cell of the matrix define the relationships between pairs of variables in each group, and the strengths of the relationships can be used in making plans for QI interventions. For example,

Table 3.5 T-Shaped Matrix—Economic Analysis of Clinic

Total Revenues	$328,149	$478,354	$264,842	$298,674	$342,139
Total Expenses	$287,138	$294,189	$163,247	$112,190	$116,329
Clinic	Pediatrics	Family Practice	Internal Medicine	Obstetrics	Gynecology
Total Visits	3536	3894	2115	1804	1266
Average Visits/mo	589	649	353	300	211

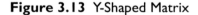

					Operating Room Efficiency Measures				
X	X	X	M		Starting Time Adherence	X	M	X	X
0	0	M	X		Cost per Case	0	0	M	M
M	0	X	X		Time per Case	X	X	M	X
0	0	0	M		Charge Capture Ratio	0	0	0	X

X = strong relationship
0 = no relationship
M = minor relationship

Figure 3.13 Y-Shaped Matrix

physician time per case is strongly related to *starting time adherence* and *time per case*; moderately related to *cost per case,* the *supply delivery* rate, the *environmental preparation* rate, *patient transport*, and *staff scheduling*; and unrelated to *charge capture ratio.* Complex relationships can thus be readily modeled using a Y-shaped matrix.

X-Shaped Matrix The final entry into the "alphabetical matrix" category is the X-shaped matrix, which relates four groups of variables in 1×2 groupings. An X-shaped matrix is illustrated in Table 3.6, which compares physician networks and product lines with product types and laboratory management packages for a managed care organization. Evident in the table is the wealth of information that can be contained in a relatively compact format. For example, MD network 1 (*MD Net 1*) participates only in the health

Table 3.6 X-Shaped Matrix

Indemnity	PPO	POS	HMO		Lab Package 1	Lab Package 2	Lab Package 3	Lab Package 4
X				Product 1				X
	X			Product 2			X	
		X		Product 3		X		
			X	Product 4	X			
X				Product 5				
X			X	MD Net 1	X	X		
X	X		X	MD Net 2	X		X	X
X	X		X	MD Net 3	X	X	X	
X		X	X	MD Net 4	X			X
X		X		MD Net 5	X	X	X	X

PPO, preferred provider organization; POS, point of service; HMO, health maintenance organization; Net, network.

maintenance organization (*HMO*) and *indemnity* product lines, and they are willing to deal with only two of the plan's laboratory management packages. Other networks of providers are more willing to participate in more of the plan's products, so unless *MD Net 1* has some special characteristic that requires its continuation, the plan may want to concentrate efforts on improving relationships with the networks that are more willing to deal with other products and lab plans. Similarly, the product lines could be strengthened contractually by increasing the number of laboratory plans offered through each product line.

Although X-shaped matrices are more complicated to create, the extra time is often repaid by the wealth of information that can be presented. When complex reports need consolidation, the X-shaped matrix presents relationships in a straightforward manner and can improve the appearance and simplicity of the report.

Specialized Matrices

Decision Matrix More specialized matrices are used for specific applications, and the decision matrix is one of the most valuable of this group. The primary function of the decision matrix is to help prioritize and evaluate a list of choices using criteria developed by the QI team. It usually involves such issues as effectiveness, system capability, cost, implementation time, and acceptance of the choice by customers, management, and staff. Several situations lend themselves to the use of decision matrices: selection of the best choice from a group of options, narrowing a list of problems or solutions to critical choices, and optimization of long lists of choices using team-generated criteria.

One of the advantages of the decision matrix approach is the assignment of numbers to the criteria, which allows calculation of ranks for each of the choices. Such numerical systems provide the improvement team with a more quantitative method for ranking choices.

A sample decision matrix can be found in Table 3.7. It deals with the problem of patient management in the emergency department, during and after the delivery of services. The matrix contains the rationale for each problem area, as well as relative scores for each variable, based on the analysis of the system performed by QI teams. The criteria identified and prioritized by the QI team are evaluated at each level of service, and a composite score for each area is calculated based on the weights provided by the criteria. The composite scores are then compared to identify the greatest need, which, for this example, is in the *postservice* category. Notably, the *preregistration* and *registration* areas follow closely behind *postservice* in need for reform. From this matrix, the QI team can begin to focus efforts on interventions for improvement.

Decision matrices have been applied not only to problem prioritization (as in the example) but also to prioritization of solutions and for comparing

Table 3.7 Decision Matrix

Choice Score	Medical Risk	Legal Risk	Effect on Other Departments	Ability to Change	Rate of Change	Score
	5	4	3	2	1	
Preregistration	Relatively high risk if serious condition not treated	If problem not treated, risk of lawsuit high	Staff usually adequate; little effect on other departments	Qualified staff easy to find	Improving facilities easy; staff increases relatively easy	
	3	4	3	2	2	34
Registration	Risk attenuated due to contact with staff	Nonmedical staff making assessments; legal risk high	Staff training could put load on HR department	Qualified staff must be trained in procedures	Qualified staff can be found quickly or transferred	
	2	3	1	1	2	34
Preservice	Triage period, risk assessed precisely	Risk of medical personnel making error	Nursing staff shortage; could hurt other units	Difficult to find staff quickly and train for ED	Slow due to shortage of nurses	
	1	3	3	3	3	27
Service	Risk assessed and treated	Risk of medical staff making error	ED medical staff well established	Staff well established; change difficult	Slow due to staff resistance	
	1	1	1	3	3	25
Postservice	Patient may not follow-up with treatment	Institution liable for lack of follow-up	Other areas would be in charge of contacts	Very hard due to extra work effort in other areas	Slow due to need to increase capacity in other areas	
	2	2	3	3	3	36

HR, human resources; ED, emergency department.

concepts for validity and acceptability. If the QI team decides to deal with the problem of postservice follow-up, they can readily adapt the decision matrix to evaluate potential solutions for the problem, prioritizing them in a similar manner and selecting the one that scores highest. Because the aggregate scores provide the basis for a decision, prioritization scores are of utmost importance in development of the criteria for the matrix.

Performance–Importance Matrix Another specialized matrix, called the performance–importance (P–I) matrix, combines the weighted scoring technique just described in the decision matrix discussion with analysis of customer perceptions. This exercise should be undertaken before any QI project is initiated so that the project can adequately serve customer needs as well as those of internal constituents. Any improvement project must ultimately address the needs of internal and external customers, and the P–I matrix ensures that external customers are not forgotten in the analysis.

The P–I matrix can also be used when customer perceptions must be collected and categorized or when the customer's perception of areas for improvement must be gauged. Note that the process for creating the P–I matrix includes surveying customer perceptions.

1. Identify customers, products, and services. Using the QI team to perform this first step will help make the process exhaustive and ensure that significant parameters are not overlooked.
2. Rank the customers based on important criteria to the organization: annual sales, key markets, industry leadership, etc.
3. Survey the top-ranked customers regarding the products and services that they use. Create a survey for each product or service that identifies attributes that customers might value and construct a rating scale for the customer to complete that assesses the performance and the importance of each major attribute. If the number of products and services for each customer is large, then the survey may be directed at answering the importance and performance questions for each product or service. (Suggested scales for each of these two measures are listed in Table 3.8.)
4. Survey internal customers with the same instrument.
5. Record comparisons and plot on the P–I matrix.

An example of a P–I matrix is presented in Figure 3.14. Customers A, B, and C, plotted on the matrix, represent three different situations. Customer A has a low performance score but a high importance score, indicating a need for substantial, rapid improvement of the product or service to meet the customer's needs. On the other hand, customer B has high scores for both performance and importance, signs that the organization is meeting this customer's needs quite well. Finally, customer C falls into the low importance, low performance category. This customer does not seem to need the organiza-

Table 3.8 Importance and Performance Scales

IMPORTANCE CATEGORIES	PERFORMANCE CATEGORIES
1 = Not important, not necessary	1 = Poor performance; regularly deficient
2 = Not necessary, but nice when available	2 = Needs improvement
3 = Neutral; somewhat valuable but not critical	3 = Adequate performance
	4 = Above average performance
4 = Important; verging on critical	5 = Top-notch performance
5 = Very important; critical	

tion's services very much, so low performance is of little significance. Customer *C* presents a problem: should the organization simply let this customer slide, or should efforts be made to increase the value of the product to the customer? The organization's strategic goals should be examined to determine a course of action in this case. The last quadrant, *quadrant 4*, indicates that the organization is performing very well, but the product or service is of little importance to the customer. In this case, the organization should consider whether such products or services should be continued or if the resources devoted to the output could be redirected to more productive products.

The same kind of analysis should be performed for internal staff as well, and the results of that survey can then be compared with the customer survey. Typically, these matrices compare customer and staff scores for each of the parameters, as in Figures 3.15 and 3.16. The importance matrix in Figure 3.15 compares staff and customer perceptions of the importance of a service that the organization provides. *A* illustrates a situation in which the staff considers the service more important than does the customer. Before discontinuing the service, the staff should be polled to ascertain the reasons for their view of the service. *B* indicates that customers and staff concur in their view of the importance of the service, and the organization need only continue trying to improve. *C* also connotes concurrence between staff and customers that a service is unimportant, and the organization should seriously examine discontinuing the service and directing resources elsewhere. Finally, a point in the fourth quadrant would specify customers valuing a service but staff disagreeing that the service is important. This conflict must be resolved so that customer perceptions of performance for an important service can be enhanced.

The performance matrix in Figure 3.16 demonstrates similar comparisons between customers and staff. At *A*, customers disagree with staff that performance by the organization meets customer needs. This area of the matrix requires substantial work to improve operations to better meet customer needs. *B* represents concordance between staff and customer perceptions of high performance and indicates the target for the organization. However, at

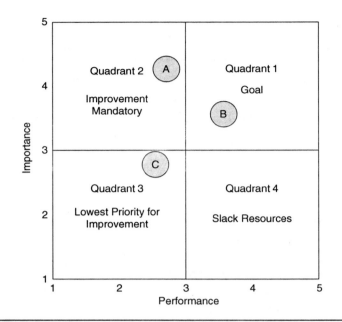

Figure 3.14 Performance–Importance Matrix

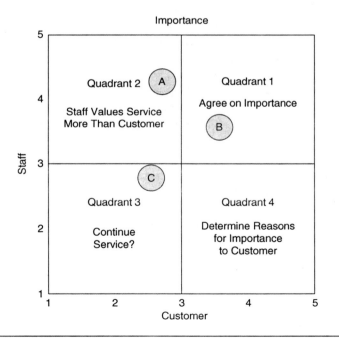

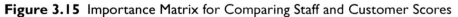

Figure 3.15 Importance Matrix for Comparing Staff and Customer Scores

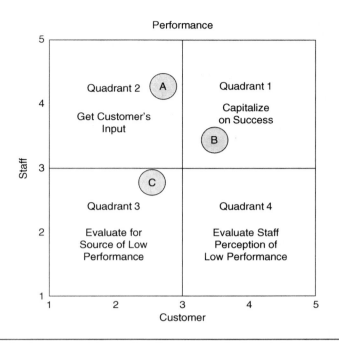

Figure 3.16 Performance Matrix for Comparing Staff and Customer Scores

C, both customers and staff agree that the performance of the organization is low, indicating that management must evaluate the service for elimination or substantial resource infusion for improvement. *Quadrant 4* again represents a relatively high customer perception of performance in the face of low staff perception of the organization's output. Staff input is important in this situation because it can portend deteriorating quality and, ultimately, customer dissatisfaction.

P–I matrices can prove highly useful for directing organizational QI efforts. Although customer perceptions may not always be correct, they must be heeded. The approach taken by the organization depends on the structure and current state of resources, but this analysis can provide management with substantial information for making appropriate, customer-focused decisions.

Kepner–Tregoe Matrix Developed primarily to isolate and identify causes of quality problems, the Kepner–Tregoe matrix (KTM; named after its creator and also called the is–is not matrix) helps managers recognize factors that underlie defects in a process. Most often used in a brainstorming environment, the KTM relates possible causes to specific categories, e.g., who, what, when, where, how, and why. The procedure for creating a KTM capitalizes on group input and an organized method of categorizing information, as discussed in the steps of the following example.

1. Characterize the problem in terms that are understandable to the QI team and that can create agreement on the nature of the predicament.
2. Create the matrix format depicted in Table 3.9.
3. Have the QI team formulate entries for each cell in the matrix, answering the questions of who, what, when, where, and how for the problem. A fundamental tenet of QI needs to be re-emphasized here: the process is the problem, not the person trying to implement or work within the process. Thus, the "who" questions are simply to help focus on process deficiencies, not to assign blame.

A pattern usually appears as the matrix is completed, particularly as the team identifies abnormal variations in the operation of the process.

Particularly important in creating the KTM is the point made in step 3, the tendency for groups to try to assign blame as the "who" part of the exercise proceeds. The QI team leader should make every effort to avoid that

Table 3.9 Kepner–Tregoe (Is–Is Not) Matrix

	IS: what actually happens now	IS NOT: what should happen but doesn't	Variations: what seems unusual about the situation
Who is involved in the process or problem?			
What inputs or outputs are involved in the problem or process?			
When does the problem occur—in what portion of the process?			
Where does the problem occur—in what part of the organization or what location?			
How important is the problem to the process? How extensive is the problem?			

situation because defensive barriers quickly arise and limit the effectiveness of the exercise.

The KTM provides an excellent means for improvement teams to find problems in processes and develop ways to resolve them. The procedure can take a fair amount of time as the team struggles with the potential causes listed in each of the categories, but the overall task is sufficiently exhaustive to ensure that process problems can be defined accurately.

Plan–Results Matrix   Evaluation of a process or a QI project should entail comparing plans with actual results, and the plan–results matrix (PRM) provides the framework for making that appraisal. Most useful in evaluating the results of interventions in a process, the PRM requires clearly defined objectives and performance measurements for a project, followed by an assessment by the QI team regarding the results. The format for a PRM is included as Figure 3.17. Because there are only four possible combinations of the two variables, plan and results, these pairs are represented in the four quadrants of the matrix. *Quadrant 1* denotes the best of all worlds, a plan that accomplished its task and produced results that were expected by the team. The second quadrant signifies a rather unlikely scenario—a good outcome without planning. Most QI professionals would deem that outcome "lucky." The third quadrant, however, indicates a poor outcome and a poor plan. Such a situation also should occur rather rarely if QI teams practice the tenets of QI and use the tools described in this book. Finally, *quadrant 4* suggests a good

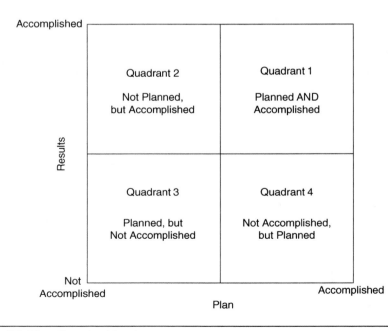

Figure 3.17 Plan–Results Matrix

plan but a poor outcome. In this scenario, the QI team must reassess the plan and determine the linkage between the plan design and the results obtained. Usually, some element of the plan can be identified as the culprit and revisions made to attain the desired goals.

Most managers create a mental version of this matrix when evaluating outcomes from QI interventions, but if the results of an intervention are more ambivalent, it is often helpful to have the QI team perform this analysis to determine the underlying causes of failure.

Requirements Matrix As processes are being designed, it is important to verify customer requirements to ensure that the output of the process meets customer demands. The requirements matrix simply tabulates specifications for internal and external customers, thus delineating the required outputs. The sample requirements matrix in Table 3.10 reveals the categories of internal and external customers that must be considered for a representative managed care health plan.

The requirements matrix can be completed for the organization as a whole or for individual product or service lines, but the most useful analysis occurs at the product or service level. As the processes for producing or administering a particular product or service are being formulated, required outputs should be continually reviewed to make certain that all needs are being satisfied as much as possible. Obviously, trade-offs between the needs of internal and external customers become necessary, but astute managers should apply expertise to be sure that the core requirements of all customers are met.

Effective–Achievable Matrix The final matrix to be discussed, the effective–achievable matrix (EAM), assists the QI team in ranking possible choices in process implementation. In most cases, the EAM is applied to a list of choices that the team has constructed through a brainstorming exercise but that have no apparent priority. With the use of a weighting system similar to that previously described for the decision matrix, each choice is

Table 3.10 Requirements Matrix

	Designation	Product Requirements	Process Requirements
External	Employers	Low cost Broad coverage Effective medical management Quality management Regular reports Minimal cost escalation on renewal	Rapid response to queries Member satisfaction with processes Efficiency to keep administrative costs low

Table 3.10 *continued*

	Designation	Product Requirements	Process Requirements
External (cont.)	Members	Broad coverage Minimal copayments and deductibles Broad access Family coverage Portability Out of network access	Rapid response to queries Understandable responses Simple explanation of rights and responsibilities Friendly staff Little or no paperwork
	Regulators	Compliance with state and federal laws Maintain adequate reserves Prudent fiscal management	Documentation of compliance Meet deadlines for report submissions Clarity of language and documentation in reports
	Accreditation bodies	Compliance with accreditation guidelines Appropriate safeguards for members and payers	Meet criteria for accreditation or certification Efficient processes that deliver value to customer
	Providers	Excellent reimbursement for services Broad, understandable coverage for members Simple product descriptions	No paperwork Rapid payment No hassles with medical management Assurance of quality
Internal	Clerical staff	Understandable benefit designs Appropriate infrastructure and support to administer products	Job security Excellent pay and benefits Reasonable working hours
	Executive staff	Board support for management activities Reasonable product prices and quality Good return on investment	Job security Excellent pay and benefits Reasonable working hours Perquisites
	Management staff	Executive support for management activities Adequate resources for managing product Simple product line structure	Job security Excellent pay and benefits Reasonable working hours Perquisites

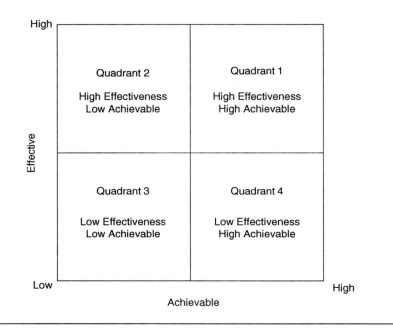

High

Effective

Quadrant 2

High Effectiveness
Low Achievable

Quadrant 1

High Effectiveness
High Achievable

Quadrant 3

Low Effectiveness
Low Achievable

Quadrant 4

Low Effectiveness
High Achievable

Low

High

Achievable

Figure 3.18 Effective–Achievable Matrix

ranked on an effectiveness scale and an achievable scale. A format for the effective–achievable matrix can be found in Figure 3.18. Typical rankings for the EAM are simply high or low on effectiveness and achievability. The choices are then placed on the matrix according to their ranking.

Evident in Figure 3.18 is the implication that choices that fall into *quadrants 3* and *4* are best ignored because they are either ineffective or both unachievable and ineffective. *Quadrant 1* points are the most successful, but if no points fall into that quadrant, then *quadrant 2* may have the best possibilities, i.e., difficult to achieve but most likely to be effective. A QI team can readily prioritize projects, interventions, and other parameters such as performance measures using the EAM. Although many managers perform this type of analysis *a priori*, the rigor of the EAM analysis usually is superior because it involves a team approach.

◆ Failure Mode and Effects Analysis—Prospective Process Review

The study of processes can be prospective or retrospective. The techniques that have been discussed so far can be used in either situation, but one prospective approach has been used for several decades by the aviation and automotive industries to prevent errors or accidents. Failure mode and effects analysis (FMEA) is applied to existing or proposed processes to anticipate errors and to design systems to avoid mistakes. Starting in 2001, the Joint Commission on Accreditation of Healthcare Organizations (JCAHO) required hospitals to implement a process to anticipate and prevent errors in patient care services. FMEA provides a means of performing this analysis, and the tools that have been discussed in this chapter can contribute to the review.

FMEA involves studying a process, either existing or proposed, to determine where a failure may occur and what effect that failure will have on the process or an outcome. One approach to FMEA involves the following steps.

1. Choose a high-risk process for review. Although QI processes typically fall into any of three categories—high risk, high cost, or high volume—FMEA projects generally are classified as high risk of error.
2. Assemble a team of people who are familiar with or use the process regularly.
3. Create a flowchart of how the process works currently. If the process is new, skip this step and proceed directly to step 4.
4. Create a flow chart that defines the optimum process (a PERT diagram may provide the best information).
5. Evaluate the process flowcharts to determine the location, type, and severity of failure modes, i.e., the potential failures that may occur at each step of the process.
6. For each failure mode, calculate a criticality index that helps prioritize action plans for change. The criticality index, also called a risk priority number, is the product of rankings for three parameters: severity ranking, occurrence ranking, and detection ranking. The criticality index for each failure mode can then be used to identify high priority items, with the highest scores receiving the highest priority.
7. Implement changes using the plan-do-study-act cycle.
8. Recalculate the criticality index for each failure mode after implementation of the improvement. Each failure mode should be re-evaluated because improvement in one part of a process may cause improvements in other parts of the process.
9. Optimize the process and make the changes part of the process.

The advantage of FMEA derives from the use of a system of quantifying the three most important attributes of a failure mode, i.e., severity, occurrence, and ability of the system to detect the failure. Each of the parameters can be scored using a modified Likert scale, as noted in Table 3.11. Although the scales are subjective, the ability to gain an estimate of the importance of each factor in the failure mode provides a powerful tool for prioritizing safety and error issues. A sample FMEA form is included as Figure 3.19. The form can be created in a word processing or spreadsheet program to simplify analysis and data recording.

Table 3.11 FMEA Scoring System

Parameter	Score	Description
Severity	1	Slight annoyance that may affect the system
	2	Moderate system effects
	3	Moderate system effects that may affect the patient
	4	Major system problems; patient not affected
	5	Major system problems; patient affected
	6	Minor injury to the patient
	7	Major injury to the patient
	8	Terminal injury to the patient
	9	Patient death
Occurrence	1	Does not occur
	2	Occurrence not probable; no data available
	3	Occurrence not probable; minimal data available
	4	Occurrence not probable; data available on incidence
	5	Moderate probability of occurrence; incidence low
	6	Moderate probability of occurrence; incidence medium
	7	High probability of occurrence; data available but not conclusive
	8	High probability of occurrence; well documented and conclusive
	9	Very high probability of occurrence, data available but not conclusive
	10	Very high probability of occurrence, conclusive data available
Detection	1	Error always detected
	2	Very high likelihood of error detection
	3	High likelihood of error detection
	4	Moderately high likelihood of error detection
	5	Moderate likelihood of error detection
	6	Moderately low likelihood of error detection
	7	Low likelihood of error detection
	8	Unlikely chance of error detection
	9	Error almost never detected

FMEA, failure mode and effects analysis.

PROCESS

PRE-INTERVENTION ANALYSIS

Function/Task	Failure Mode	Effect	Severity Score (S)	Occurrence Score (O)	Detection Score (D)	Criticality Index*	Recommended Action	Target Date

*Criticality index = S × O × D.

PROCESS

POST-INTERVENTION ANALYSIS

Function/Task	Failure Mode	Effect	Action/Completion Date	Severity Score	Occurrence Score	Detection Score	Criticality Index

Figure 3.19 FMEA Data Collection and Analysis Form

Once failure modes are identified, the approach to creating interventions to prevent errors falls into one of six categories:

1. minimizing waste and rework through elimination of process steps or items that are not used or that do not add value to the process, such as multiple data entry into a computer system;
2. improving work flow processes by gaining better coordination between related processes, minimizing the number of steps and/or individuals involved in the process, ensuring appropriate levels of competence for participating in the process, and moving more work to the customer;
3. optimizing equipment and materials by automation and integration of the supply chain;
4. improving timeliness of inputs and service delivery through integration of the supply chain, reduction in cycle time, and reducing the time to execute each step;
5. reducing variation by standardizing processes and developing plans for dealing with process variation;
6. improving the work environment by making information more accessible, providing workers who are accountable for a particular process with the authority to deal with contingencies, and ensuring proper lighting, ergonomic instrumentation, and comfortable surroundings.

FMEA has been used in health care in a number of areas, particularly to reduce medication errors (Benjamin, 2003; Grissinger and Rich, 2002; Mac-Nally, Page, and Sunderland, 1997), reducing the risk from blood transfusions (Burgmeier, 2002), and improving the reliability of maintenance of biomedical instruments (Ridgway, 2003). Because the method can anticipate and eliminate potential causes of errors, FMEA serves an important function in the improvement of quality in health care systems.

◆ Root Cause Analysis—Retrospective Process Review

Once an error has occurred, analysis of the situation to determine the underlying cause(s) of the error and making recommendations for preventing the error in the future are the subject of root cause analysis (RCA). JCAHO has required a process for investigating errors for the past several years, so hospitals and other facilities that are required to have JCAHO accreditation have implemented some version of RCA, but other health care organizations, e.g., physician offices, health plans, and other health facilities, usually lack an organized approach.

RCA involves application of the tools discussed in this chapter to identify a remediable cause of an unfavorable outcome, usually limited by time and available resources. Two important attributes of this definition deserve emphasis: the cause must be capable of being fixed, and it must be uncovered in a reasonable amount of time using a reasonable expenditure of resources. From a practical standpoint, RCA must be performed efficiently but must also demonstrate effectiveness if changes are to be acceptable to senior management and stakeholders. Once an adverse outcome or event is identified, the following procedure is typical.

1. Assemble a team of process experts to evaluate the event.
2. Create a process flow diagram if one does not already exist.
3. Examine the flowchart for the procedure that failed and led to a suboptimal outcome.
4. Use specialized flowcharts (e.g., PERT diagram, cost of quality, critical to quality, or deployment) to analyze process parameters and identify root causes for the process failure.
5. Use group techniques (brainstorming, brainwriting, nominal group technique) to refine and prioritize underlying root causes of the faulty procedure.
6. Use QI tools such as the Ishikawa diagram, relationship diagrams, and tree diagrams to help relate data to specific root causes.
7. Redesign the process using group techniques and list reduction techniques (e.g., multivoting) to optimize the group's decisions.
8. Implement the changes in a pilot project, if possible, prior to generalizing the change to all areas of the organization.

Commercial software packages have been created to guide the analysis process (see "Root Cause Analysis—Commercial Packages" in the reference section). Because RCA is such an important component of a quality assurance program and efficiency is key to making needed changes in processes, a commercial package may be a worthwhile investment.

Successful RCA culminates in the identification of underlying causes of problems in a process. The key to effective RCA, however, is a thorough understanding of the process and underlying factors, so the QI team must ensure that a process analysis has been performed as the starting point using the tools described in this chapter.

◆ Continuous QI—Concurrent Process Review

The tools described in this chapter and the statistical approaches in the next three chapters also can be used to concurrently evaluate processes in a health care organization. Ongoing monitoring of health care processes, both clinical and administrative, can detect issues and trends for which early intervention can prevent adverse outcomes and reduce the costs of rework and error recovery.

In addition to using them as part of a professional approach to continually enhance their efficiency and effectiveness, many health care organizations have established quality monitoring systems in response to regulatory or accreditation requirements (Bates, et al., 1998; Halpern, 1996). Using techniques such as the balanced scorecard and statistical process control, health care organizations can detect process improvement opportunities early and intervene with enhancements to improve outcomes and reduce cost. Because these efforts are ongoing, they are termed "continuous" QI (CQI). Many of the measures are also tracked at regional and national levels by agencies such as the Centers for Medicare and Medicaid Services (CMS) in the *Statements of Work for Quality Improvement Organizations* (Centers for Medicare and Medicaid Services, 2003) and organizations such as the NCQA, which promotes the use of HEDIS measures for health plans (National Committee for Quality Assurance, 2003). Efforts to standardize specific measures across institutions will permit comparison of health care organizations, as well as provide baseline measures for quality assurance.

◆ Relationship of Quality Assurance Approaches

The three approaches to quality assurance described in this chapter, CQI, FMEA, and RCA, are designed for application in a systems approach to health care. These three methods of ensuring quality should be integrated into the organizational performance improvement system, as noted in Figure 3.20. As processes are being designed, proactive FMEA can anticipate problems and preclude errors. The CQI approach maintains, manages, and improves quality as a process function within the organization, and RCA can be used to address process failures or aberrant outcomes. This combination of approaches serves as the foundation of a performance improvement system for any health care organization.

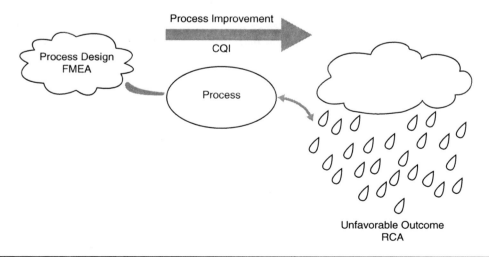

Figure 3.20 Relationship of FMEA, CQI, and RCA in a Performance Improvement System

CQI, continuous quality improvement; RCA, root cause analysis

◆ Data Requirements in Quality Management

An old saying in QI circles can be stated simply: "In God we trust; all others bring data." The QI paradigm demands valid data throughout the process, from analyzing quality problems to determining causes and designing solutions and then measuring the efficacy of the intervention with performance measures. Obtaining data is fraught with problems in health care because data sources can be varied and sometimes produce conflicting information. Because some data require arduous work to collect, a few basic principles are helpful in deciding what data to gather.

First, there must be a clear understanding of why particular information needs to be collected. Do not collect data items simply to be thorough or exhaustive, but select only those data elements that will be used in the analysis. Second, collect all data elements that will be necessary for the analysis. The worst outcome of a study is to lack data elements for the analysis and have to return to collect more data. Also, use the least invasive methods for data collection. If data that are collected in the normal course of business will suffice for the analysis, use that information, rather than collect more data.

Be certain that the operational definition of the data is agreed upon prior to starting the collection. The second worst outcome of a study is if the wrong data are collected because the data collectors did not understand the requirements of the study. Ensure that the data collected are in a format that is appropriate to the proposed analysis. If numeric data are required for the analysis, then collect numeric data. Finally, before starting data collection, review the study and be certain that the data requirements are clearly delineated to eliminate errors. By following these guidelines, the QI team can eliminate data collection errors and reduce impositions on staff members and customers.

QI studies generally use analytic statistics to evaluate data. Analytic statistics apply to time series of data; the other major approach to data analysis, enumerative statistics, is more traditional in health care and involves studying a process at only one or two points in time. Because QI implies continuous re-evaluation of a process to ascertain improvement, the analytic statistical approach is more useful for QI projects. Thankfully, analytic statistics include the most basic of statistical parameters, i.e., mean, variance, and standard deviation, to perform data analysis. The actual application of this approach is the subject of Chapter 4, "Statistical Process Control: Basic Principles," but the implication for data collection is that most QI data will be collected over time, rather than at just a single point in time.

Data Sources and Collection Methods in Health Care

Although data abound in the health care industry, access to the data is highly restricted as a result of the sensitive nature of the information. Clear guidelines exist regarding access to information on individual patients, and any analysis that is performed on large databases must conform to the rules governing patient privacy. Thus, most organizations restrict analysis of patient data to a few individuals who are trained in protecting patient confidentiality. Sources of data in health care can be divided into a few general categories:

◆ claims data submitted to insurance companies
◆ Medicaid data submitted to state Medicaid agencies or managed care organizations
◆ Medicare data submitted to the federal government or fiscal intermediaries
◆ transaction data in physician and institutional billing systems
◆ patient chart data
◆ surveys
◆ state birth certificates and death certificates
◆ data from pharmaceutical companies and pharmaceutical benefit managers
◆ data repositories

Each of these data sources will be examined in more detail.

Claims Data from Insurance Companies

Perhaps the most frequently used data source in health care consists of the information that insurance companies collect to process medical bills. Providers of all types—physicians, hospitals, home health agencies, skilled nursing facilities, etc.—submit information to insurers to be paid for services. The information can be sent on specific forms, such as the HCFA-1500 form or the UB-92 form, or it can be submitted electronically for direct entry into the information system of the insurer. The data consist of specific information about a patient encounter. In the United States, these data elements include

◆ patient identifying and demographic information
◆ type of service rendered, including general categories such as accident-related and birth control services
◆ place where the service was rendered
◆ diagnosis using the international classification of diseases (ICD)-9-CM coding system
◆ procedures and services provided using the current procedural terminology (CPT) coding system
◆ duration of service
◆ charge for the service
◆ provider of the service

These data elements are then entered into the insurer's computer system and processed for payment after a modicum of data validation (such as making sure that 100-year-old men are not admitted to the hospital with a diagnosis of term pregnancy). The insurer's computer system also checks each claim record against eligibility files to verify that the patient is a member of the health plan. Any claim that does not meet the data validation criteria is rejected or "pended" to a holding file. Insurance company staff members then usually adjudicate these claims to determine if an error has occurred and notify the billing organization of any errors that they find. The process has become highly efficient in the past few years, but in spite of the improvements in claims processing, many problems persist with the data that the insurance companies use to make decisions.

Probably the most crucial problem with the insurance company data is the paucity of information that it contains about patient care. The data elements that are collected have diagnosis codes that are frequently only approximations of the patient's actual diagnosis because the ICD-9-CM coding system lacks the robustness to accurately code all medical diagnoses. Some insurers can record only a few of the diagnosis codes in the claims system, meaning that patients with multiple clinical conditions may have only a few listed in the computer. Finally, the procedure codes submitted by providers contain no information about results of tests performed on patients, so the insurance company database contains only the fact that a patient had a test, not the critical information—the results of the test.

Another shortcoming of insurance company databases stems from the inconsistent way that providers are paid. Different providers are paid different amounts for the same procedure. For example, an orthopedist may be paid substantially more for reducing a dislocated elbow in a child than a pediatrician performing the same procedure. Providers quickly learn of these inequities, and because insurance companies rarely eliminate these irregularities, providers become "creative coders." Thus, a simple examination may become "unbundled" into a series of procedure codes, all of which describe a single service rendered. Insurers struggle mightily to stamp out these coding practices, with little success. The net result of these problems is a lack of consistency in coding by providers across the continuum of care. In addition to these reimbursement inequities, insurers and providers both have "coding dyslexia," i.e., use of different codes for the same condition based solely on the requirements of the insurer or the perception of the provider.

Insurers promote inadequate coding in other ways, as well. Physicians who are capitated for providing services to groups of patients are paid only a single amount per patient, regardless of the services that are provided to the patient. HMOs, in particular, employ this form of payment for primary care services. Sending bills to insurance companies adds costs to provider overhead, so if providers are not paid based on the information submitted for the care rendered the patient, then providers often do not submit that information. Thus, the insurer's database lacks substantial portions of the data that would normally be submitted when providers are paid a fee for each service delivered to patients. For HMOs, such data problems require access to other data sources, such as the patient chart, to determine levels of service for their members. Costly examinations of patient records in physician offices ensue, adding to the administrative burden of the insurer and the provider. In spite of these additional data sources, however, the claims database of the insurer still lacks fundamental information for decision making.

Finally, the data in claims databases tend to be inconsistent from company to company. Insurers collect different data for paying claims, and because payment schedules are not uniform between insurance companies, providers may have different methods of coding for different insurers. Added to that complication is the variation in how insurers filter and process data for claims payment, limiting comparability of data analysis between plans. On the other hand, organizations such as the NCQA and the Foundation for Accountability have produced operational definitions of specific measures that force health insurers to perform standardized analyses of their data to improve comparisons between health plans. The contribution of the NCQA to this issue, as mentioned earlier in the chapter, is called HEDIS, and it consists of over 50 measures of clinical effectiveness and administrative efficiency. With time, more of these measures should be identified, reducing the problem of comparing information between health plans.

Medicaid Data

Medicaid data submission practices vary tremendously across the country. Some states have traditional claims-paying systems, whereas many others have converted some or all of the Medicaid population in their state to managed care. In those states with traditional systems, the state or an intermediary acts as an insurance company and receives provider claims, performs filtering and screening on the information, and then pays the claims in batches. All of the typical fee-for-service claims-paying problems thus apply to these systems because providers have learned coding techniques to maximize their financial returns. In those states that have converted their Medicaid-eligible citizens to managed care, nearly all have contracted with managed care companies to provide the HMO services. The insurers assume responsibility for processing claims, leading to disparate claims systems that have different data management techniques. These states require managed care organizations to submit their claims data in specific formats to the state computer systems for storage and analysis, but the interface between the managed care organization systems and the state systems remains tenuous at the present time. As with any technology, these problems will ultimately be overcome, but in the interim period, QI analysts must exercise care when analyzing data from these sources.

Data from Medicaid systems that have converted to managed care is subject to the same foibles as other managed care systems, including failure to submit claims in a capitated environment, creative coding to enhance financial return, and unbundling services. These databases tend to be exceedingly large, as well, both because the number of members in the Medicaid programs is huge and because of the tremendous volume of services that this population customarily consumes. Special approaches to data analysis beyond the scope of this book are necessary to ensure that the data are validated and properly coded if quality analyses are to be effective.

Medicare Data

Medicare is undergoing changes similar to those in the Medicaid program. As Medicare+Choice programs proliferate around the country, billing data are changing to reflect the new managed care focus in this federal insurance program for the aged and disabled. Just as other managed care plans have had problems with data collection and reporting, the Medicare+Choice plans will have similar difficulties.

At the present time, however, Medicare claims are submitted to the federal government through intermediaries for direct fee-for-service claims payment. After the data are collected and processed, the federal government makes portions of them available for public use over the Internet (*http://cms.hhs.gov/researchers/statsdata.asp*). Subsets of the data provide information about utilization of hospital services, enrollment, provider utilization, payment rates, and a host of other databases. Of course, the data have been filtered to remove patient-specific identification information, but these databases provide a rich source of information about the Medicare population.

Transaction Data in Provider Billing Systems

Provider computer systems are the source of insurance company, Medicaid, and Medicare data. Nearly all providers now have computerized billing systems, so all of the data required to bill for a patient encounter are contained in medical office and hospital computers. This information can be used for analysis in the same way that information in the computers of payers is used. Beyond relatively simple reports such as aged accounts receivable and provider productivity reports by CPT or ICD code most provider computer systems are not tapped for QI information. As this rich source of data is increasingly recognized, however, and as providers are increasingly called upon to provide QI information across all payers, programs will be developed to analyze provider databases.

The problems with coding persist at this level as well. Because providers may unbundle services and creatively code to maximize financial return, the same caveats apply to analyzing these data sources that exist in insurance company databases. Patients with the same clinical characteristics may be coded differently based solely on the payment schedules of the insurer. This incongruity is especially pronounced in hospital systems that have installed specialized software to optimize diagnosis and procedure codes to maximize financial returns. Data from these systems can be internally consistent, however, and can serve as a good source of information for QI projects.

Clinical Information in Patient Charts

The sole source of complete clinical data remains the patient chart. As patient charts are converted from bulky and unmanageable paper-based systems to computerized systems, the utility of patient clinical data will soar. At the present time, skilled chart reviewers, most often trained nurses, pore over patient records seeking specific data elements for QI studies. The chart audit process is time-consuming and costly, and problems with consistency between nurse reviewers plague the data analysis. When data are stored electronically, many of these problems will disappear.

Several other difficulties occur with medical chart data. Physicians vary substantially in the amount of information that they record about their patient interactions. Some physicians are meticulous in their recordkeeping habits; others are quite terse. Patients with similar or the same diagnoses may be described differently by two different physicians, so the medical chart may lead nurse reviewers to conclude that similar patients are different clinically. Additionally, other factors may intervene in the interpretation of the patient chart, such as missing data, poor handwriting, failure to follow specific data recording conventions, etc. Figure 3.21 is a page from a patient chart that demonstrates the difficulty that nurse reviewers face when evaluating chart data. Thus, even though the medical chart should be the primary source of clinical data, it is not the perfect resource for QI data.

Surveys

Increasingly, health care analysts survey patients and providers to obtain information about the efficiency and effectiveness of the system. From simple one- or two-question surveys to long instruments like the Consumer Assessment of Health Plans Survey (CAHPS), consumers and providers are increasingly being polled on their perceptions of the health care system. Several important issues surround surveys, however, particularly if they are to be used for QI activities.

First, the survey questions must be written to actually measure the issue of interest. Frequently, a survey may be written and administered without any validation of survey questions to be certain that the questions actually ask for the correct information. Without such validation, surveys may lead to erroneous conclusions and produce actions that reduce quality rather than create improvements.

Second, a survey question should not suggest the answer to the question. For example, a question such as "Have you been taking your medicine like your doctor said you should?" will invariably receive a yes answer, making the query not only ineffective but also potentially dangerous if patient care relies on the responses. Survey questions should be phrased in such a way that the respondent can answer honestly without fear of retribution or humiliation.

Third, answers to some survey questions should not suggest answers to other questions. Most people try to appear consistent in their responses to

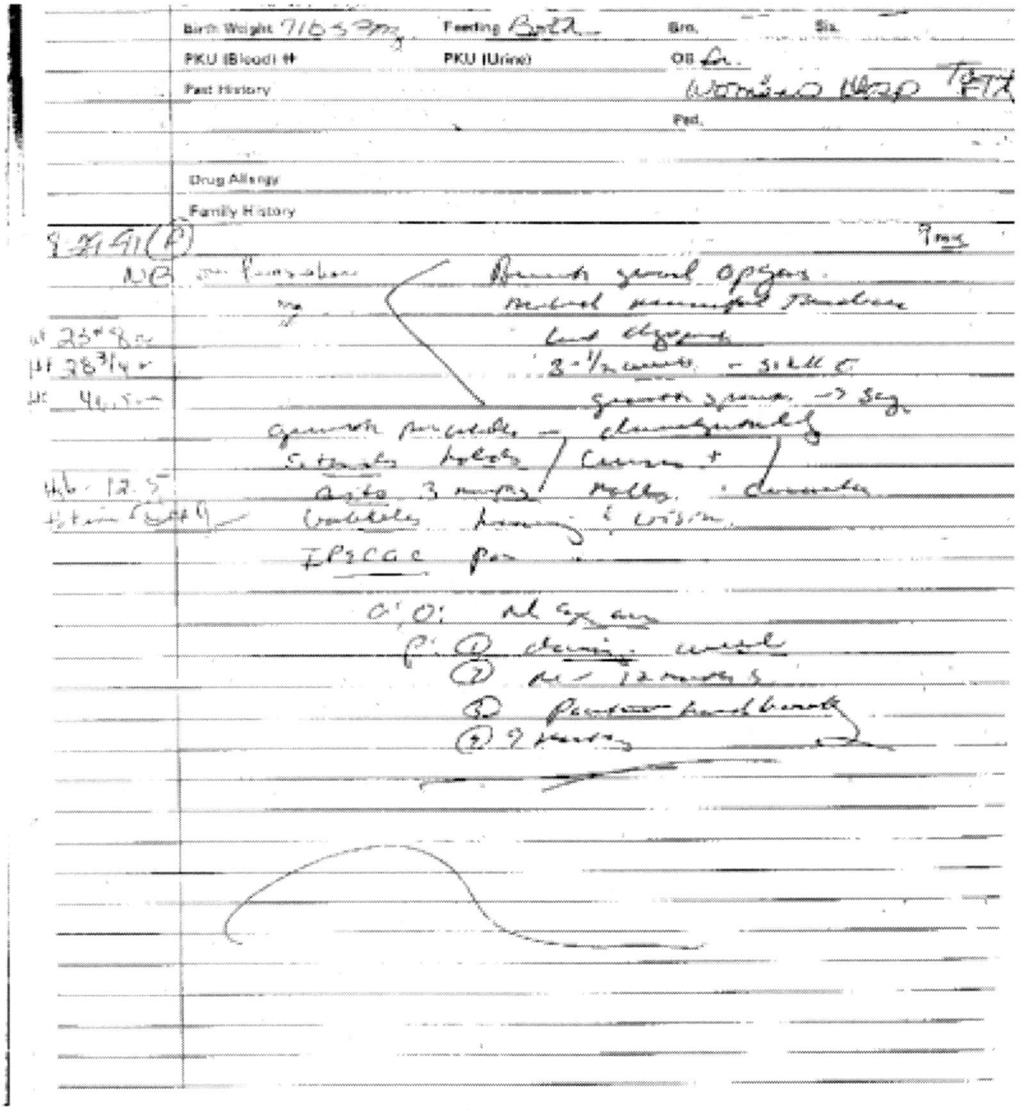
Birth Weight
Feeding
Bro.
Sis.
PKU (Blood) #
PKU (Urine)
OB
Past History
Ped.
Drug Allergy
Family History

Figure 3.21 Sample Entry in Patient Chart

survey questions, so if the questions seem to be related and require correlation, errors can occur as respondents try not to seem contradictory in their answers.

Finally, survey questions need to be tailored to the understanding of the respondents. If questions are phrased in such a way that the respondent cannot comprehend their meaning, then the survey results will be erroneous.

These are just a few of the problems that can arise from using surveys for QI activities. A number of validated, standardized patient satisfaction surveys are available, e.g., the SF-36 and SF-12 instruments and the CAHPS survey used in Medicare and Medicaid plans. For population analyses, these surveys may be most appropriate. For individual QI activities in organizations, these instruments may prove too general for meaningful analysis. However, if the organization decides to produce a survey specific to its own needs, a consultant can often help ensure that the instrument is valid and accurate. Numerous disease- or condition-specific instruments are also available for use, either with or without associated fees (Bowling, 1995).

Other Data Sources

A number of other data sources can be of use in analyzing quality improvement activities. Most states have computerized databases of birth and death certificate information that can be correlated with clinical information to perform studies that assess mortality and provide more precise birth information than do many provider and payer data sets. Public health departments usually serve as the source for this information.

Pharmaceutical companies are collecting large volumes of data on drug utilization patterns that will provide no patient-specific information but which can be used to assess drug usage in populations divided into any number of demographic distributions. Similar to pharmaceutical companies are pharmacy benefits managers that contract with health insurers to administer pharmacy benefits for large health plans. These companies have patient-specific data, and often these databases are among the most accurate for measuring individual drug utilization.

Finally, many data repositories are appearing that provide information that does not contain patient identification but does provide specific patient information. Many health plans, for example, are combining information from various sources besides claims management systems into large data warehouses from which extracted data can be used to perform sophisticated studies of quality and utilization. The Internet is a good source for these databases, and a number of these sites are listed in the bibliography.

Health Insurance Portability and Accountability Act and Data Sources

The promulgation in 2003 of data privacy rules required by the Health Insurance Portability and Accountability Act (HIPAA) has changed methods of data collection, analysis, and reporting throughout the health care industry. Passed in 1996, HIPAA was designed to provide people who were changing jobs with continuous health insurance coverage regardless of their clinical condition, but another feature of the act was intended to streamline the transfer of data between providers and payers by standardizing data sets and then protecting the information in those data sets to protect consumers. Although the US Congress was tasked with creating rules to effect these processes, CMS ultimately assumed responsibility for creating and implementing the rules and regulations to implement the law, first by standardizing transaction sets for data interchange (Transaction Rule, 2002), then ensuring privacy of patient information (Privacy Rule, April 2003), and finally in upcoming rules for security and a system for a national provider identifier that are being formulated as of this writing.

The privacy rule affects the use of data sets for QI activities. The rule defines protected health information as any information created (in any format) or received (in any format) by a health care organization regarding a patient's past, present, or future health (physical and mental) condition. However, that information can be used by a health care organization for treatment, payment, or health care operations, which includes QI and assurance purposes. The law provides for severe penalties for inadvertent or purposeful disclosure of protected health information to unauthorized parties, so some health institutions have implemented more stringent rules to ensure compliance, which may influence the use of protected health information for improvement activities. Because these local rules may require special authorization for use of health care information, it becomes an important part of the task of any QI team to ensure that all salient rules regarding data collection, analysis, and reporting are evaluated prior to undertaking a performance improvement project. CMS has provided a resource for the HIPAA rules at *http://cms.hhs.gov/hipaa*.

◆ Discussion Points

1. Describe the health care delivery system in terms of processes. Are there any exceptions to considering health care systems as processes?
2. A flowchart can be constructed to describe nearly every process. Create a flowchart depicting the care of a nonemergent patient in a typical emergency department. Draw a flowchart for the care of a critically injured patient in the emergency department.
3. Choose a process in your own work setting and create a program evaluation and review technique (PERT) diagram to describe resource utilization and the critical path.
4. Evaluate the flowchart in discussion point 2 using critical to quality analysis.
5. A quality improvement team at a hospital is given the task of reducing the postoperative infection rate for hysterectomies. Describe the approach to the project in detail, including possible data sources, methods of evaluating current practice patterns, and the staff involved in the quality improvement project.
6. A managed care plan is about to embark on a quality improvement project to improve mammography rates in women between 40 and 65 years of age. The health plan's health maintenance organization spans the entire state and includes 250 hospitals and 2350 physicians. Outline an

approach to the project, including possible interventions, data sources, performance measures, and outcome measures.

7. A physician's office has noticed that laboratory data have become increasingly difficult to obtain from the hospital reference laboratory. The physician uses the hospital laboratory for all but simple laboratory tests, which she performs in her office. A courier picks up the samples for analysis from her office three times a day, and in the past, laboratory reports were available on the same day that the test was sent to the laboratory. For the past 3 months, however, laboratory test results have taken from 2 to 4 days to return from the laboratory. Brainstorm possible reasons for the delays and potential solutions. Create a flowchart to show current patterns according to your hypothesis and a work flow diagram to indicate potential actions for improvement. Describe how the office staff can determine the cause of the problem.

8. The quality improvement team at the ABC Home Health Agency wants to evaluate its present approach to handling patients with decubitus ulcers. Describe an approach to the analysis, as well as a method of collecting data and the types of analysis tools that can be of help in the evaluation.

9. Choose a product or service from your organization and create a performance–importance matrix. Poll your coworkers and evaluate their responses with the performance matrix and the importance matrix.

10. Describe several sources of data for quality improvement studies in a health care organization and critique each source for data accuracy, precision, and validity.

11. Describe the effect that the Health Insurance Portability and Accountability Act has had on the use of data for quality programs and projects throughout the health care industry.

◆ Notes

Bates D. W., Pappius E. M., Kuperman G. J., Sittig D., Burstin H., Fairchild D., et al. (1998). Measuring and improving quality using information systems. *Medinfo, 9*(2), 814–818.

Benjamin D. M. (2003). Reducing medication errors and increasing patient safety: Case studies in clinical pharmacology. *Journal of Clinical Pharmacology, 43*(7), 768–783.

Bowling A. (1995). *Measuring disease*. Bristol, PA: Open University Press.

Burgmeier J. (2002). Failure mode and effect analysis: An application in reducing risk in blood transfusion. *Joint Commission Journal on Quality Improvement, 28*(6), 331–339.

Centers for Medicare and Medicaid Services. (2003). *Statement of work*. Retrieved August 2003, from *http://cms.hhs.gov/qio/2b.pdf*

Grissinger M., and Rich D. (2002). JCAHO: Meeting the standards for patient safety. *Journal of the American Pharmacists Association (Wash), 42*(5 Suppl 1), S54–S55.

Halpern J. (1996). The measurement of quality of care in the Veterans Health Administration. *Medical Care, 34*(3 Suppl), MS55–MS68.

Hayes B. E. (1998). *Measuring customer satisfaction: Survey design, use, and statistical analysis methods.* Milwaukee, WI: ASQC Press.

MacNally K. M., Page M. A., Sunderland V. B. (1997). Failure mode and effects analysis in improving a drug distribution system. *American Journal of Health Systems Pharmacy, 54*(2), 171–177.

McLaughlin C. P., and Kaluzny A. D. (1994). *Continuous quality improvement in health care: Theory, implementation, and applications.* Gaithersburg, MD: Aspen.

National Committee for Quality Assurance. (2003). *NCQA releases HEDIS 2004, 10 new measures address public health, service issues.* Retrieved August 2003, from *http://www.ncqa.org/communications/news/Hedis2004.htm*

Ridgway M. (2003). Analyzing planned maintenance (PM) inspection data by failure mode and effect analysis methodology. *Biomedical Instrumentation and Technology, 37*(3), 167–179.

◆ ## Additional Reading

Schaeffer R. L., et al. (1996). *Elementary survey sampling.* Belmont, CA: Wadsworth.

Tague N. R. (1995). *The quality toolbox.* Milwaukee, WI: ASQC Press.

◆ ## Web Sites

Medicare Information Clearinghouse. Accessed July 2003, from *http://cms.hhs.gov/researchers/statsdata.asp*

Medicaid Statistics. Accessed July 2003, from *http://cms.hhs.gov/medicaid/mcaidsad.asp*

National Technical Information Service: Federal Data Resources. Accessed July 2003, from *http://www.ntis.gov/products*

University of Virginia Clinical Data Repository: an example of a robust data set for use by medical school faculty. Accessed July 2003, from *http://www.hsc.virginia.edu/cdr*

Utah Office of Health Data Analysis. Accessed July 2003, from *http://health.utah.gov/html/health_data.html*

◆ ## Root Cause Analysis—Commercial Packages

Apollo Root Cause Analysis: *http://www.apollorca.com*

Root Cause Analyst software: *http://www.rootcauseanalyst.com*

TapRooT Root Cause Analysis: *http://www.taproot.com*

Chapter 4

Statistical Process Control: Basic Principles

DONALD E. LIGHTER

◆ Introduction

One of the most powerful tools available to a quality improvement team is statistical process control. Statistical process control tools have evolved over the past 70 years to include highly sophisticated analytic approaches that evaluate the efficacy of processes over time. The underlying statistical analysis for statistical process control is remarkably straightforward, using such familiar statistical parameters as the mean and standard deviation. In fact, statistical knowledge is not a critical factor for using the techniques of statistical process control because computer software now performs all the necessary calculations. A more important concept is that of statistical thinking, a term attributed to W. Edwards Deming and used to describe the need to understand the nature of the data sets that are providing information for interventions and to apply the proper statistical process control tools to produce useful information (Leitnaker, et al., 1995). This chapter will deal with the conceptual basis of statistical process control, starting with basic concepts of statistical thinking.

◆ Data Analysis Models

One of the fundamental tenets of quality improvement (QI) can be stated: "In God we trust; all others bring data." No improvement initiative can succeed without some type of data collection and analysis because the very concept of improvement implies measurement of the effect of an intervention. Another of the famous bits of QI dogma is "You can't manage what you can't measure," suggesting that any system that requires management also requires some method of measurement. Collection and analysis of data are central to the function of QI in any organization, and there are several different models for data analysis, including

- ◆ research
- ◆ inspection
- ◆ micromanagement

◆ benchmarking
◆ outcomes for personal gain
◆ improvement

Each of these data analysis models has a different focus, and each approach can have significant implications for an organization using the information.

The research approach to data analysis usually involves evaluation of an intervention on a controlled set of variables at a specific time. Research studies are very important to health care because new drugs and therapies must be tested in highly controlled conditions prior to general usage, primarily to determine potential for harm. Because they can have such a devastating effect on patients, drugs and medical therapies must be thoroughly scrutinized to determine both therapeutic and adverse effects before they are released to the public. Controlled experiments, discussed in more depth in Chapter 7, "Advanced Statistical Applications in Continuous Quality Improvement," provide an environment in which the effect of the drug or therapy can be assessed at a specified level of scientific confidence. Only by controlling environmental variables can these effects be adequately assessed. Understandably, the research approach to data collection and analysis can be very expensive, and in most cases, the expense and risk to the system necessitate the use of pilot projects and trials on subsets of a population to make predictions about the effects of an intervention.

Unfortunately, however, data collection and analysis can also be used counterproductively. The inspection approach exemplifies this issue. One of Deming's 14 QI principles is the elimination of inspection as an approach to QI. That principle is based on the concept that the entire organization has been transformed into one in which quality is incorporated into every facet of operations. Deming placed a great deal of responsibility on management to create the optimal environment for worker productivity, empowering employees to "drive out waste" (Deming, 1986). When management has performed well, workers function optimally, and the need for inspection disappears. Most organizations that do use the inspection approach tend to concentrate on finding the person(s) who created defects, ignoring Deming's admonition to "drive out fear." Use of data for recrimination is shortsighted and self-defeating because time and materials are wasted ensuring compliance to management goals rather than on improving the quality of the product or services and the processes used in production. The failure of managed care organizations in the 1990s to substantively change patterns of care through oversight and inspection provides the most salient example of the inability of the inspection approach to improve the health care delivery system (Halterman, Camero, and Maillet, 2003). Although some health care organizations still rely on inspection tactics, a more effective approach in the future will suffuse QI values throughout the organization and eliminate the perceived need for inspection.

Some managers remain inherently distrustful of workers in spite of good performance. These "micromanagers" use data collection and analysis to direct employee activities down to the most specific task, removing the incentive for the employee to be innovative or productive. Employees in these situations usually direct all of their energy to satisfying the boss's detailed instructions rather than finding ways of improving quality or productivity. In most cases, workers are the best arbiters of the most effective way of performing a task for which they have been trained, and successful managers learn this fact early in their careers. As outlined in Chapter 2, the group process can be a powerful tool for achieving organizational improvement goals, but it requires an essential trust in the ability of employees to do their jobs. Data analysis for micromanagement usually entails finding ways that employees are not conforming to a manager's directions, rather than seeking the underlying worth of an employee's efforts.

Benchmarking can fit into the same category with micromanagement and inspection. Effective benchmarks are performance measurements of world-class industry leaders, mostly from the same industry (in this case health care), but in some cases from similar industries with comparable services, e.g., the hospitality industry. Ineffective benchmarks often are just productivity values set by management to be met by workers, without regard to barriers and inherent process capacities. Benchmarking has become more widely used in health care, but when incorrectly applied, benchmarks become difficult to justify. Benchmarks that are set by management may have no relationship to the actual productivity capabilities of workers and may instead be based on the economic goals of the company. When productivity goals are adopted from an outside source, they often have little connection with the population or environment in which the company operates. An example of such a problem exists with national standards such as the Health Plan Report Card (National Committee for Quality Assurance, 2003). Health plans submit data to the National Committee for Quality Assurance (NCQA), which then summarizes and reports the data for standard Health Plan Employer Data and Information Set (HEDIS) measures. Although seemingly a useful method of comparing health plans, the data submitted by the health plans come from large transaction databases that can contain errors, which has led the NCQA to instigate an auditing process, in effect since 2000, to reduce that source of error. Additionally, aggregate data from plans with differing populations makes comparison to the population of a particular health plan potentially error prone because some health plans consist of populations with a larger disease burden than others. For example, pregnancies in a cohort of health plan members from a disadvantaged population often require substantially different management techniques than a cohort of pregnant patients from a health plan with predominantly middle or upper class members. More information regarding population characteristics helps to determine if using Health Plan Report Card data to compare an individual health plan's performance makes sense. In general, benchmarking can be fraught with errors if applied inappropriately.

Outcomes measurement in health care has become exceedingly important over the past few years, primarily because society and payers want to ensure that they are receiving value. Outcome measures can be subverted, however, into self-serving objectives that do not enhance quality. From individuals to groups and entire organizations, outcome measures can become targets that undermine organizational values to achieve artificial goals. For example, a health plan may report only those performance measures that show the plan in a positive light, concealing those that are suboptimal. A medical group may release information regarding the cost of care only if it validates the group's assertion of being a low-cost provider of services. A hospital could publish data showing its top 10 surgical procedure complication rates, rather than revealing all of its results. Use of data to produce outcome measures must not become construed as a means of promoting an individual, organization, or group; rather, the purpose of outcome measures must be to identify opportunities for improvement.

Finally, the improvement approach to data collection and analysis differs from these other approaches in a number of ways. The object of study in the improvement approach is the process of care, rather than just an intervention. Improvement studies start with analysis of an underlying process over a period of time, thus differing from most research studies that measure variables at only a few points in time. Additionally, the improvement approach generally will not have the highly controlled environment characteristic of research studies. Variables will generally be observed many times during a specified period, with measures of variation noted during the analysis. Effective improvement studies also carry no punitive overtones. Data obtained in an improvement approach are used for gaining insight into a process, with an ultimate goal of improving the process. The effect of interventions can be assessed by formulating appropriate performance measures, chosen not for improving the image of the organization but rather to gain better information about how interventions can improve the process. The improvement approach to data collection and analysis fulfills Deming's 14 criteria for QI by focusing on the process and empowering workers to find solutions to productivity problems.

Obviously, the improvement approach is designed for QI, and avoiding the pitfalls of using data analysis for personal recrimination or self-aggrandizement makes the outcome of a study or intervention much more useful to an organization over the long term. The QI team must be alert to the misuse of data and maintain the goal of improving performance through enhanced quality.

◆ Process Problems and Statistical Process Control

Process problems generally fall into the following categories:

- ◆ lack of knowledge about how a process should work
- ◆ lack of knowledge about how a process actually works

- ◆ errors in executing correct procedures
- ◆ inability to recognize errors
- ◆ inability to correct errors
- ◆ inadequate preventive measures
- ◆ need for reworking the product, service, or process being studied
- ◆ process variation (common and special cause)

Each of these problems can impede process optimization, adding to cost and diminishing quality. Statistical thinking and the use of statistical process control (SPC) tools have the potential to identify the underlying causes of process malfunction, and the problem categories help define approaches for process improvement.

Most managers start with a basic belief that they know how a process should work, based on previous experience or education. Although this assumption may be substantially correct, almost any system will have nuances that can produce suboptimal performance, and in most cases, workers who routinely deal with the system will have in-depth knowledge of these variations. Effective managers help uncover these variations and devise methods to optimize the process. SPC techniques can be applied to study these variations and then measure the results of efforts to minimize untoward variance in the process. For example, a run chart helps identify trends and specific types of variation that may need immediate attention. Other QI tools, such as those discussed in Chapter 3, help characterize a system more thoroughly so that performance measures can be chosen and specific interventions designed. Using these methods, a QI team can create an optimal process description that serves as the goal for improvement efforts.

Another common error in studying processes for QI involves failing to understand how a process is actually performing. Understanding the current state of a system requires examination of processes over a period of time sufficient to gain a longitudinal view of performance and trends, and it is not sufficient just to make some quick measurements of a process at a single point in time. One of the early tasks in this analysis is to identify appropriate performance measures to use. For example, in the effort to evaluate diabetes complications such as foot ulcers or retinopathy, using the rates of these complications may not be sufficient because the incidence of these events may need to be studied over several months or years to discern a valid rate. Instead, shorter term measures, e.g., hemoglobin A1c levels or urinary studies for microalbuminuria, may be necessary to define areas for intervention in a system of care. Once appropriate performance measures are defined, then proper baseline analysis can be performed to describe the system.

Another source of variation in systems involves proper procedures executed incorrectly. The first thought that comes to the minds of most managers is that workers are at fault. Deming stresses in his writing that only rarely are workers truly at fault for poor performance; in most cases, the system is not conducive to optimal performance. For example, the instructions for the procedure could be incorrect or difficult to understand, or the configuration of equipment used in the procedure may not conform to the description given in the manual. Health care workers face these situations frequently, such as when a particular piece of equipment has controls placed where natural usage causes a mistake. When there is an apparent digression from a proper procedure, managers must resist the impulse to blame workers. The source of the problem will most often be found in the environment.

Perhaps even more difficult to manage is the problem of unrecognized errors. As a health service is being performed, errors may be difficult to detect until they have caused serious complications. One of the more serious problems facing the health care industry is prevention of adverse drug events. Nearly all physicians have had the experience of an incorrect drug or dosage being administered to a patient, sometimes with tragic consequences. If such errors could be detected or anticipated before administration of the drug, then adverse outcomes could be avoided, with an overall improvement in quality. The failure modes and effects analysis approach discussed in Chapter 3 helps anticipate errors in a process, but tracking risky processes to detect errors such as these is an important application of SPC.

Once devastating errors have occurred, correction of the error is almost always costly, both economically and in terms of comorbidity. Some errors cannot be corrected, and the end result for patients is often long-term disability or death. Costs to the health care delivery system are immense because care of these debilitations generally requires substantial resources, and the cost of subsequent legal actions often can devastate providers and add unproductive expense throughout the system. Uncorrected errors in health care can be difficult to manage and should always prompt QI efforts. Statistical methods of tracking the precursors of these problems can help avoid these misfortunes.

The best approach to such problems is prevention. Prevention has demonstrated efficacy in systems as disparate as auto mechanics and cardiovascular health. Some medical systems, however, do not emphasize preventive interventions enough. Many QI projects have been implemented to prevent diseases or the complications of diseases (Sisk, et al., 1997; Smith, et al., 1998; Wagner, et al., 1996). The concept of prevention lends itself to all areas of the health care industry. Various types of risk in QI environments will be discussed in Chapter 10, "Making Continuous Quality Improvement Work: Care Management," and preventive approaches are of great value in attenuating these risks.

Rework describes any repetition of a process to replace defective output. American industry recognized the problem of rework decades ago, when W. E. Deming, J. M. Juran, and Philip Crosby introduced different methods of reducing waste in production lines. With statistical process control, output from a process can be tracked over time to determine untoward variation and deviation from desired output. Control charts provide a scientific method for following processes over time to detect deterioration in procedures and outputs. Rework is costly in economic as well as human terms, and the use of tools such as SPC to reduce rework can improve the quality of patient care.

Finally, the concepts of common cause and special cause variation are central to SPC. Common cause variation describes variability in a process that is inherent in the design of the process, whereas special cause variation entails variability resulting from some extraordinary event that changes a performance measure or process output beyond common cause limits of ±3 standard errors from the mean. An example of common cause variation can be found in the varying numbers of visits to an emergency department over a period of time. A special cause in that situation would occur in the face of a major disaster such as a plane crash. Normal variation in the visit rate would be apparent on a control chart until the disaster, when a substantial increase in visits would be observed. Common cause variation requires approaches such as process re-engineering, whereas special cause variation may only need to be noted as the reason for a specific point that exceeds control limits. Special causes, in spite of their exceptional circumstances, often can be eliminated more easily than common cause variation, which can require substantial, expensive revisions in a process.

◆ ## Statistical Basis of SPC

Evaluating quality in health care can be complicated. Processes are complex, procedures sophisticated, and outcomes difficult to measure. However, QI science provides techniques for dissecting any process into smaller components for analysis, then using tools to provide ongoing assessment of the process. Control charts and their associated techniques constitute important tools for quality analysis.

The first important concept for SPC involves the difference between a sample and a population. Sometimes the distinction is rather difficult, but in general a population is the entire group of individuals of concern to an organization. A sample is a subset of that group, usually consisting of a manageable group of individuals selected at random from the population. In some systems, the population size is so large that data collection and analysis are too expensive and logistically prohibitive. Thus, a sample must be selected for the analysis that is representative of the population. Sampling can be a complex task, and entire textbooks are devoted to different sampling techniques (Scheaffer, Mendenhall, and Ott, 1996). For the most commonly used control charts, however, specific sampling rules apply and will be discussed with each type of chart.

As mentioned, the distinction between a population and a sample can sometimes become blurred. For example, for a health plan, all of the members of the plan would constitute the plan's population. However, for the state insurance commission, with responsibility for overseeing insurance services for all citizens in a state, all of the individuals in the state will comprise the population, and the members of an individual health plan may be a sample of the state's population. Thus, for the health plan, the membership is the population, but for the state insurance commission, the health plan's membership is a sample. Similarly, a physician's practice population is all of the patients that are registered for care with that practice, but this group represents a sample of the community population. At times, the distinction can be of importance because the mathematical treatment of samples and populations is different.

Another important issue with the application of SPC is that of the type of variable to be analyzed. Two types of variables are usually identified: discrete and continuous. Discrete variables are those that have distinct numeric values with no intermediate values between each number. Counts of events are considered discrete variables because they are integers with no intermediate values. Continuous variables are also numeric, but they have an infinite number of possible values between any two numbers. An example of a continuous variable could be height measurements in a population. Although measurement of height will be accurate only to about two decimal places, the range of values between two height measurements is, at least theoretically, infinite. The type of variable used for the control chart analysis is also important for determining which type of chart to use.

A few basic statistical parameters are important to control charting and are listed in Table 4.1. Sample statistics are estimates of their counterparts in the population. When the population mean or standard deviation is unknown, the sample mean and standard deviation can be used as a substitute if the sample was chosen at random from the population. The population mean is defined by the following equation.

(4.1)
$$\mu = \frac{\sum x_i}{n}$$

where μ = population mean
x_i = each individual measurement in the population, and
n = the total number of individuals in the population.

The population mean provides information about the central tendency of the data set. Sample means are calculated in the same manner, except that

Table 4.1 Statistical Parameters Used in Control Charts

TYPE	DESCRIPTION	SYMBOL
Population	Mean	μ
	Standard Deviation	σ
Sample	Mean	$\bar{x}$
	Standard Deviation	s

the value of n is the number of individual observations in the sample. Sample means measure the central tendency of the sample but also tend to approximate the population mean. Although a useful measure, the central tendency indicates nothing about the variability of a data set, which can be very large or very small, as in Table 4.2. Note that *data set 1* ranges from a low value of 7 to a high value of 69, whereas *data set 2*, with the same mean, ranges from a low of 28 to a high of 34. Thus, two data sets with the same mean have substantially different variation measures.

One method of describing this variation between two data sets is the standard deviation, which is defined by the following equation:

(4.2)
$$\sigma = \sqrt{\frac{\sum(x_i - \mu)^2}{N}}$$

where σ is the population standard deviation,
$\quad x_i$ is the individual observations in the population,
$\quad \mu$ is the population mean, and
$\quad N$ is the total number of individual observations in the population.

The population standard deviation is frequently unknown and must be approximated by a sample standard deviation (sometimes called a standard error), using the following

(4.3)
$$s = \sqrt{\frac{\sum(x_i - \bar{X})^2}{n-1}}$$

where s is the sample standard deviation,
$\quad x_i$ is the individual observations in the sample,
$\quad \bar{X}$ is the sample mean, and
$\quad n$ is the number of individual observations in the sample.

Table 4.2 Disparate Data Sets Have the Same Mean

DATA SET 1	DATA SET 2
69	34
48	28
12	29
32	31
7	34
18	30
$\bar{x} = 31$	$\bar{x} = 31$

The sample standard deviation is often used as an estimate for the population statistic in QI because data for entire populations are often unavailable.

Data can be analyzed by the frequency with which a value or range of values appears in the data set. These evaluations are termed distributions, a subject that will be discussed in some detail in Chapter 7, "Advanced Statistical Applications in Continuous Quality Improvement." For the purposes of this discussion, however, most data sets in QI studies tend to approximate the normal distribution, the well-known bell curve of statistical theory. When a data set does not seem to conform to the normal distribution, some analytic techniques can be applied to determine the type of distribution, and in some cases, mathematical transformations of the data can be performed that allow use of the normal distribution.

The key underlying issue, however, is the need for the data set to approximate a normal distribution, and most software programs can perform a quick graphic estimate of the distribution's closeness to the normal distribution (see Figure 4.1).

A normal probability plot is another method incorporated into most statistical software and spreadsheet programs. Using this graph, the conformance of a data set to a normal distribution can be assessed by determining if a plot of the data set arranged in quantiles matches a predicted normal distribution. In Figure 4.2, the data set is shown as the plot points, and the predicted normal distribution is shown as the thin line.

Because the plot points lie close to the thin line, the data set in the figure closely approximates a normal distribution. With this type of analysis, performance measures from a process can be evaluated to determine if they are fairly close to being normally distributed, allowing application of the tech-

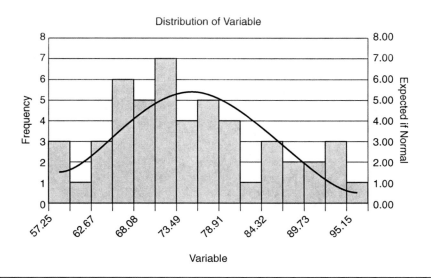

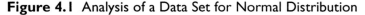

Figure 4.1 Analysis of a Data Set for Normal Distribution

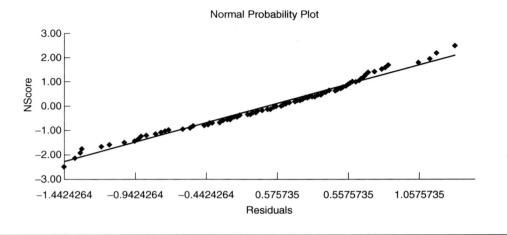

Figure 4.2 Normal Probability Plot

niques of SPC. Data sets that are not normally distributed may require different analyses.

Control Charts

Control charts are time–series analysis tools that track the consistency of data of calculated statistics through time. Control charts can be used for numerous applications in the health care industry in order to evaluate the quality of processes and monitor the results of QI interventions. The use of control charts to monitor and evaluate quality encompasses a large part of the science of SPC. Following is an example of one application of SPC in a health care organization.

Example 4-1

The infection control officer of the state health department is concerned that the number of reported postsurgical nosocomial infections seem to have increased over the past several months in the state's 150 hospitals. To try to substantiate her theory, she obtains the monthly number of nosocomial infection cases for the last 4 years for all of the hospitals, as displayed in Table 4.3.

After examining the data, she decides to group the data by quarters during each calendar year, thereby defining a sample size of three (3 months per quarter). By considering each quarter's three data points as a subgroup, a measure of variability—the range—can be calculated, as well as a measure of central tendency—the average—for each quarter. By doing so, she is able to evaluate any changes in the average and range in nosocomial infections from one quarter to the next. This analysis of the data provides her with

Table 4.3 Historical Nosocomial Infection Data for Example 4-1

MONTH	n	MONTH	n
1	60	25	91
2	100	26	12
3	80	27	19
4	40	28	54
5	33	29	44
6	54	30	62
7	96	31	29
8	42	32	92
9	101	33	46
10	20	34	80
11	53	35	71
12	61	36	92
13	20	37	10
14	34	38	91
15	91	39	68
16	34	40	110
17	37	41	34
18	61	42	41
19	40	43	32
20	82	44	54
21	32	45	59
22	64	46	84
23	53	47	92
24	44	48	83

information about the average and the variability (range) in post-operative nosocomial infection rates from one quarter to the next.

To summarize the data even further, she graphs the averages and ranges so that patterns in the statistics can be visualized throughout the 4-year time period. Graphs of the averages and ranges for the nosocomial data can be found in Figure 4.3. As seen in the figure, there appears to be a substantial amount of variation in the numbers and ranges of infections from quarter to quarter, but is that level of variation significant? A control chart can help provide the answer. To transform the data in Table 4.3 into a control chart, three basic components must be added to the graphs: a centerline representing the overall average; an upper control limit ; and a lower control limit.

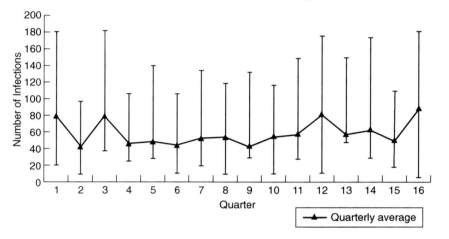

Figure 4.3 Numbers of Nosocomial Infections by Quarter

Control chart data points can be the actual sample data or calculated statistics such as $\overline{X}$ (average) values (such as the average number of infections per quarter), ranges between the points in a data set, standard errors, or standard deviations. A more detailed description of the different types of control charts and how to match control charts with data sets can be found in Chapter 5, "Statistical Process Control Approaches: Basic Theory and Use of Control Charts." Regardless of the type of data being plotted, control charts display an overall average or "centerline" for the plotted values, which, in this case, provides a way of comparing each subgroup of data with the central tendency of all the data collected. Using these principles, the control chart in Figure 4.4 was constructed from the nosocomial infection data. Note that the control chart in the figure consists of two graphs, one (the $\overline{X}$ chart) for the average value for each subgroup (or quarter) and the other an analysis of the range values. More about the interpretation of these two types of charts is presented in Chapter 5.

Placing the data and centerlines on both charts certainly reveals more information than before, but doing so also raises a few questions, such as

◆ Is the X value in *quarter 16* significantly higher than the overall average (shown as the centerline) of 68?
◆ Are *quarters 2* and *9* significantly lower compared with other quarters?
◆ Is the higher variability displayed on the range chart in *quarter 13* a source of concern?

These questions are unanswerable without the knowledge of the expected "normal" variation in the data points. Upper and lower control limits,

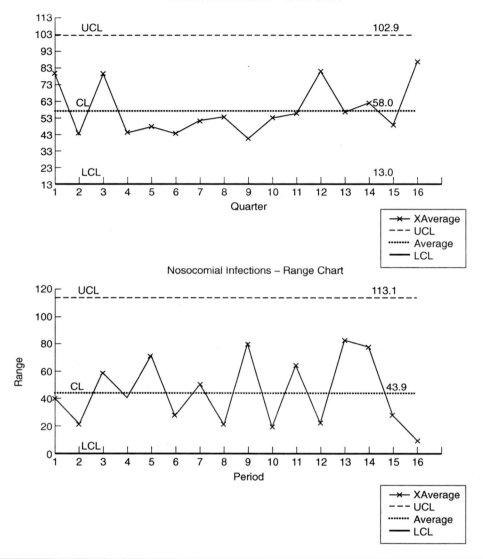

Figure 4.4 Nosocomial Infection Control Charts for Example 4-1

designated on the graphs as UCL and LCL, can provide answers to these questions.

Control limits are based on variation in the data set, and they are calculated with the help of the normal distribution. The normal curve allows close approximation of the expected variation in a data set; for example, for a data set that conforms to the normal distribution (i.e., is normally distributed), 99.7% of all data points fall within ±3 standard deviations from the average. Thus, there are only 3 chances in 1000 that a false positive error is made or of erroneously inferring that a specific data point has an attributable (special) cause when it actually is due to inherent variation in the process (common cause). The control limits of a control chart are calculated as three standard deviations above and below the chart's centerline (±3 sigma). Control limits are valuable because they allow assessment of the consistency and stability (control) of data and provide answers to questions such as

◆ Are the data consistent from one subgroup to another?
◆ How much variation is considered normal for the data set?
◆ Does the average change substantially from one subgroup to the next?
◆ Does the variability (represented by ranges or standard deviations) change significantly from one subgroup to the next?

In most cases, the population standard deviation (σ) is not known, and as in many statistical analyses, it must be estimated. Control chart constants are available in standard tables and can be used to calculate upper and lower control limits as described in Chapters 5 and 6. The power of control charts lies in the ability to detect significant, real-time changes in a process. If a significant change has occurred (i.e., a data point falls outside the upper or lower control limits), then action can be directed at eliminating a detrimental cause of the change or incorporating a favorable assignable cause into the process.

After creating the control charts in Figure 4.4, all of the data points appear to be within control limits for the state's hospitals. Thus, the variability represented by the range values, as well as the averages, is within the normal bounds of expected variation for the process. If there were points that fell outside control limits, those points would indicate that some unusual change had occurred in the process. Because all the points in this analysis fall within control limits, the infection control officer can be reassured that there are no indications of an unusual increase in the incidence of nosocomial infections. Although *quarter 16* reveals a higher number of nosocomial infections, the control chart demonstrates that the increase is not statistically significant.

It is important to distinguish between control limits and specifications. Control limits are statistical predictions of normality made with the use of process data; specifications are requirements obtained from external sources. For example, in Example 4-1, the infection control officer could have been directed to maintain nosocomial infections below an average of 50 infections per quarter. That specification would not be used to calculate control limits for the control charts but rather would be an indicator used by the infection control officer to determine if current numbers of postoperative infections were acceptable or not. Control limits, on the other hand, provide a means of defining normal variation in a process, even if the process results in unacceptable products or services. If the specification limit for nosocomial infections in Example 4-1 were set at 50 per quarter, then most of the points in the data set would be out of compliance but within the normal bounds of variability.

Run Charts

Run charts can also be used to evaluate trends in performance measures. Figure 4.5 is a sample run chart for the nosocomial data in Table 4.3. Run charts are relatively simple time plots of the median and the data, and runs are defined as groups of consecutive points above or below the median. Points on the median are not counted as part of the run, and when the data line crosses the median, a new run is begun. Runs for the nosocomial infection data are circled in Figure 4.5. Although each single point above or below the median also defines a run, those runs have not been circled in the figure in order to simplify the chart.

Although the concept of the run chart appears simple, interpretation of the chart is somewhat more complex. Rules for interpreting the chart are presented in Table 4.4. The four rules that constitute analysis of a run chart emanate from statistical theory regarding runs testing. A means of determining the probability that a series of observations is indeed random, a runs test evaluates the number of runs for each of two events (above the median and below the median), according to the following series of equalities

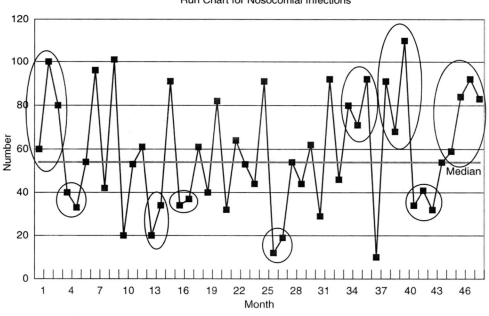

Figure 4.5 Run Chart for Nosocomial Infections

(4.4)
$$\bar{\mu} = \frac{2n_1 n_2}{n_1 + n_2} + 1$$

where $\bar{\mu}$ is the expected number of runs, if they are randomly distributed,
$\quad$ n_1 is the number of runs of type 1, and
$\quad$ n_2 is the number of runs of type 2;

(4.5)
$$\sigma^2 = \frac{2n_1 n_2 \left(2n_1 n_2 - n_1 - n_2\right)}{\left(n_1 + n_2\right)^2 \left(n_1 = n_2 - 1\right)}$$

where σ^2 is the variance of the expected number of runs,
$\quad$ n_1 is the number of runs of type 1, and
$\quad$ n_2 is the number of runs of type 2.

Using these equations for the mean and variance, the probability that the sequence is random can be calculated by a Z statistic

(4.6)
$$Z = \frac{\mu - \bar{\mu}}{\sigma}$$

where Z is the standard normal test statistic for determining the randomness of the sequence,
$\quad$ μ is the actual number of runs,
$\quad$ $\bar{\mu}$ is the expected value of runs from equation 4.4, and
$\quad$ σ is the standard deviation of the expected number of runs, i.e., the square root of the variance determined from equation 4.5.

Rules for interpreting run charts can be found in Table 4.4.

Table 4.4 Rules for Interpreting a Run Chart

	RULE
1	A run of over 8 points indicates a special cause, most likely a mean that varies over time
2	Seven or more consecutive points moving in the same direction signify a special cause
3	The probability that the sequence is random, as determined by the calculations in Equations 4.4 through 4.6 should exceed 95% or a level corresponding to the sensitivity of the analysis.
4	A repeating pattern of points or at least 14 points alternating up and down may indicate bias in data collection or sampling

Using the Z statistic, the probability that the sequence is random can be found in a two-tailed Z table. Referring again to 4.5, the following information can be used to calculate the Z statistic

Total number of runs $(\mu) = 28$
Total runs above the median $(n_1) = 14$
Total runs below the median $(n_2) = 14$

$$\bar{\mu} = \frac{2(14)(14)}{(14+14)} - 1 = 13$$

$$\sigma^2 = \frac{\left[2(14)(14)\right]\left[2(14)(14) - 14 - 14\right]}{(14+14)^2(14+14-1)} = 6.741$$

$$\sigma = 2.60$$

$$Z = \frac{28 - 13}{2.60} = 5.77$$

Consulting a standard two-tailed Z table such as that in Appendix 4.1, it can be seen that a Z-score of 5.77 exceeds the range of the table and represents a p-value (probability) of almost 1, meaning that the sequence is random. The rules for evaluating run charts are derived using this type of analysis.

Approach to Control Chart Analysis

Control charts provide exceptional insight into processes. Properly applied, they have the potential to assist health care organizations with maintaining quality standards through ongoing surveillance and rapid correction of anomalies in business and medical processes. However, control charting can be misused as well, leading to erroneous inferences and detrimental interventions. For example, mislabeling a common cause variation as a special cause can prompt the organization to intervene inappropriately, often worsening the problem or creating an unfavorable outcome. Thus, the approach to control charting must involve the following steps to improve the chance of success:

1. Define the process to be evaluated.
2. Using a flowchart, outline each step in the process.
3. Evaluate the flowchart for potential quality problems or opportunities for improvement.
4. Determine potential interventions for the steps in the process that require improvement.
5. Define performance measures to monitor the progress of improvement.
6. Implement the intervention and observe the effects.

7. Evaluate the results and refine the intervention to continually improve the process.

These procedures follow Shewhart's familiar plan-do-study-act cycle (McLaughlin and Kaluzny, 1994), as illustrated in Figure 4.6. Control charts are instrumental in evaluating the process and monitoring interventions as they are implemented. By differentiating common and special causes, the QI team should be able to intervene only when necessary and optimally manage scarce resources.

Each of the steps in the Shewhart framework is described in greater detail in other chapters, but the importance of an organized approach cannot be emphasized enough. Cogent application of QI efforts can potentially allocate health care resources to improve the quality of care, as well as

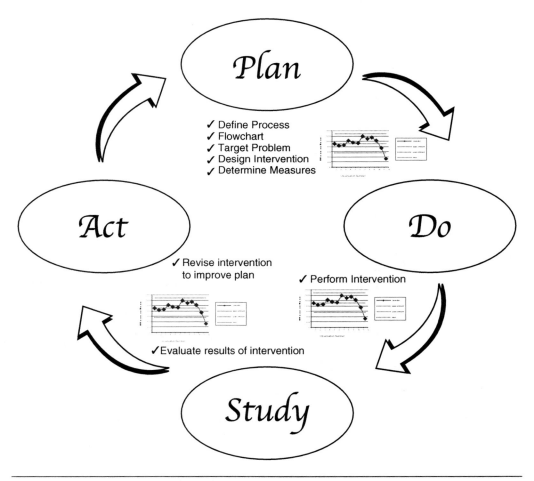

Figure 4.6 Shewhart Cycle Related to Control Charting

reduce costs. Adequate planning will optimize those efforts, and an organized QI team can have an immense impact on organizational efficiency and effectiveness.

◆ Conclusion

SPC has significant potential for directing and monitoring change in the health care industry. By adding the SPC scientific approach to a QI plan, the validity of the program can be improved, making the efforts of the team more attractive to providers. Because the concept of statistical process control has been validated over many years in the industrial sector, ample evidence exists to justify the approach in health care. The next two chapters describe SPC in more detail, including examples of how these techniques can be applied in health care.

◆ Discussion Points

1. What is the meaning of the phrase "You can't manage what you can't measure?"
2. How is benchmarking used in the health care industry? Does benchmarking provide a useful approach for most applications?
3. What is the value of assessing outcomes in a health care process? Are outcomes measures easy to define? Why or why not?
4. How does the quality improvement approach to data collection and analysis differ from traditional methods of data analysis in health care? What advantages does the QI approach provide?
5. Describe the concepts of common cause and special cause variation. What approach is required to remedy each type of variation?
6. Differentiate between discrete and continuous variables and provide examples from your experience.
7. What statistical distribution serves as the basis for standard control chart analysis? Why does that distribution describe most data sets?
8. Describe the basic components of a control chart. What type of control chart is most commonly used?
9. When interpreting a control chart, what is the importance of the range or standard deviation chart?
10. What are the differences between control charts and run charts? How is a runs analysis useful in evaluating a control chart?
11. Describe the approach to using control charts. Why is it necessary to understand the process before using a control chart?

◆ Notes

Deming W. E. (1986). *Out of the crisis*. Boston, MA: MIT Press.

Two tailed Z table. Retrieved August 2003, from *http://www.marymt.edu/~psychol/exper/Ztable.html*

Halterman S., Camero C., Maillet P. *The consumer driven approach: Can it pick up where managed care left off?* Retrieved August 2003, from *http://www.aon.com/about/publications/pdf/issues/cdhp_10apr03.pdf*

Leitnaker M. G., Sanders R.D., Hild C. (1995). *The power of statistical thinking: Improving industrial processes*. Reading, MA: Addison–Wesley.

McLaughlin C., and Kaluzn A. D. (1994). *Continuous quality improvement in health care: Theory, implementation, and applications.* Gaithersburg, MD: Aspen.

National Committee for Quality Assurance. (2003). *Health plan report card*. Retrieved July 2003, from *http://hprc.ncqa.org/index.asp*

Scheaffer R. L., Mendenhall W., Ott L. (1996). *Elementary survey sampling* (5th ed.). New York: Duxbury Press.

Sisk J. E., Moskowitz A. J., Whang W., Lin J. D., Fedson D. S., McBean A. M., et al. (1997). Cost-effectiveness of vaccination against pneumococcal bacteremia among elderly people. *Journal of the American Medical Association, 278*(16), 1333–1339.

Smith S., et al. (1998). Smoking cessation: What's new since the AHCPR guideline? *Journal of Respiratory Diseases, 19*(5), 412–426.

Wagner E. H., Austin B. T., VonKorff M. (1996). Improving outcomes in chronic illness. *Managed Care Quarterly, 4*(2), 12–25.

◆ Additional Reading

Carey R. G. (1995). *Measuring quality improvement in healthcare: A guide to statistical process control applications.* New York: Quality Resources.

Wheeler D. J. (1998). *Building continual improvement*. Knoxville, TN: SPC Press.

Appendix 4.A
Two-Tailed Z Table

Appendix 4.A Two-Tailed Z Table

Z	P	Z	P	Z	P	Z	P	Z	P	Z	P	Z	P	Z	P
0	0.5	0.41	0.659	0.82	0.794	1.23	0.891	1.64	0.949	2.05	0.98	2.46	0.993	2.87	0.998
0.01	0.504	0.42	0.663	0.83	0.797	1.24	0.893	1.65	0.951	2.06	0.98	2.47	0.993	2.88	0.998
0.02	0.508	0.43	0.666	0.84	0.8	1.25	0.894	1.66	0.952	2.07	0.981	2.48	0.993	2.89	0.998
0.03	0.512	0.44	0.67	0.85	0.802	1.26	0.896	1.67	0.953	2.08	0.981	2.49	0.994	2.9	0.998
0.04	0.516	0.45	0.674	0.86	0.805	1.27	0.898	1.68	0.954	2.09	0.982	2.5	0.994	2.91	0.998
0.05	0.52	0.46	0.677	0.87	0.808	1.28	0.9	1.69	0.954	2.1	0.982	2.51	0.994	2.92	0.998
0.06	0.524	0.47	0.681	0.88	0.811	1.29	0.901	1.7	0.955	2.11	0.983	2.52	0.994	2.93	0.998
0.07	0.528	0.48	0.684	0.89	0.813	1.3	0.903	1.71	0.956	2.12	0.983	2.53	0.994	2.94	0.998
0.08	0.532	0.49	0.688	0.9	0.816	1.31	0.905	1.72	0.957	2.13	0.983	2.54	0.994	2.95	0.998
0.09	0.536	0.5	0.691	0.91	0.819	1.32	0.907	1.73	0.958	2.14	0.984	2.55	0.995	2.96	0.998
0.1	0.54	0.51	0.695	0.92	0.821	1.33	0.908	1.74	0.959	2.15	0.984	2.56	0.995	2.97	0.999
0.11	0.544	0.52	0.698	0.93	0.824	1.34	0.91	1.75	0.96	2.16	0.985	2.57	0.995	2.98	0.999
0.12	0.548	0.53	0.702	0.94	0.826	1.35	0.911	1.76	0.961	2.17	0.985	2.58	0.995	2.99	0.999
0.13	0.552	0.54	0.705	0.95	0.829	1.36	0.913	1.77	0.962	2.18	0.985	2.59	0.995	3	0.999
0.14	0.556	0.55	0.709	0.96	0.831	1.37	0.915	1.78	0.962	2.19	0.986	2.6	0.995	3.01	0.999
0.15	0.56	0.56	0.712	0.97	0.834	1.38	0.916	1.79	0.963	2.2	0.986	2.61	0.995	3.02	0.999
0.16	0.564	0.57	0.716	0.98	0.836	1.39	0.918	1.8	0.964	2.21	0.986	2.62	0.996	3.03	0.999

z	P	z	P	z	P	z	P	z	P	z	P	z	P	z	P
0.17	0.567	0.58	0.719	0.99	0.839	1.4	0.919	1.81	0.965	2.22	0.987	2.63	0.996	3.04	0.999
0.18	0.571	0.59	0.722	1	0.841	1.41	0.921	1.82	0.966	2.23	0.987	2.64	0.996	3.05	0.999
0.19	0.575	0.6	0.726	1.01	0.844	1.42	0.922	1.83	0.966	2.24	0.987	2.65	0.996	3.06	0.999
0.2	0.579	0.61	0.729	1.02	0.846	1.43	0.924	1.84	0.967	2.25	0.988	2.66	0.996	3.07	0.999
0.21	0.583	0.62	0.732	1.03	0.848	1.44	0.925	1.85	0.968	2.26	0.988	2.67	0.996	3.08	0.999
0.22	0.587	0.63	0.736	1.04	0.851	1.45	0.926	1.86	0.969	2.27	0.988	2.68	0.996	3.09	0.999
0.23	0.591	0.64	0.739	1.05	0.853	1.46	0.928	1.87	0.969	2.28	0.989	2.69	0.996	3.1	0.999
0.24	0.595	0.65	0.742	1.06	0.855	1.47	0.929	1.88	0.97	2.29	0.989	2.7	0.997	3.11	0.999
0.25	0.599	0.66	0.745	1.07	0.858	1.48	0.931	1.89	0.971	2.3	0.989	2.71	0.997	3.12	0.999
0.26	0.603	0.67	0.749	1.08	0.86	1.49	0.932	1.9	0.971	2.31	0.99	2.72	0.997	3.13	0.999
0.27	0.606	0.68	0.752	1.09	0.862	1.5	0.933	1.91	0.972	2.32	0.99	2.73	0.997	3.14	0.999
0.28	0.61	0.69	0.755	1.1	0.864	1.51	0.934	1.92	0.973	2.33	0.99	2.74	0.997	3.15	0.999
0.29	0.614	0.7	0.758	1.11	0.867	1.52	0.936	1.93	0.973	2.34	0.99	2.75	0.997	3.16	0.999
0.3	0.618	0.71	0.761	1.12	0.869	1.53	0.937	1.94	0.974	2.35	0.991	2.76	0.997	3.17	0.999
0.31	0.622	0.72	0.764	1.13	0.871	1.54	0.938	1.95	0.974	2.36	0.991	2.77	0.997	3.18	0.999
0.32	0.626	0.73	0.767	1.14	0.873	1.55	0.939	1.96	0.975	2.37	0.991	2.78	0.997	3.19	0.999
0.33	0.629	0.74	0.77	1.15	0.875	1.56	0.941	1.97	0.976	2.38	0.991	2.79	0.997	3.2	0.999
0.34	0.633	0.75	0.773	1.16	0.877	1.57	0.942	1.98	0.976	2.39	0.992	2.8	0.997	3.21	0.999
0.35	0.637	0.76	0.776	1.17	0.879	1.58	0.943	1.99	0.977	2.4	0.992	2.81	0.998	3.22	0.999
0.36	0.641	0.77	0.779	1.18	0.881	1.59	0.944	2	0.977	2.41	0.992	2.82	0.998	3.23	0.999
0.37	0.644	0.78	0.782	1.19	0.883	1.6	0.945	2.01	0.978	2.42	0.992	2.83	0.998	3.24	0.999
0.38	0.648	0.79	0.785	1.2	0.885	1.61	0.946	2.02	0.978	2.43	0.992	2.84	0.998	3.25	0.999
0.39	0.652	0.8	0.788	1.21	0.887	1.62	0.947	2.03	0.979	2.44	0.993	2.85	0.998	3.26	0.999
0.4	0.655	0.81	0.791	1.22	0.889	1.63	0.948	2.04	0.979	2.45	0.993	2.86	0.998	3.27	0.999

Two-tailed Z table available from *http://www.marymt.edu/~psychol/exper/Ztable.html*.

Chapter 5

Statistical Process Control Approaches: Basic Theory and Use of Control Charts

DOUGLAS C. FAIR

Introduction

Perhaps no statistical tool is more closely identified with quality improvement than a control chart. Although most control chart applications are relatively straightforward, variations in the technique have been refined over the past 50 years, producing many different methods for evaluating data sets. The control chart chosen for an analysis depends on the questions that the user is trying to answer as well as the data type and the nature of the parameter being evaluated. This chapter covers basic control charts as well as an approach to determining the appropriate chart that one should use.

Overview of Data Types

As discussed in Chapter 4, data can be divided into two different types: discrete (sometimes called attributes) and continuous, most often referred to as variables data. Variables data can be evaluated along some type of measurement scale, such as a ruler to measure heights. Although the scale on the ruler has discrete values, the actual height measurement has an infinite number of possible values between any two points on the scale and thus is considered a continuous variable. Examples of variables data include actual time to perform an arthroscopic surgery or procedural costs measured in dollars and cents. To properly evaluate variables data in time series, typically some version of a Shewhart $\bar{X}$ and range (R) chart is used.

Attributes data result from counting individual items that fall into one or more categories. Examples include the number of defects in a manufactured product or the number of late or missed office appointments for a clinic. These data cannot be measured along a continuous scale. They either fit one category or they fit another. Patients in a clinic are either late or they are not. An error has either occurred or it has not. A manufactured product either has a defect or it does not. Furthermore, attributes data can take two different forms: categorical attributes and counts attributes.

With categorical attributes, the data fit only one of two categories: Good or bad, late or on-time, pass or fail, conforming or nonconforming, etc. That is, categorical data represent a collection of information that either fits or does not fit some examination criteria. A generic term for describing a failure of examination criteria is to call the failure event a "nonconformity" or a "nonconforming item." The term "nonconformity" generically describes a situation where an event has failed to occur as expected. A nonconformity could represent the number of missed appointments for a clinic or the proportion of postoperative deaths out of 1000 surgical procedures. The number of nonconformities cannot exceed the total number of items in the study. For example, the number of patients arriving late to appointments cannot exceed the number of appointments that have been scheduled. Either p-charts or np-charts are used to assess the statistical control of categorical attributes data.

Counts data, on the other hand, represent the number of failure events that occur over a given time, area, or space. For example, say an office is interested in determining the severity of insurance claim errors. An error might be a misspelled name, a missing identification number, an incorrect diagnosis or procedure code, or any number of problems. Fifty claims are checked each day for several weeks and the total number of errors is tallied each day. In this example, the number of errors is not limited to 50 per day, nor are they categorized as either good or bad. Instead, when an error is found, it is noted and logged. It is possible that each claim may have more than one error. In fact, given a sample of 50 claims, the error rate could be in the hundreds or even thousands. Theoretically, an unlimited number of errors could occur for the area, space, or time that has been identified for inspection. Either c-charts or u-charts are used to asses the statistical control of counts attributes.

◆ Charts for Categorical Attributes

p- and np-charts are used for evaluating the consistency of categorical attributes through time. The "p" in p-chart stands for "proportion." This word is used because the plotted points on a p-chart represent the proportion of nonconforming items in a subgroup. The items in the subgroup are inspected and are found to either meet or fail some requirement or criteria. For each subgroup, the number nonconforming is noted, and a proportion nonconforming is calculated and then plotted on a time-series chart. If the subgroup size changes during the period of study, p-charts must be used so that the plot points can be fairly compared to one another.

Consider an office manager who wishes to better understand the rate of missed patient appointments by week. It is unlikely that the number of physician appointments is the same from week to week. Instead, the number of appointments will vary, sometimes dramatically. By plotting the weekly proportion of missed appointments, the office manager is able to fairly compare one week's performance to the next.

Although similar to *p*-charts, *np*-charts are used to evaluate the actual number of nonconforming rates through time. Because the number of nonconforming items is plotted on *np*-charts, they may only be used when subgroup size is constant. In actuality, when subgroup size is unchanging, one has the choice of using either the *p*-chart or the *np*-chart, depending on preference. If team members are more comfortable discussing actual numbers of events, then the *np*-chart is more appropriate. If those same people are more comfortable analyzing proportions data, then the *p*-chart is the right chart to use. However, when subgroup size varies, the *p*-chart must be used.

The "*n*" in *np* represents subgroup size, and the "*p*" characterizes the proportion nonconforming. When multiplied together, $n \times p$ represents the actual number of nonconforming items in an *np*-chart's subgroup. As a general rule, *p*-charts and *np*-charts are best used when the product of $n \times p$ is greater than 5, and the value of *p* is no larger than 10. When using one of these two charts, the average proportion nonconforming ($\bar{p}$) must be calculated. Additionally, $\bar{p}$ serves as the centerline on *p*-charts, but it is also used (when multiplied by *n*) to calculate the centerline on *np*-charts.

p-Charts

The centerline and control limits for *p*-charts are as follows:

$$(5.1) \quad \bar{p} = \frac{\text{total number of nonconforming items}}{\text{total number of items in study}}$$

$$(5.2) \quad UCL_p = \bar{p} + 3\sqrt{\frac{\bar{p}(1-\bar{p})}{n}} \quad \text{and}$$

$$(5.3) \quad LCL_p = \bar{p} - 3\sqrt{\frac{\bar{p}(1-\bar{p})}{n}}$$

where *n* is subgroup size,
$\bar{p}$ is the average proportion of nonconforming items, and
UCL and *LCL* are the upper and lower control limits.

Example 5-1

The operating room committee of St. Anywhere Hospital has been tracking postoperative mortality over the past 30 months. They have collected the data shown in Table 5.1, which include the number of postoperative deaths after a major procedure, as well as the total number of major procedures that are performed each month. New

Table 5.1 p-Chart: Postoperative Mortality St. Anywhere Hospital

Month	Number of Postoperative Mortalities	Subgroup Size	Proportion Nonconforming (Mortalities/Subgroup Size)
1	8	493	0.0162
2	3	485	0.0062
3	6	490	0.0122
4	8	492	0.0163
5	9	483	0.0186
6	3	493	0.0061
7	2	487	0.0041
8	9	478	0.0188
9	5	476	0.0105
10	3	481	0.0062
11	8	483	0.0166
12	4	494	0.0081
13	8	487	0.0164
14	3	493	0.0061
15	5	491	0.0102
16	7	487	0.0144
17	8	493	0.0162
18	3	489	0.0061
19	8	491	0.0163
20	9	493	0.0183
21	4	492	0.0081
22	3	474	0.0063
23	4	482	0.0083
24	3	499	0.0060
25	5	487	0.0103
26	6	494	0.0121
27	8	501	0.0160
28	0	478	0.0000
29	3	483	0.0062
30	5	494	0.0101

physicians have joined the staff in the last year, and the committee wants to know if the observed mortality rate has changed. Because the patient fits only one of two categories (survived or did not survive) and because the number of monthly operations varies, the p-chart is used for analysis.

By plotting the proportion of monthly mortalities and applying control limits, the p-chart in Figure 5.1 was created. The average of 0.0109 indicates that, on average, 1.09% of the monthly operations resulted in a mortality. Because there appear to be no indications of trends, shifts, or other special causes, the committee concluded that there did not seem to be a significant increase in the proportion of mortalities during the study. Note that the control limits change for each month because the subgroup size (number of monthly operations) varies.

As indicated in Figure 5.1, the variation in the postoperative mortality rate can be attributed to common cause variation. In a situation such as this, decreasing postoperative deaths would require further study to determine the underlying causes of death and the contribution that the hospital's current processes may make in those deaths, followed by targeted interventions for improvement.

Creating a p-Chart

The procedure for creating a p-chart is as follows:

1. Collect categorical attributes data that are defined as either conforming or nonconforming compared with some requirement. At least 20 subgroups should be collected. The data should include the number

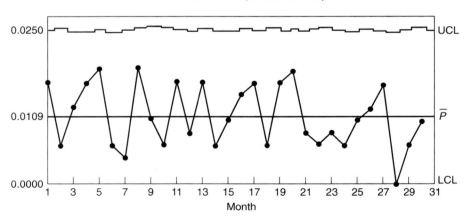

Figure 5.1 *p*-Chart: Postoperative Mortality St. Anywhere Hospital
UCL, upper control limit; *LCL*, lower control limit.

of nonconforming items and the total number of items inspected for each subgroup.

2. Calculate the proportion nonconforming (p) for each subgroup.
3. Plot each of the p-values on a chart in time order.
4. Calculate the average proportion nonconforming ($\bar{p}$) for the data set according to formula 5.1.
5. Create a horizontal line across the chart to represent $\bar{p}$.
6. Apply formulas 5.2 and 5.3 to calculate the UCL and LCL for each subgroup.
7. Create horizontal control limit lines for each subgroup on the chart. If the LCL is a negative value, then the LCL is considered to be zero.
8. If the team chooses to use a p-chart when subgroup size is constant, then only one UCL and one LCL will be necessary for all the data.
9. Optionally, create a Pareto chart to display the frequency of nonconforming items.

In Figure 5.1, the UCL on the p-chart varies from one subgroup to the next, and unique control limits are calculated separately for each subgroup; i.e., because control limits are a function of n, when the number of monthly operations changes, the corresponding control limits on the p-chart also change. Varying control limits can be avoided by specifying an unchanging sample size for each subgroup in the study. Alternatively, if subgroup sizes are not significantly different, average subgroup size ($\bar{n}$) may be used in place of n in formulas 5.2 and 5.3. For the St. Anywhere data, the largest sample size was 501 and the smallest was 474. Assuming this difference is not significant, the average subgroup size ($\bar{n} = 488$) could be used to calculate unchanging control limits for an np-chart. When subgroup size is constant, either an np-chart or a p-chart may be used, and the decision to use one chart over the other is purely at the discretion of the team performing the analysis.

np-Charts

Centerline and control limit formulas for np-charts are as follows:

$$(5.4) \quad n\bar{p} = \frac{\text{total number of nonconforming items}}{\text{total number of subgroups}}$$

$$(5.5) \quad UCL_{np} = n\bar{p} + 3\sqrt{n\bar{p}(1-\bar{p})} \quad \text{and}$$

$$(5.6) \quad LCL_{np} = n\bar{p} - 3\sqrt{n\bar{p}(1-\bar{p})}$$

The data used for constructing the np-chart can be found in Table 5.2. Note that Table 5.2 uses the same data as in the *number of postoperative*

Table 5.2 *np*-Chart: Postoperative Mortality St. Anywhere Hospital

MONTH	NUMBER OF POSTOPERATIVE MORTALITIES
1	8
2	3
3	6
4	8
5	9
6	3
7	2
8	9
9	5
10	3
11	8
12	4
13	8
14	3
15	5
16	7
17	8
18	3
19	8
20	9
21	4
22	3
23	4
24	3
25	5
26	6
27	8
28	0
29	3
30	5

np-Chart with average subgroup size ($\bar{n}$).

mortalities column found in Table 5.1. Instead of plotting the proportion non-conforming (the far right column in Table 5.1) as was done with the *p*-chart, the raw numbers of mortalities are plotted. When the centerline and control limits for the *np*-chart are applied to the raw data, the result is an *np*-chart as displayed in Figure 5.2. On this chart, the team can see that the average number of monthly postoperative mortalities is 5.333 and that the normal high could be a little over 12 per month.

Although the difference between *p*- and *np*-charts is usually simply a matter of scale, the *np*-chart can be misleading if the *n*-values vary significantly from one subgroup to the next. In most cases, the use of *p*- and *np*-charts depends on what information is most meaningful for the quality improvement (QI) team. If the actual count of the parameter being studied is important and best understood, then the *np*-chart will be more useful, given the appropriate precautions regarding sample size. On the other hand, *p*-charts may be more helpful when the rate or proportion nonconforming is of interest.

Creating an **np**-*Chart*

The procedure for creating an *np*-chart is as follows:

1. Collect categorical attributes data that are defined as either conforming or nonconforming compared with some requirement. At least 20 subgroups should be collected. The data should include the number of nonconforming items and the total number of items inspected for each subgroup.
2. Confirm that subgroup size (n) is constant.
3. Plot the number nonconforming for each subgroup on a chart in time order.
4. Calculate $n\overline{p}$ (the *np*-chart centerline) according to formula 5.4.

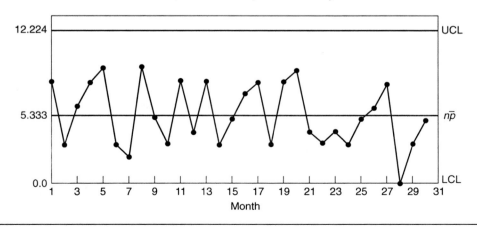

Figure 5.2 *np*-Chart: Mortality Data

5. Create a horizontal line across the chart to represent $n\overline{p}$.
6. Apply formulas 5.5 and 5.6 to calculate the *UCL* and *LCL*.
7. Create horizontal control limit lines on the chart. If the *LCL* is a negative value, then the *LCL* is considered to be zero.
8. Optionally, create a Pareto chart to display the frequency of nonconforming items.

◆ Charts for Counts Attributes

c-charts and *u*-charts are of greatest use in the quest to understand counts attributes data, where the number of nonconformities per inspection unit is counted. Recall that *p*- and *np*-charts are used for evaluating categorical attributes data where the number or proportion of nonconforming items fails some examination criteria. Each item inspected is deemed to have either passed or failed some requirement. However, when tracking nonconformities, the nonconformity is either present or it is not. If a nonconformity is present, it does not necessarily mean that the item inspected has failed, nor is the item necessarily categorized as defective. Instead, the error is either present or it is not. The goal is not to determine the number of "good vs. bad." Instead, the goal is to understand the rate of nonconformities (errors, flaws, defects, etc.) over some area of time or space, often called an inspection unit.

An inspection unit is the area, time, or space over which nonconformities are counted. Depending on the situation, an inspection unit might be defined as the number of problems uncovered during a 24-hour period in 10,000 square feet of inspected floor space or the number of errors in 50 insurance claims. If the severity of housekeeping errors is of interest, then depending on the situation, an inspection unit might be defined as a single room or an entire hospital floor. The job of an inspection unit is to define the breadth and depth of the ongoing inspections so that the results may be properly reported and interpreted.

c-Charts

The use of *c*-charts assumes that the inspection unit is equal to one and unchanging from one subgroup to the next. If the inspection unit varies in size from one subgroup to the next, then a *u*-chart should be used rather than a *c*-chart. The *c*-chart control limit formulas follow:

$$(5.7) \quad \overline{c} = \frac{\text{total number of nonconformities}}{\text{total number of inspection units}}$$

$$(5.8) \quad UCL_c = \overline{c} + 3\sqrt{\overline{c}}$$

$$(5.9) \quad LCL_c = \overline{c} - 3\sqrt{\overline{c}}$$

The data sets for these analyses conform to the Poisson distribution (see Chapter 7, "Advanced Statistical Applications in Continuous Quality Improvement") for which the mean and variance are equal.

Example 5-2

The XYZ Clinic has a total of five examination rooms that are cleaned daily by a maintenance contractor. Each morning, the office manager inspects the examination rooms for any of several omissions in the cleaning process: failure to properly dispose of the "red bag" wastebaskets, dust left on floor, counters not cleaned, etc. These defects are tallied for each room and then summed for a total number of nonconformities each day. In this case, the daily inspection unit is always five examination rooms. The inspection is performed for 50 consecutive days. The data collected are found in Table 5.3.

The inspection unit is identical for each subgroup, so the actual number of nonconformities is plotted, resulting in the graph in Figure 5.3. On average, 7.12 defects are found each day for all five examination rooms inspected. The *UCL* of 15.125 signifies that it is normal for around 15 defects to be found each day. More than 15 would be considered significantly higher than normal and would suggest the presence of some special cause. In fact, *days 4, 24, 34,* and *36* indicate statistically higher levels of defects compared with the other days in the study. Because of this, further investigation was performed to help uncover unusual circumstances that may have been present for each of those days. Based on the investigation, it was determined that on each day that a special cause was present, the clinic had closed late due to the large volume of patients. This left the cleaning crew with less time for completing their job, ultimately resulting in more nonconformities being found. To help reduce nonconformities due to these special causes, the clinic manager worked out a notification system that allowed the cleaning team to adjust its hours on those days when the clinic stayed open late.

By using the control chart in this manner, identification of special causes can help direct improvement energies toward correcting atypical process problems; i.e., those issues that are not a part of everyday processes can be attacked and eliminated, further reducing the defect level and making visible other causes that adversely impact defect levels.

Creating a c-Chart

The procedure for creating a *c*-chart is as follows:

1. Identify a constant inspection unit.
2. Collect counts attributes data for each inspection unit. At least 20 subgroups should be collected.

Table 5.3 *c*-Chart: Room Cleaning Nonconformities St. Anywhere Hospital

Day	Number of Cleaning Room Errors	Day	Number of Cleaning Room Errors
1	8	26	2
2	3	27	14
3	6	28	1
4	17	29	4
5	4	30	8
6	5	31	10
7	8	32	12
8	12	33	5
9	3	34	16
10	8	35	13
11	5	36	16
12	6	37	5
13	0	38	3
14	4	39	8
15	2	40	4
16	6	41	8
17	8	42	2
18	1	43	9
19	9	44	6
20	6	45	4
21	7	46	5
22	4	47	3
23	8	48	9
24	19	49	12
25	15	50	3

3. Plot each of the *c*-values on a chart in time order.
4. Calculate the average number of nonconformities ($\bar{c}$) for the data set according to formula 5.7.
5. Create a horizontal line across the chart to represent $\bar{c}$.
6. Apply formulas 5.8 and 5.9 to calculate the *UCL* and the *LCL*.
7. Create horizontal control limit lines on the chart. If the *LCL* is a negative value, then place the *LCL* at zero.
8. Optionally, create a Pareto chart to display the frequency of nonconformities.

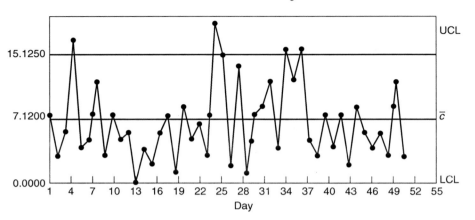

Figure 5.3 Room Cleaning Errors XYZ Clinic Cleaning Study

u-Charts

When the number of inspection units varies, the c-chart cannot be used. These situations arise when the number of units produced varies from one plot point to the next. Take the example where insurance claims are checked for errors. In some weeks, 100 forms might be checked, whereas other weeks, only 80 or 50 might be checked. In order to fairly compare one week's performance to the next, the data must be normalized or "unitized." By unitizing the data, weeks with differing numbers of claims can be placed on the same chart. Not only does unitizing allow users to compare plot points with differing subgroup sizes, but it also serves as the basis for the u-chart's name because each plot point represents a "unitized count" of nonconformities.

The calculated u-value adjusts for the number of inspection units by dividing the count of defects (c) by n, the number of inspection units present in each subgroup. Once calculated, each subgroup's u-value is plotted on the control chart. u-Values are calculated with formula 5.10.

$$(5.10) \quad u = \frac{c}{n}$$

where c is the number of nonconformities in the subgroup, and
　　　　n is the number of inspection units present in the subgroup.

u-Chart control limits are calculated in the same manner as those for c-charts but are adjusted for n, the number of inspection units in the subgroup

$$(5.11) \quad \bar{u} = \frac{\text{total number of nonconformities}}{\text{total number of inspection units}}$$

$$(5.12) \quad UCL_u = \bar{u} + 3\sqrt{\frac{\bar{u}}{n}}$$

$$(5.13) \quad LCL_u = \bar{u} - 3\sqrt{\frac{\bar{u}}{n}}$$

n = the number of inspection units from which the nonconformities were found.

Like the p-chart with varying n, control limits on the u-chart are calculated for each subgroup of data. Thus, the u-chart is a special version of the c-chart, adjusted for a variable number of units within which nonconformities are counted.

Example 5-3

The food service department at St. Anywhere Hospital was trying to determine the level and type of food complaints so that they could better serve their patients' needs. They kept a count of the total number of meals prepared each day and logged the number and type of food complaints that were encountered. Because the number of meals prepared each day varied based on the number of patients and a single meal could potentially generate numerous complaints, a u-chart (Figure 5.4) was chosen for the analysis.

Counts of nonconformities were collected for each of 28 days. Five sections of the hospital participated in the study. The number of meals served and the number and type of complaints were noted each day, along with the section from which the meals were served.

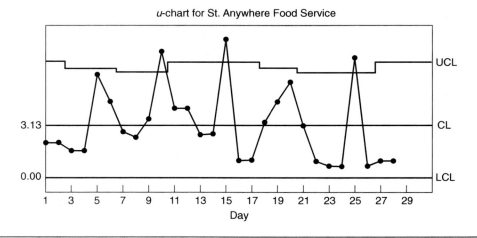

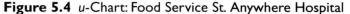

Figure 5.4 *u*-Chart: Food Service St. Anywhere Hospital

To make the analysis and interpretation of the results simpler, the team decided upon an inspection unit of 100 meals. The data are found in Table 5.4. Control limits will be different for each subgroup based on its unique number of inspection units.

Table 5.4 *u*-Chart: Meal Nonconformities St. Anywhere Hospital

Day	Number of Meal Complaints (c)	Agreed-Upon Inspection Unit	Number of Meals Served	Inspection Units per Subgroup (n)	Unitized Count (u = c/n)
1	4	100	200	2.0	2.00
2	4	100	200	2.0	2.00
3	4	100	250	2.5	1.60
4	4	100	250	2.5	1.60
5	15	100	250	2.5	6.00
6	11	100	250	2.5	4.40
7	8	100	300	3.0	2.67
8	7	100	300	3.0	2.33
9	10	100	300	3.0	3.33
10	22	100	300	3.0	7.33
11	8	100	200	2.0	4.00
12	8	100	200	2.0	4.00
13	5	100	200	2.0	2.50
14	5	100	200	2.0	2.50
15	13	100	200	2.0	6.50
16	5	100	200	2.0	2.50
17	2	100	200	2.0	1.00
18	8	100	250	2.5	3.20
19	11	100	250	2.5	4.40
20	14	100	250	2.5	5.60
21	9	100	300	3.0	3.00
22	3	100	300	3.0	1.00
23	2	100	300	3.0	0.67
24	2	100	300	3.0	0.67
25	21	100	300	3.0	7.00
26	2	100	300	3.0	0.67
27	2	100	200	2.0	1.00
28	2	100	200	2.0	1.00

Interpreting the u-*Chart*

Overall, the average number of unitized meal complaints was 3.13, meaning that for every 100 meals served, approximately 3 complaints were logged. Subgroup (day) numbers 10, 15, and 25 were found to be outside control limits, indicating the presence of some special causes of variation. Those causes acting on the system resulted in significantly higher levels of complaints for the three subgroups. In fact, the team noted that subgroup numbers 5 and 20, although not outside control limits, also seemed to be fairly large in comparison with the other unitized counts. The level of unitized complaints in subgroups 5 and 20 did not indicate statistically significant events by themselves, but when the team considered that all subgroups divisible by 5 had consistently larger levels of complaints per 100 meals served, it did seem odd. Therefore, the team decided to look closely at what might be happening every 5 days that could explain the higher complaint levels.

Additionally, the team took the actual complaints themselves and created a Pareto chart, which graphically displays the frequency of defects from highest to lowest occurrence. An overall Pareto chart is found in Figure 5.5. Overall, 25 complaints were lodged because *food*

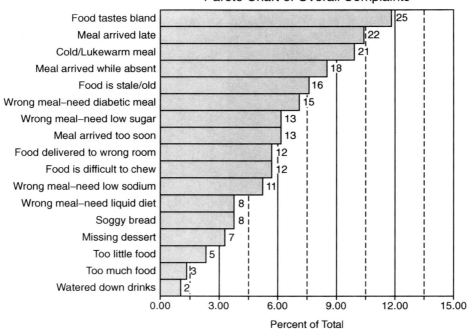

Figure 5.5 Food Service Nonconformities St. Anywhere Hospital

tastes bland, 22 complaints were *meal arrived late,* and so forth. By studying this overall Pareto chart, the team gained critical information that can steer them in the direction of problem solving and troubleshooting.

However, because the team also collected information concerning the hospital section number from which the meal was delivered, they took the same complaint data and created a Pareto chart that displays the complaints by section. The Pareto chart in Figure 5.6 shows the same data as Figure 5.5, only categorized by hospital section number. This way, the team was able to break down the meal complaints by origination of the defect. Overall, Figure 5.6 shows that *sections 2* and *4* had the highest levels of complaints compared with the other three sections. In fact, the total of 72 complaints in *section 2* was 36% higher than in *section 4* and was more than twice the level of *sections 1, 3,* and *5*. Therefore, the team was able to identify not only which defects were more prevalent (from figure 5.5) but were steered in the direction of hospital *section 2* (by Figure 5.6 data) as the place to focus their efforts.

However, they were not satisfied with the information. The team wanted to better understand the type of meal complaints that were being lodged for *section 2* and *section 4*. Therefore, they created a multilevel Pareto chart to display not only the total number of meal complaints by section but also to display what those complaints were. Figure 5.7 displays the multilevel Pareto chart that was created. Note that the total number of complaints shown in *section 2* of the chart is still displayed as 72, and *section 4* still shows a total of 53. However, the smaller, darker Pareto directly below each section

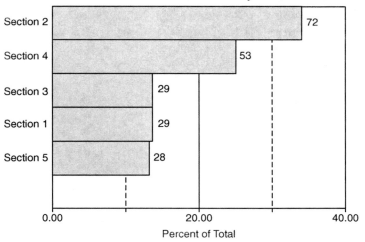

Figure 5.6 Nonconformities Summarized by Hospital Section Number

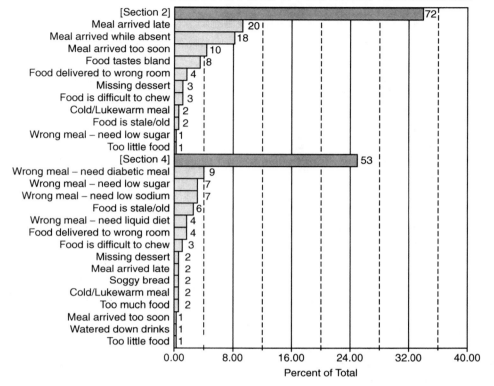

Figure 5.7 Multilevel Pareto Chart: Nonconformities Per Hospital Section Number

total represents the type of meal complaints that were lodged for each section. Note that the predominant complaints noted in *section 2* included *meal arrived late, meal arrived while* [the patient was] *absent,* or *meal arrived too soon.* For *section 4*, the overriding complaints were of wrong meals being delivered to patients. This information gave the improvement team specific directions in terms of what complaints to look for, where to look for them, and the type of actions that should be taken for each section number.

Control charts help teams to identify special causes with respect to time, and Pareto charts help those same teams to understand where to look and what improvement actions are best to take.

Creating a u-Chart

The procedure for creating a *u*-chart is as follows:

1. Identify a meaningful inspection unit on which the team can agree.

2. Collect counts attributes data for each subgroup. At least 20 subgroups should be collected.
3. For each subgroup, calculate the number of inspection units (n) by dividing the actual number inspected by the agreed-upon inspection unit.
4. For each subgroup, calculate the unitized count of nonconformities (u) by dividing the counts of nonconformities (c) by the number of inspection units per subgroup (n).
5. Plot each of the u-values on a chart in time order.
6. Calculate the average number of unitized nonconformities ($\bar{u}$) for the data set according to formula 5.11.
7. Create a horizontal line across the chart to represent $\bar{u}$.
8. Apply formulas 5.12 and 5.13 to calculate the UCL and LCL for each subgroup.
9. Create horizontal control limit lines on the chart for each subgroup. If the LCL is a negative value, then place the LCL at zero.
10. Optionally, create a Pareto chart to display nonconformity frequency.

◆ Analysis of Variables Data

As discussed previously in this chapter, variables data are the result of measuring some product, service, or result. Examples of variables data include the measurement of a patient's height or weight, the cost associated with tracking down insurance information, or the time necessary to complete a step in the medical care process. Regardless of the measurement, variables data are very different from attributes data and likewise require different statistical tools and interpretations.

Although variables and attributes data are different, the foundation of their respective control charts is not; i.e., like attributes control charts, variables control charts display plotted statistics on a time-series chart and have a centerline and upper and lower control limits based on three standard deviations from the mean. However, two control charts must be constructed when analyzing variables data: one to observe subgroup central tendency and another chart for understanding subgroup variation.

Over the years, many different variables data control charts have been created to manage the challenges that confront their use in industry. It is vital that the correct control chart be chosen to ensure proper analysis and conclusions. The following section deals with these important issues and presents a method for selecting the proper control chart for each application.

Selection of Variables Data Control Charts

If selected and used correctly, control charts are powerful tools for evaluating the consistency of data over time. Although control charts all share fundamental assumptions and are constructed in a similar manner, users can choose among a wide variety of chart types to analyze data. The control chart decision tree shown in Figure 5.8 has been developed to aid in the selection of the appropriate control chart for a particular situation. Typically, the type of variable control chart selected for an analysis is based on the answers to three questions.

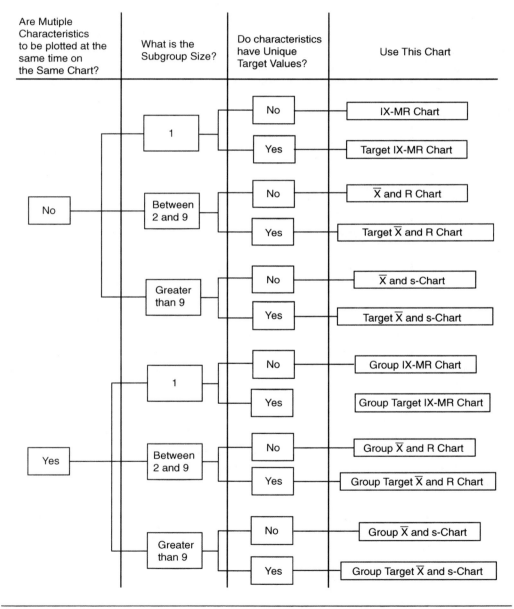

Figure 5.8 Control Chart Decision Tree for Continuous Variables

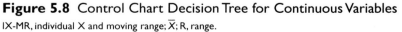

IX-MR, individual X and moving range; $\overline{X}$; R, range.

Question 1. Are multiple characteristics to be analyzed at the same time on the same chart?

Most companies have many different indicators of performance and quality. For organizations interested in evaluating the consistency of a single characteristic, traditional control charts such as the $\overline{X}$ and R can be employed. In some situations, users may want to compare multiple characteristics on a single chart. This can be accomplished by using a group chart. For example, a surgical unit with several different subspecialties may be interested in comparing some characteristic that is common between them all. Rather than create a separate chart for each specialty, a group chart could plot, analyze, and track all of the specialties on a single chart. Group charts are excellent tools for the user who wishes to compare several different quality indicators on a single chart.

Question 2. What is the subgroup size?

For the most part, when variables data control charts are employed, their subgroup size is typically one, between two and nine, or greater than nine. For a subgroup size of one, the individual X (IX) and moving range (MR) chart (IX-MR) should be used for the analysis. For subgroup sizes between two and nine, $\overline{X}$ and range charts are most appropriate. Finally, $\overline{X}$ and s-charts are best suited for subgroup sizes that are greater than nine.

Question 3. Do characteristics have different target values?

Sometimes a performance characteristic is of interest to all organizations, even though the organizations are very different, and although they may all perform analyses and create reports for that characteristic, each organization may require a different outcome or expect their performance to be different in some way. That is, each organization's performance target for the characteristic may be dissimilar even though the quality characteristic is the same. For example, average length of stay (ALOS) is certainly of interest to every hospital; however, each hospital may have a different target for ALOS. Because of their different targets, ALOS data from two hospitals could not be plotted on the same chart. The problem is one of scaling. However, these scaling issues can be alleviated with a special type of control chart. Target charts are designed to "normalize" data based on each individual data point's deviation from its target. By doing so, the target value is treated as a zero point, and all chart plot points are positive and negative numbers around the target of zero. By normalizing data in this way, multiple characteristics with different target values can be tracked on the same chart.

Commonly Used Control Charts

Many different control charts will be discussed in this text. However, they are all variations on three traditional variables data control charts: *IX-MR*,

$\bar{X}$ and R, and $\bar{X}$ and s. This section will discuss these common charts and provide some examples of their use.

IX-MR *Charts*

CRITERION	VALUE
Multiple characteristics on the same chart?	No
Subgroup size?	1
Unique target values for characteristics?	No

IX-MR charts are used for evaluating the consistency of variables data where a single characteristic is tracked with a subgroup size (n) of 1. On the *IX* chart, the individual data point that is plotted on the chart represents the best estimate of a data set's central tendency. Even though individual data values are plotted on the *IX* chart, its main purpose is to indicate central tendency and estimate an overall average.

As a companion to the *IX* chart, the *MR* chart displays the variability component of the individual data points. As with every variables data control chart, the consistency of central tendency as well as dispersion need to be evaluated for a true picture of process performance. Knowledge of a data set's average is not sufficient; the underlying variability between the individual data points also provides substantial information. The *MR* chart fulfills the requirement of the analysis of the variability of a data set.

Although some readers may not be familiar with the *MR* statistics, they might recognize the R statistic. The range is traditionally calculated as the difference between the largest and the smallest value in a subgroup of measurements. However, when using the *IX-MR* chart, variability in the form of the range is calculated as the absolute difference between two successive individual (*IX*) values. For example, assume that four individual measurements are taken 1 week apart and they are as follows: 15, 25, 16, and 42. The range between the first two numbers is the absolute value of the difference between them: $|15 - 25| = 10$. The absolute value of the range between successive "moving" pairs of numbers provides the remainder of the values for the *MR*, i.e., $|25 - 16| = 9$ and $|16 - 42| = 26$. For each *MR* value, a plot point is placed on the corresponding *MR* chart. The *MR* chart allows users to evaluate the consistency of variability through time. Once the *MR* chart is found to be consistent, its average *MR* value is used in calculating control limits for the *IX* chart.

Typically, *IX-MR* charts are used to

◆ evaluate the consistency of time-ordered variables (measurements) data,
◆ track the consistency of data that occurs infrequently (such as monthly sales, financial data, occupancy, or other infrequently occurring data), and

◆ plot and display each and every data point that is collected.

Use of the *IX-MR* chart is governed by several criteria that must be met so that the statistical analysis will be valid.

◆ The subgroup size is one.
◆ Measurements are normally distributed.
◆ Measurements are independent of one another.
◆ Only one characteristic of interest at a time is to be placed on the chart.

The use of *IX-MR* charts for tracking small samples of data is particularly important because this technique can be applied to data sets of individual values, such as the ALOS analysis mentioned earlier. Because ALOS can assume any of an infinite number of values, and because it is usually calculated monthly, it is a continuous variable for which only a single data point will be available each month. Thus, an *IX-MR* chart would be ideal for analyzing this type of data. *IX-MR* control chart formulas are found in Exhibit 5-1, and constants for calculating control limits (D_3, D_4, and A_2) are found in the Appendix.

Example 5-4

To better understand how long patients were staying at their institution, St. Anywhere Hospital carefully gathered data each month to determine the length of stay for all of their patient visits. Then, from all of those visits, the ALOS for each month was calculated for 24 months. The ALOS was calculated from a range of services for

---

Exhibit 5-1 *IX-MR* Chart Formulas

	Moving Range	**Individual X**
Plot Point	MR = absolute difference between two successive *IX* values	IX = individual measurement
Average (centerline)	$\overline{MR} = \dfrac{\sum MR}{k-1}$	$\overline{IX} = \dfrac{\sum IX}{k}$
UCL	$UCL_{MR} = D_4\,\overline{MR}$	$UCL_{IX} = \overline{IX} + A_2\,\overline{MR}$
LCL	$LCL_{MR} = D_3\,\overline{MR}$	$LCL_{IX} = \overline{IX} - A_2\,\overline{MR}$

MR, moving range; *IX,* individual *X; k,* number of subgroups; *UCL,* upper control limit; *LCL,* lower control limit.

myocardial infarction provided in critical care and cardiac surgery units. There has been no case-mix adjustment performed on the data. The ALOS data is provided in Table 5.5.

By only looking at the data in the table, it is difficult to determine if the ALOS for any one month was significantly better or worse than another. For example, month 8 shows an ALOS of 13.83 days, the longest average stay of the 24 months. Conversely, during month 12, the ALOS was only 11.30 days, the lowest ALOS of them all. So the question becomes, Are they different? Should there have been an inquiry into why the 8th month showed such poor performance

Table 5.5 ALOS Data for St. Anywhere Hospital

MONTH	ALOS	MR
1	11.80	—
2	11.76	0.04
3	11.26	0.50
4	11.31	0.05
5	13.28	1.97
6	12.66	0.62
7	13.64	0.98
8	13.83	0.19
9	11.84	1.99
10	11.90	0.06
11	12.82	0.92
12	11.30	1.52
13	12.07	0.77
14	12.78	0.71
15	12.01	0.77
16	13.57	1.56
17	13.34	0.23
18	12.55	0.79
19	12.21	0.34
20	13.37	1.16
21	12.13	1.24
22	13.10	0.97
23	12.49	0.61
24	12.53	0.04

ALOS, average length of stay.

while the 12th month showed a much better value? Similar questions apply to the 1.99 *MR* value between months 8 and 9 and the 0.04 *MR* between months 1 and 2. To answer these questions, a control chart can be employed. Alternately, the questions might be stated in this manner: Is there a statistically significant difference between the ALOS in month 8 *vs.* month 12? Are the two *MR*s of 1.99 and .04 significantly different from each other to warrant concern or additional action?

Obviously the two *IX* numbers are different—13.83 is higher than 11.30—but are they so different as to merit an investigation as to why they are so unusual? Likewise, can one conclude that the *MR* values of 1.99 and 0.04 are so very different that those involved with the study should be concerned with the increase (or decrease) in variation? The control chart will answer these questions and provide a context for either taking action or concluding that the numbers simply are due to the normal variation found in the data set.

Calculations for the *MR* chart were made according to the formulas in Exhibit 5-1.

$$\overline{MR} = \frac{\sum MR}{k-1} = \frac{18.03}{23} = 0.784$$

$$UCL_{MR} = D_4\,\overline{MR} = 3.267(0.784) = 2.561$$

$$LCL_{MR} = D_3\,\overline{MR} = 0(0.784) = 0$$

Calculations for the *IX* chart were also performed according to the formulas in Exhibit 5-1.

$$\overline{IX} = \frac{\sum IX}{k} = \frac{299.55}{24} = 12.481$$

$$UCL_{IX} = \overline{IX} + A_2\,\overline{MR} = 12.481 + 2.660(0.784) = 14.566$$

$$LCL_{IX} = \overline{IX} - A_2\,\overline{MR} = 12.481 - 2.660(0.784) = 10.396$$

When the data in Table 5.5 are plotted with the control limits and centerlines from these calculations, the *IX-MR* chart in Figure 5.9 is obtained.

Because the control limits of an *IX* chart are calculated with the centerline of the *MR* chart, the *MR* chart should be interpreted before the *IX* chart. On the *MR* chart, each subgroup should be

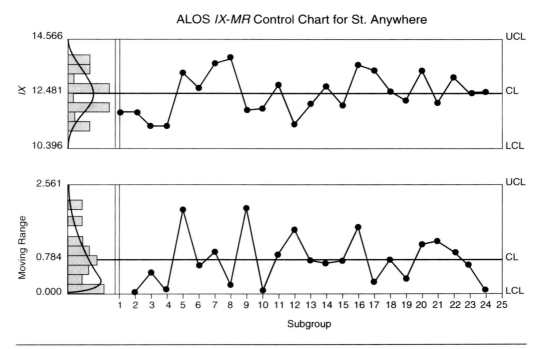

Figure 5.9 *IX-MR* Control Chart: St. Anywhere ALOS

ALOS, average length of stay.

compared with the centerline (average *MR*) of 0.784. The centerline (as with all control charts) serves as a primary point of comparison for any data set because it provides a consistent value with which all points on the graph can be assessed. The centerline of the *MR* chart indicates that for all 24 months of ALOS values, the average difference between any two successive ALOS values was 0.784 days.

In addition to comparing each plot point to the centerline, each plot point should also be compared with the *MR* chart control limits. As with all control charts, control limits define the 99.7% bounds of normal variability as ±3 standard deviations from the average. In this example, the *UCL* and *LCL* for the *MR* chart were calculated, respectively, as 2.561 and zero, meaning that the *MR* values have a 0.997 probability of falling between zero and 2.561. Thus, it would not be unusual to find a *MR* value as small as zero or as large as 2.561. Therefore, the largest and smallest *MR* values of 1.99 and .03 should not be considered unusual because they fall within the normal limits of variability. Nothing out of the ordinary should be attributed to the values of 1.99 or 0.03. They are simply indicative of the normal variation within the process and should be treated no differently than any other *MR* value between zero and 2.561.

When interpreting the *IX* chart, it can be seen that no data points fall outside the control limits, and there also appear to be no shifts, trends, or patterns. In other words, unless something significant and dramatic changes, it is normal to see the month-to-month ALOS vary between 10.4 and 14.6 days with an overall average of about 12.5 days. Therefore, the lowest and highest ALOS values within the data set (11.30 and 13.83) are considered normal because they too fall within the control limits of the *IX* chart.

Overall, the *IX-MR* control chart clearly shows that the ALOS, as well as the variation in the ALOSs (highlighted by the *MR* chart) was consistent, stable, predictable, and unchanged over the 24-month period of the study. From the control chart, the hospital administrators could discern no indications of special cause because the points in question were within the range of common cause variation. Although the control chart showed consistent ALOS values, they determined that the overall average ALOS was unacceptably high. Therefore, the team endeavored to uncover systemic sources of variation that would potentially reduce the overall ALOS average.

$\overline{X}$ *and* R *Charts*

CRITERION	VALUE
Multiple characteristics on the same chart?	No
Subgroup size?	2–9
Unique target values for characteristics?	No

$\overline{X}$ and range (R) control charts are variables data control charts whose plot points are calculated statistics rather than individual data values. The *IX-MR* charts described in the previous section require that only a single measurement be taken before a point is placed on the chart. When constructing $\overline{X}$ and R charts, several measurements are sampled from a population. The typical $\overline{X}$ and R chart has a fixed sample size, usually consisting of between two and nine individual measurements. The sampled data are typically called a subgroup, and the number of measurements within a subgroup is called the subgroup size or n.

Once each subgroup of data has been gathered, two statistics: the average ($\overline{X}$) and range are calculated and used as plot points on the $\overline{X}$ and R control charts. The $\overline{X}$ value is used as an indicator of central tendency for the population, and the range is used to describe the variability of the population. R values, because of the simplicity of their calculation, serve as a convenient, simple, and expedient way of estimating the variability of a data set. Additionally, sample R values can be used to estimate the overall standard deviation for the population.

Like all variables data control charts, the $\overline{X}$ and R chart is used to evaluate the consistency of some quality characteristic over time. To use these charts, data must be fairly abundant because each subgroup must have at least two and no more than nine data values. Additionally, each subgroup must have the same number of samples, be independent of one another, and be normally distributed. Formulas for $\overline{X}$ and R charts can be found in Exhibit 5-2. Applications for these charts abound in health care, and one such instance is presented in the next example.

Example 5-5

The financial manager at XYZ Clinic has been concerned lately with what seems to be a decrease in cash flow. Since being hired almost 2 years ago, the manager has been calculating a measure called "weekly receivables" (WR) each Friday using the following equation:

WR = total receivables/weekly sales

Calculated in this way, the week's receivables indicate how long it takes to collect monies owed to the practice for services rendered, which in turn could have an impact on overall cash flow.

In order for XYZ Clinic to achieve its long-term growth plans, cash flow must be improved to fund short-term growth efforts. Before making any hasty decisions about how to do this, the manager is interested in first understanding how the WR have been behaving since her arrival. The manager wants to know if the WR are increasing (as some speculate), decreasing, or remaining constant. To factually evaluate the situation, the manager decides to construct an $\overline{X}$ and R chart. By doing so, the office will be able to determine if receivables are increasing and if alternative methods of funds collections are required to meet their plans for growth.

The manager has computed WR for each of the last 80 weeks and subgrouped the data by month. The results are found in Table 5.6. Calculation of control limits and the centerline for the range chart follow:

$$\overline{R} = \frac{\sum R}{k} = \frac{110.69}{20} = 5.535$$

$$UCL_R = D_4 \overline{R} = 2.282(5.535) = 12.631$$

$$LCL_R = D_3 \overline{R} = 0(5.535) = 0$$

Calculations for the $\overline{X}$ chart are as follows:

$$\overline{\overline{X}} = \frac{\sum \overline{X}}{k} = \frac{113.94}{20} = 5.697$$

$$UCL_{\overline{X}} = \overline{\overline{X}} + A_2\overline{R} = 5.697 + 0.729(5.535) = 9.732$$

$$LCL_{\overline{X}} = \overline{\overline{X}} - A_2\overline{R} = 5.697 - 0.729(5.535) = 1.662$$

The control limits and centerlines above were used to construct the control chart in Figure 5.10. The chart reveals no special cause because all plot points fall within the control limits. Specifically, the

Table 5.6 WR Data for XYZ Clinic

MONTH	WEEK 1	WEEK 2	WEEK 3	WEEK 4	RANGE	AVERAGE
1	6.60	7.16	3.12	6.03	4.04	5.73
2	8.81	4.98	6.38	5.76	3.83	6.48
3	0.51	4.56	4.68	7.74	7.23	4.37
4	5.05	5.82	5.47	3.45	2.37	4.95
5	9.64	8.57	6.31	6.35	3.33	7.72
6	0.85	10.00	1.95	4.03	9.15	4.21
7	5.68	8.34	5.69	9.60	3.92	7.33
8	5.47	4.11	1.73	7.23	5.5	4.64
9	2.46	4.46	2.22	6.97	4.75	4.03
10	6.05	2.04	5.44	7.81	5.77	5.34
11	4.72	4.84	4.22	10.53	6.31	6.08
12	7.12	6.35	6.44	0.50	6.62	5.10
13	6.60	0.88	8.99	7.07	8.11	5.89
14	7.86	5.93	3.09	6.82	4.77	5.93
15	11.32	8.57	5.62	4.21	7.11	7.43
16	4.38	2.50	8.43	7.21	5.93	5.63
17	7.51	6.13	2.14	9.84	7.7	6.41
18	6.60	7.16	3.12	6.03	4.04	5.73
19	8.83	4.99	4.77	1.54	7.29	5.03
20	4.42	7.34	5.11	6.77	2.92	5.91

WR, weekly receivables.

average range of 5.535 indicates that the average difference between any four WR were different, on average, by 5.535 weeks, whereas the *UCL* of 12.631 specifies that for any month, WR could normally be as different as 12.631 weeks. Thus, the range of WR could be anything less than 12.631 weeks and still be within normal limits. Overall, the *R* chart displays consistent variation in the WR, with no special causes or any indication of significant increases or decreases in variation between WR. Therefore, the standard deviation of WR is not changing significantly from one time period to the next. So, for the last 20 months since the office manager was employed, there has been no significant difference in the variation in WR.

The $\overline{X}$ chart tells a similar story. For the last 20 months, the average WR is about 5.7 weeks. The upper and lower control limits indicate that, normally, the average WR during any single month could be as high as 9.7 weeks or as low as 1.6 weeks. There are no averages outside of the control limits that would signal special causes, and there are no trends or unusual patterns in the data points. This visual representation of averages indicates that nothing unusual has occurred in the last 20 months with respect to the average WR. Therefore, the speculation that WR have recently been increasing is

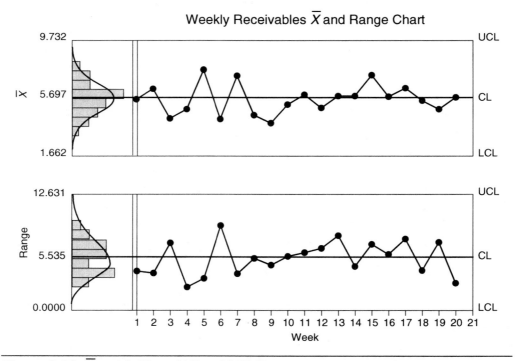

Figure 5.10 $\overline{X}$ and *R* Chart: WR at XYZ Clinic

WR, weekly receivables.

incorrect. Because no special causes exist and because the system has been operating within its expected range, the financial manager must consider common cause approaches to the problem of cash flow, i.e., those that examine the system and improve processes.

The $\overline{X}$ and R control chart is used for subgrouped data with between two and nine data points per sample. Subgrouping is preferable when there are plenty of data to analyze and the subgroup size can be fixed and unchanged throughout the period of analysis. Additionally, subgrouping has the added benefit of being able to more quickly detect significant changes in the overall average than an IX chart. In fact, the larger the subgroup size, the more sensitive the $\overline{X}$ chart becomes and the more quickly it will be able to detect significant changes in the process average.

The WR example illustrates the utility of control charts in clarifying problems. The original presumption was that the cash flow was being adversely affected by an increase in WR; however, the control chart showed no special causes that would indicate this to be true. The lack of special causes indicates that the financial system has not significantly changed. Thus, the WR will continue to vary between the control limits unless a significant change occurs in the financial processes, so the question to ask now is: "Although the week's receivables average is consistent, is it acceptable to the practice?" If not, then changes would have to be made either to the billing or payment processes to positively affect the WR data and resulting cash flow. To more closely evaluate the acceptability of the data, a comparison can be performed between the individual data points and the acceptable limit. The following example demonstrates a method of making this comparison.

Example 5-6

The practice manager and board of directors of XYZ Clinic have set the maximum WR at 7 weeks. A histogram can illustrate the relationship between the maximum allowable WR and the clinic's performance measure. The graph is presented in Figure 5.11. The histogram consists of all 80 individual data values from the 20 subgroups in Table 5.6. Even though the overall average WR of 5.697 falls below the target of 7 weeks, about 30% of the WR falls above the target. In this case, although the average and variation are consistent over the last 20 months, the percentage of time they are above 7 weeks receivables is unacceptable. Although this number may be unacceptable, this condition should be expected to continue if nothing is done to change the processes measured by the WR performance measure; i.e., the practice can expect to have approximately 30% of the WR above the acceptable target of 7 weeks unless significant corrective action is taken. The variation in the process, although considered normal on the control chart, is still excessive.

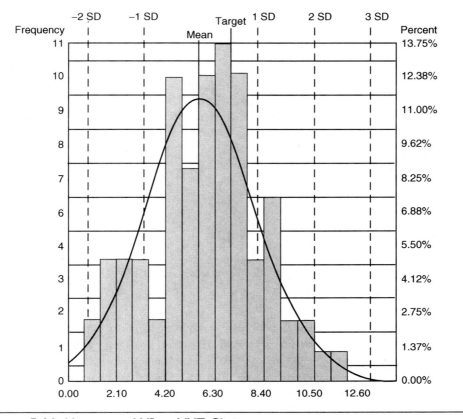

Figure 5.11 Histogram: WR at XYZ Clinic

SD, standard deviation.

Like the *IX-MR* chart, the $\overline{X}$ and R chart was developed to separate special cause variation from common cause variation, thereby allowing a context for problem solving and corrective action. The primary difference between *IX-MR* charts and $\overline{X}$ and R charts is that the latter require subgrouping and the plotting of subgroup statistics instead of individual data values. Additionally, the $\overline{X}$ and R chart, because of its subgrouping nature, results in much higher sensitivity to small changes in the overall process average. When a change in the process average could adversely affect important business measures or have dire consequences, greater sensitivity to process average changes is a significant benefit that $\overline{X}$ and R charts provide their users.

An important variation of the $\overline{X}$ and R chart proves useful when subgroup sizes vary. The charts discussed thus far assume that subgroup size remains constant, but in some situations, subgroup size can vary substantially. For example, in a rapid-cycle improvement project, the relatively short time frame of an improvement cycle can lead to varying subgroup sizes, because less control can be exercised on the study. When subgroup sizes vary, the $\overline{X}$ and R charts can still be used, but the variations in subgroup size must be

Exhibit 5-2 $\bar{X}$ and R Chart Formulas

	Range	$\bar{X}$
Plot Point	R = absolute difference between largest and smallest subgroup value	$\bar{X} = \dfrac{\sum X}{n}$
Average (centerline)	$\bar{R} = \dfrac{\sum R}{k}$	$\bar{\bar{X}} = \dfrac{\sum \bar{X}}{k}$
UCL	$UCL_R = D_4 \bar{R}$	$UCL_{\bar{X}} = \bar{\bar{X}} + A_2 \bar{R}$
LCL	$LCL_R = D_3 \bar{R}$	$LCL_{\bar{X}} = \bar{\bar{X}} - A_2 \bar{R}$

R, range; n, subgroup size; k, number of subgroups over which control limits will be calculated.

reflected in the formulas for calculating control limits. Basically, three approaches can be used with $\bar{X}$ and R charts when subgroup size varies.

◆ The average sample size ($\bar{n}$) can be used to calculate control limits. If the sample sizes are not greatly different (e.g., within 15% of mean sample size), then $\bar{n}$ can be calculated and used in the control limit calculation.

◆ Control limits can be calculated separately for each data point based on its subgroup size. Rather than computing a single $\bar{R}$ value across all subgroups, the formula in Exhibit 5-2 is applied, using the individual subgroup R for each subgroup. This value is then used to calculate control limits for each subgroup on the $\bar{X}$ and R charts.

◆ Normalize the $\bar{X}$ values and plot them as Z-scores. Calculate the estimated standard deviation for each sample, then divide it into the $\bar{X}$ value of each subgroup. The resulting statistic represents the distance, in sigma units, that each mean deviates from the overall average. Control limits will remain constant at ±3.

The following example illustrates a situation in which subgroup size varies.

Example 5-7

The anesthesia division at St. Anywhere has been asked to evaluate a new technique for induction of and recovery from anesthesia during cholecystectomies (gall bladder removal). They hope to determine the efficacy of the new technique in reducing stays in the recovery room. The division will adopt the technique if significant reductions can be demonstrated in recovery room time postoperatively, and they would like to have the results within a month. Three of the hospital's ten nurse anesthetists have volunteered to participate in the study that will be conducted over a period of 4 weeks. The time in recovery will be recorded for each patient undergoing a cholecystectomy using this new technique, and the data will be tracked with a control chart. Data from the study are shown in Table 5.7 and control charts in Figure 5.12. The charts in Figure 5.12 display control charts with varying control limits based on the changing subgroup sizes. Figure 5.13 illustrates the control charts resulting from the first approach described previously; i.e., using the average sample size ($\bar{n}$) for computing control limits. Figure 5.14 presents the Z-score chart for the same data. With use of the variable limits chart in Figure 5.12, the R chart

Table 5.7 Anesthesia Project Data St. Anywhere Hospital

DAY	t1	t2	t3	t4	t5	t6	t7	n
1	1.5	1.2	1.8	1				4
2	1.9	1.6	3.4	2.1	1.2	0.75		6
3	3	2.1	1.8					3
4	1.3	1.7	1.6	1.6	1			5
5	2.1	1.9	1.2	0.6	0.95			5
6	1.5	1.4	1.2					3
7	1.8	1.6	1.5	0.7	0.8	1.6	1	7
8	1.1	2.1	1.6	1.5				4
9	1.2	1.3	1	1.7	1.4			5
10	1.3	3.2	1.4	1.3				4
11	2	2.1	1.3					3
12	1.2	1.4	1.5	1.6	1.3	1.4		6
13	1.1	1.7	1.4	1.3	1.8	1.5	1.2	7
14	1.5	1.6	1.75	1.4				4
15	1.3	1.7	1.4	1.6	1.5	1.4		6
16	1.1	2.6	1.6	1.8				4
17	0.8	0.9	1.1	2.7				4
18	2.6	1.4	1.7	1.7	1.9	1.5		6
19	1.2	2.1	1.3	1.5	1.8	1.4	1.8	7
20	2.1	1.8	2.2					3

t = time spent in recovery.
n = subgroup size (the number of patients evaluated) each day.

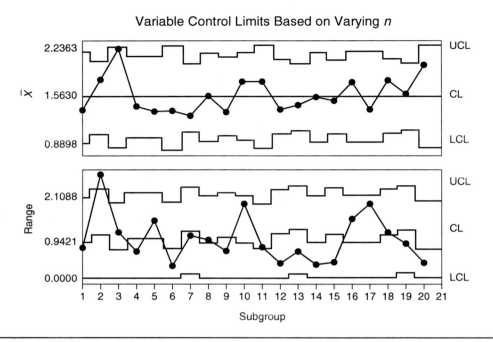

Figure 5.12 Control Chart: St. Anywhere Anesthesia Project—Variable Limits

appears to be out of control, with the second point exceeding the *UCL*. The chart in Figure 5.13 supports a similar conclusion because the second point is above the *UCL* on the *R* chart. Finally, the *Z*-score chart in Figure 5.14 indicates that the process is in control and does not include an *R* chart because the measures are normalized for the $\overline{X}$ values only.

The results of these analyses indicate that the procedure requires further study because the variability of the process was initially out of control. Because the process stabilized later in the study, the out-of-control point in the early stages may not recur; however, the nurse anesthetists in the anesthesia group opted to continue to study the new process for another 2 weeks.

$\overline{X}$ and *R* charts are powerful commonly used control charts that help users indicate the presence of assignable causes of variability and identify opportunities for improvement. They are flexible enough to be used with relatively small samples of data (between two and nine sample points) and can be used with varying subgroup sizes as well as those that are constant. As subgroup sizes increase and the abundance of available data increases above nine, the predictive value of the variability measure improves even more, as demonstrated in the next section.

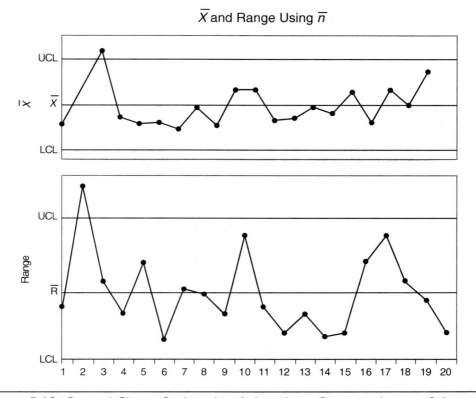

Figure 5.13 Control Charts: St. Anywhere's Anesthesia Project—Average Subgroup Size

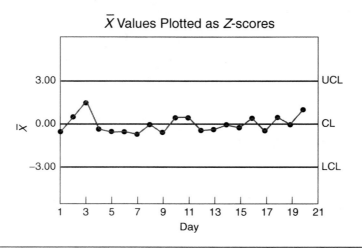

Figure 5.14 Control Charts: St. Anywhere Hospital Anesthesia Project—Z-Score

$\overline{X}$ and s-Charts

CRITERION	VALUE
Multiple characteristics on the same chart?	No
Subgroup size?	>9
Unique target values for characteristics?	No

$\overline{X}$ and s-control charts are continuous variable control charts with plot points comprised of calculated subgroup statistics where subgroup size (n) is typically 10 or larger. Although similar to the $\overline{X}$ and R chart in that it relies on the calculation of a central tendency and a variability statistic for each subgroup, the variability statistic of the $\overline{X}$ and s-chart is very different from the range statistic. The difference between the $\overline{X}$ and s-chart and the $\overline{X}$ and R chart is that the sample standard deviation (s) is used to estimate process variability in place of the range.

The sample standard deviation is a very efficient and powerful means of characterizing variation. For example, consider a subgroup of seven measurements: 3, 4, 5, 6, 7, 8, and 9. In order to characterize how much variation is present in the numbers, the range of the data set could be calculated by subtracting the smallest value in the data set from the largest. In the subgroup, the range would be 9 – 3 = 6. This range value indicates only that the difference between the largest and smallest value is six units. Notice that although the range is easy to calculate, it uses only two of the seven individual measures (the high and the low value) in its estimate of variation. Now consider a second subgroup of data so that the two subgroups are

subgroup 1: 3, 4, 5, 6, 7, 8, 9
subgroup 2: 3, 3, 3, 3, 3, 3, 9

The two subgroups are vastly different from each other: in subgroup 1, the seven values are all evenly spaced between 3 and 9, whereas in subgroup 2, all of the values are identical except for the last one. Yet, if calculated, the range is the same for each subgroup because the largest and smallest values in each subgroup are identical. Although the variation characteristics of both subgroups are very different, the range cannot detect the difference.

For larger subgroup sizes, e.g., n = 100, the range still only uses two values in its calculation. As subgroup size becomes larger, the range statistic uses an ever-smaller percentage of the existing subgroup values in its calculation. As long as the subgroup size is small (e.g., n < 10), the range can appropriately be used for control charts, but when the subgroup size increases such that n > 10, then s is a more reliable and accurate estimate of variability than the range statistic.

As illustrated in Chapter 4, the formula for calculating sample standard deviation specifies that all of a subgroup's data points are used to calculate s.

Not only are all of the individual data points used in the standard deviation calculation, but the average $(\bar{X})$ is also used in the numerator of the formula. Specifically, the average is compared to and subtracted from every single individual measurement in a subgroup. The resulting differences highlight the distance between the average and the individual values within the subgroup. This deviation from the average is a way of describing the raw magnitude of variation within the data set. Then, each deviation from the average is squared and the squared differences between the $\bar{X}$ values and the subgroup's average are summed. For the example subgroups, the average $(\bar{X})$ is 6. Given the average of 6 and a subgroup size (n) of 7, the sample standard deviation statistic is calculated as follows:

$$s = \sqrt{\frac{\sum (3-6)^2 + (4-6)^2 + (5-6)^2 + (6-6)^2 + (7-6)^2 + (8-6)^2 + (9-6)^2}{n-1}}$$

$$= \sqrt{\frac{28}{6}} = 2.16$$

Thus, the average distance that each individual value deviates from $\bar{X}$ is ~2.16. The standard deviation value is reported in the same units as the original measurements so that if the original units were reported in milligrams per deciliter, then the standard deviation is also reported in milligrams per deciliter.

Like all variable control charts, the $\bar{X}$ and s-chart is used to evaluate the consistency of variables data over some period of time. Typically, $\bar{X}$ and s-charts are used to track the consistency of variables data when large amounts of data can be economically collected. The $\bar{X}$ and s-chart requires a constant subgroup size of 10 measurements or more. As with the other $\bar{X}$ charts discussed in this chapter, the measurements must be independent and normally distributed. Formulas for calculating the $\bar{X}$ and s control limits and centerlines and statistics are found in Exhibit 5-3. The use of $\bar{X}$ and s-charts requires large volumes of data, as demonstrated in the following example.

Example 5-8

Because of the many potential infectious airborne diseases that can be transmitted in hospitals, keeping air flowing and filtered is critical. For St. Everywhere Hospital, a 120-bed hospital located in Knoxville, Tennessee, airflow has continually been monitored for the last year in nine different wings. The hospital administration is considering replacing the current air transportation and filtering system with one that is reported to dramatically improve air movement and, therefore, air quality. Recently there have been concerns about the old system and whether it has been performing up to standards.

Exhibit 5-3 $\bar{X}$ and s-Chart Formulas

	s	$\bar{X}$
Plot Point	$s = \sqrt{\dfrac{\sum(x_i - \bar{X})^2}{n-1}}$	$\bar{X} = \dfrac{\sum X}{n}$
Average (centerline)	$\bar{s} = \dfrac{\sum s}{k}$	$\bar{\bar{X}} = \dfrac{\sum \bar{X}}{k}$
UCL	$UCL_s = B_4 \bar{s}$	$UCL_{\bar{X}} = \bar{\bar{X}} + A_3 \bar{s}$
LCL	$LCL_s = B_3 \bar{s}$	$LCL_{\bar{X}} = \bar{\bar{X}} - A_3 \bar{s}$

n, subgroup size; k, number of subgroups over which control limits will be calculated.

Before moving forward and making a multimillion dollar investment in new airflow systems for each wing, hospital administration wishes to determine how the current systems are performing. Their strategy is to first understand if the current airflow system in each wing is still meeting the mandated airflow requirements, then, if necessary, approve capital expenditures to replace the systems.

The hospital administration is interested first in measuring current airflow rates and determining their consistency over time, as well as comparing performance to engineering specifications. To do so, airflow rates have been acquired for the obstetrics wing. Ten randomly selected airflow measurements have been gathered for each of the last 20 days. For purposes of the control chart analysis, each day has been treated as a subgroup to calculate an average and standard deviation. The data values and subgroup statistics are reported in Table 5.8. Like the $\bar{X}$ and R chart, the $\bar{X}$ and s-chart does not use any of the individual data values for plot points. Instead, the $\bar{X}$ and s-statistics from each subgroup are used as plot points. The individual data points can be used later for conformance analysis, process capability, and other analyses. Once the averages and s-values have been plotted, then the centerlines and control limits are calculated from the formulas found in Exhibit 5-3. The calculations for control limits and centerlines for the $\bar{X}$ and s-chart are as follows:

$$\bar{s} = \frac{\sum s}{k} = \frac{77.2414}{20} = 3.8621$$

$$UCL_s = B_4\bar{s} = 1.716(3.8621) = 6.6274$$

$$LCL_s = B_3\bar{s} = 0.284(3.8621) = 1.0968$$

$$\bar{\bar{X}} = \frac{\sum \bar{X}}{k} = \frac{673.27}{20} = 33.664$$

$$UCL_{\bar{X}} = \bar{\bar{X}} + A_3\bar{s} = 33.664 + 0.975(3.8621) = 37.430$$

$$LCL_{\bar{X}} = \bar{\bar{X}} - A_3\bar{s} = 33.664 - 0.975(3.8621) = 29.898$$

Once the calculations are complete the centerlines and control limits are then placed on the chart along with the plot points. The control charts are shown in Figure 5.15.

Because there are no points outside control limits, no runs, trends, or other patterns on the *s*-chart, the standard deviation of airflow has remained consistent. The control limits of the *s*-chart indicate that the standard deviation of airflow could normally be as large as 6.6274 cubic feet per minute (cf/min) or as small as 1.0968 cf/min. Any standard deviation value larger than the UCL or smaller than the LCL would be an indication of a significant change in airflow variability.

Table 5.8 Airflow Data St. Everywhere Hospital

	DAY 1	DAY 2	DAY 3	DAY 4	DAY 5	DAY 6	DAY 7
	35.5	28.2	30.7	36.9	36.6	30.3	35.5
	38.1	31.7	36.5	34.9	32.8	31.2	38.1
	29.7	33.5	37.6	37.0	33.5	34.6	29.7
	36.2	31.2	40.0	34.7	37.7	35.1	36.2
	35.2	27.2	36.3	20.6	36.4	36.1	35.2
	32.1	36.5	42.0	41.0	29.1	38.3	32.1
	35.5	28.1	34.4	37.8	42.0	29.6	35.5
	33.4	35.0	30.4	33.5	37.9	37.6	33.4
	30.3	31.3	35.9	31.0	32.9	36.7	30.3
	29.1	32.7	33.9	31.5	33.8	35.7	29.1
$\bar{X}$	33.51	31.54	35.77	33.89	35.27	34.52	33.51
s	3.0798	3.0511	3.6637	5.5487	3.5938	3.0875	3.0795

continues

Table 5.8 *continued*

	DAY 8	DAY 9	DAY 10	DAY 11	DAY 12	DAY 13	DAY 14
	42.1	30.5	32.8	24.3	35.2	29.2	33.8
	28.5	33.1	36.5	33.5	36.4	36.6	30.2
	39.8	28.1	35.8	34.2	40.8	31.5	30.6
	28.7	26.4	40.7	37.2	31.8	36.3	34.4
	30.7	32.6	25.7	39.9	33.4	36.1	25.2
	44.9	27.4	37.0	32.1	26.8	26.2	33.7
	32.5	31.1	29.4	33.9	33.5	29.1	32.3
	35.6	30.7	29.7	32.1	28.9	31.0	38.4
	31.8	37.1	34.3	32.8	30.8	32.0	35.1
	28.1	35.1	29.5	30.7	27.0	25.8	31.1
$\overline{X}$	34.27	31.21	33.14	33.07	32.46	31.38	32.48
s	6.0647	3.3900	4.5498	4.0871	4.3750	3.9749	3.5355

	DAY 15	DAY 16	DAY 17	DAY 18	DAY 19	DAY 20
	30.9	31.4	31.0	34.7	35.0	30.4
	35.8	41.0	37.2	40.1	40.4	29.7
	31.8	33.1	36.2	34.2	42.0	27.9
	35.8	37.0	30.4	29.7	33.6	32.3
	36.4	37.9	26.2	37.6	40.6	34.5
	28.8	36.1	29.4	37.2	26.5	39.3
	34.5	32.3	39.8	33.4	37.4	34.4
	30.0	33.6	32.5	35.6	35.0	39.8
	36.9	39.5	35.7	37.6	36.2	34.4
	32.7	32.0	33.0	40.0	30.8	33.3
$\overline{X}$	33.36	35.39	33.14	36.01	35.75	33.60
s	2.9056	3.3857	4.1018	3.1782	4.7486	3.8404

The overall average airflow for the last 20 days is 33.664 cf/min (the centerline on the $\overline{X}$ chart). The upper and lower control limits for the $\overline{X}$ chart indicate that, normally, the average airflow movement through the obstetrics wing could be as high as 37.430 cf/min or as low as 29.898 cf/min. Although no $\overline{X}$ values fall outside the control limits, there is a run of seven plot points below the centerline for

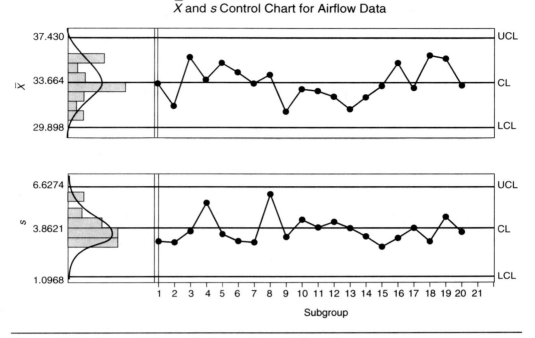

Figure 5.15 Control Charts: St. Everywhere Airflow Data

days 9 through *15*. This is an indication that the average airflow was significantly lower over these 7 days compared with any other time period on the chart. When maintenance was notified, they reported that they had just performed their monthly maintenance on the filtering system. The semiclogged filtering system was the most likely special cause for the seven plot points below the average. At the request of hospital administration, maintenance agreed to change the air filters every 3 weeks instead of the more customary 4-week interval. Doing so should eliminate the monthly run of seven points below the average as well as improve overall airflow in obstetrics.

After uncovering the special cause for the airflow reduction for *days 9* through *15*, hospital administration asked to see the individual data points compared with the airflow system specifications. In obstetrics, the airflow requirements are no more than 45 cf/min, no less than 28 cf/min, with a target value of 36.5 cf/min. These requirements are treated, respectively as the Upper Specification Limit (*USL*) and the Lower Specification Limit (*LSL*). The control chart was used to assess the consistency of the average and standard deviation through time, but a histogram had to be used to compare the individual airflow values to their requirements.

The histogram in Figure 5.16 shows that not all of the data points fall within the stated specifications for airflow rates. Additionally, the

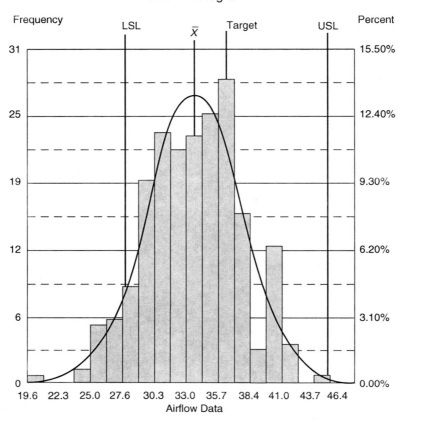

Figure 5.16 Histogram: St. Everywhere Hospital Airflow Data

average airflow ($\overline{X}$) is lower than the stated airflow target value. Because the $\overline{X}$ control chart demonstrated a runs-based special cause, the lack of consistency indicates that future behavior of the airflow rates in obstetrics cannot be accurately predicted. If the control chart had shown no signs of special causes, then the airflow rates could be confidently predicted to continue within the same set of control limits until some significant change had occurred. The histogram indicates that about 7% of the airflow values actually fell below the lower specification limit of 28 cf/min. In turn, the lower airflow rates could possibly relate to a higher incidence of airborne infectious diseases in the obstetrics unit. As a result of this study, the administration is now seriously considering the purchase of a new air filtering and movement system for the obstetrics wing.

The $\overline{X}$ and s-chart is used to subgroup data and plot statistics instead of individual data points. Using an $\overline{X}$ and s-chart is preferable to using an $\overline{X}$

and R chart when there is a wealth of data to analyze, when the data is inexpensive to gather, and when the subgroup size is 10 or larger. Additionally, the use of a larger subgroup size makes the $\overline{X}$ and s-chart more sensitive to subtle process changes. Generally, the larger the subgroup size, the better it is for quickly detecting process shifts, trends, and changes.

Like the $\overline{X}$ and R chart, the $\overline{X}$ and s-chart was developed to separate special cause variation from common cause variation, thereby allowing a context for problem solving and corrective action. When a change in the process average could adversely affect important business measures or have dire consequences, greater sensitivity to changes in the process average is a significant benefit provided by $\overline{X}$ and s-charts.

◆ Runs Testing in Control Charts

The analysis in Example 5-8 alluded to a runs analysis of the $\overline{X}$ control chart. Although similar to the evaluation of run charts detailed in Chapter 4, a runs analysis in control charting has a few notable nuances. Control charts are often divided into zones based on distance from the mean, as shown in Figure 5.17. *Zone A* represents values that are 2–3 standard deviations from the mean, *zone B* has values that are 1–2 standard deviations from the mean, and *zone C* contains those points with values that are less than 1 standard deviation from the mean. Patterns of points in these zones can also indicate special causes of process variation. The rules for performing runs analysis on control charts are listed in Table 5.9. If a pattern of points conforms to any of these rules, the process should be evaluated for assignable causes.

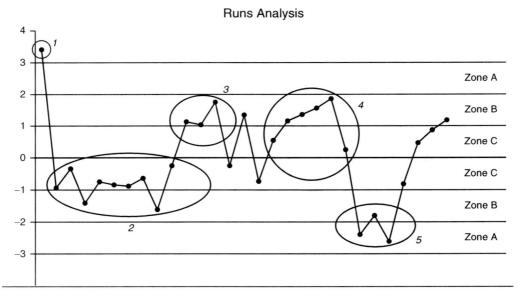

Figure 5.17 Runs Analysis of Control Chart

Table 5.9 Runs Analysis Rules and Indications of Special Causes

RULE	DESCRIPTION
1	Points above the *UCL* or below the *LCL*
2	More than 7 consecutive points either above or below the centerline
3	Four of five consecutive points in Zone B or Zone A (greater than two standard deviations)
4	More than 5 points either steadily increasing or decreasing
5	Two of three consecutive points in Zone A (between 2 and 3 standard deviations)

◆ The Power of Control Charts

The most common control charts in use by QI professionals are described in this chapter. *IX-MR,* $\overline{X}$ and *R*, and $\overline{X}$ and *s*-charts represent the vast majority of control charts used by industry today, and they can be applied to many situations in health care. In some situations, however, data sets may not be structured for these tools, and other specialized control charts may be required. The selection and application of these other types of control charts is the subject of Chapter 6, "Advanced Statistical Process Control."

◆ Discussion Points

1. Control charts provide substantial power for analyzing time sequenced data sets. What general requirements must data sets satisfy for control chart analysis?
2. Differentiate between attribute data and continuous variables. How is the statistical analysis of each of these types of variables different?
3. Describe the use of *p*- and *np*-charts. How are the charts different, and what is the advantage (if any) of using one over the other?
4. *c*-charts and *u*-charts have specific applications for attributes data. Describe these applications and give examples.
5. Define and describe the concept of control limits. What values are used for control limits, and why are these values used?
6. What three issues are important in selection of a control chart? Explain how to use the decision tree presented in this chapter to select the individual *X* and moving range (*IX-MR*) chart.
7. Under what conditions is the *IX-MR* chart appropriate? Give an example from the health care industry.
8. Explain the significance of a point that falls above the upper control limit. How does it differ from one that is within control limits? How do points within control limits differ from one another?

9. When is it appropriate to use the $\overline{X}$ and R chart? What statistical parameter is estimated by the range?
10. How can a histogram be used to analyze the distribution of data? How should data be grouped for histogram analysis?
11. Describe three methods of analyzing a data set with unequal sample sizes. Is one method preferable? Why?
12. How can an $\overline{X}$ and s-chart be used? What conditions must be met for the chart to be valid?
13. How is the $\overline{X}$ and s-chart superior to the $\overline{X}$ and R chart?
14. Describe the concept of runs analysis of control charts. What is the value of performing runs analysis?

◆ Notes

Balestracci D., and Barlow J. (1996). *Quality improvement: Practical applications for medical group practice.* Englewood, CO: Center for Research in Ambulatory Health Care Administration.

Ryan T. (1989). *Statistical methods for quality improvement* (pp. 182–188). New York: John Wiley & Sons.

Wise S., and Fair D. (1998). *Innovative control charting: Practical SPC solutions for today's manufacturing environment.* Milwaukee, WI: ASQ Press.

Zimmerman S., and Icenogle M. (1999). *Statistical quality control using Excel.* Milwaukee, WI: ASQ Press.

Appendix 5.A

Tables of Statistical Factors

Table 5A.1 Factors for Computing 3s Control Limits: $\overline{X}$ and R Charts

n	A_2	D_3	D_4	d_2
1	2.660	0	3.267	1.128
2	1.880	0	3.267	1.128
3	1.023	0	2.574	1.693
4	0.729	0	2.282	2.059
5	0.577	0	2.114	2.326
6	0.483	0	2.004	2.534
7	0.419	0.076	1.924	2.704
8	0.373	0.136	1.864	2.847
9	0.337	0.184	1.816	2.970
10	0.308	0.223	1.777	3.078
11	0.285	0.256	1.744	3.173
12	0.266	0.283	1.717	3.258

n = subgroup size.

Chapter 6

Advanced Statistical Process Control

DOUGLAS C. FAIR

◆ Introduction

Although traditional control charts can uncover a wealth of information, specialized applications of control charts have been developed for specific situations. Control charts provide decision support for determining the nature of a quality problem in a process, but they also serve a monitoring function to determine the effect of interventions to improve quality. In the quality improvement cycle discussed in previous chapters, performance measures provide the link between preintervention process management and the results from a quality improvement project. Selecting the appropriate control chart is key to ensuring that interpretation of the effect of an intervention is correct. This chapter presents a number of other types of control charts as presented in the selection diagram introduced in Chapter 5 and reprinted as Figure 6.1.

◆ Using the Control Chart Selection Diagram

The nodes on the decision tree rely on three specific questions.

1. Are multiple characteristics to be plotted at the same time on the same chart?
2. What is the subgroup size?
3. Do characteristics have unique target values?

These issues were discussed in Chapter 5 and will not be repeated here, but by answering these three questions, the appropriate control chart for a given situation can be determined. For example, if the data set being analyzed has multiple characteristics, 10 samples per subgroup, and no unique target values, then the appropriate tool is the group $\overline{X}$ and s-chart. The remainder of this chapter will be devoted to discussing each of these different charts.

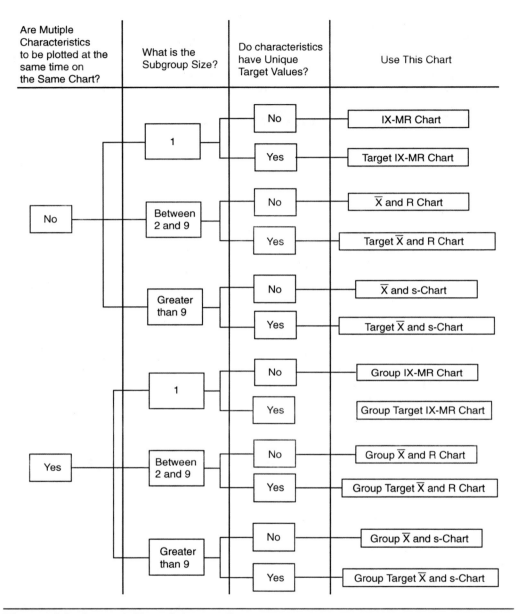

Figure 6.1 Control Chart Selection Diagram

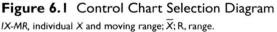

IX-MR, individual *X* and moving range; $\overline{X}$; R, range.

Target Charts

Target charts are best applied when (1) the practitioner wants to place several similar but different characteristics on the same chart, and (2) the characteristics have unique target values. For example, say a physician is treating three different groups of patients for the same ailment, asthma. Depending on the age of the patient, the doctor prescribes different treatment regimens. The performance measurement of interest is peak expiratory flow (PEF), but the target PEF is unique based on patient age.

PATIENT GROUP	TARGET PEF
1 (Ages 4–7)	250
2 (Ages 8–10)	300
3 (Ages 11–13)	350

Separate traditional control charts would be needed to evaluate PEF performance for each patient group because the charts would have unique scales and because the target values are different. However, the scale of the data can be normalized for all patient groups. Normalization is performed by subtracting from the measurements their unique target values. The target value becomes the zero point, and the resulting normalized data takes on the form of either a negative or a positive number. If the actual measurement is the same as the target, the result is zero. Table 6.1 shows how the deviation from target normalization is performed for the PEF example.

By performing this simple normalization, the data now share the same scale and can be placed on the same chart. Coding of data in this manner allows the analysis and comparison of different treatments, medications, or patients on the same chart.

In addition to the plot points on the chart, target charts also display a zero line representing the different target values. Additionally, vertical lines separate the different characteristics of interest on the chart (the different patient groups and their performance relative to their PEF targets), as shown in Figure 6.2. The advantage of having all three categories on the same chart should be apparent: Patterns in the process can be readily

Table 6.1 Target Normalization for PEF Example

PATIENT GROUP	TARGET PEF	ACTUAL PEF	DATA NORMALIZATION (ACTUAL PEF—TARGET PEF)
1	250	264	14
1	250	244	−6
2	300	305	5
2	300	299	−1
3	350	341	−9
3	350	338	−12
3	350	358	8

PEF, peak expiratory flow.

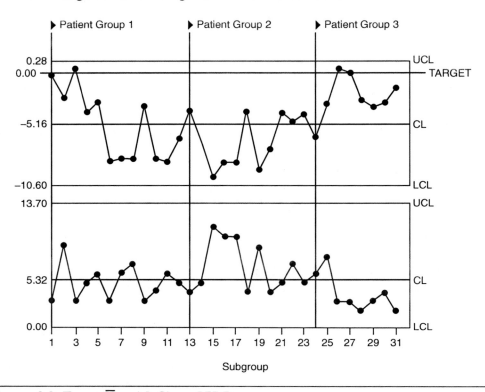

Figure 6.2 Target $\overline{X}$ and R Chart: PEF Data

Three different patient groups with different target values are shown. PEF, peak expiratory flow; *UCL*, upper control limit; *LCL*, lower control limit.

detected, and if any particular problems are associated with one of the categories, the pattern should be discerned easily. Thus, when one area of the control chart is out of control, the pattern should indicate whether the problem has occurred because of a particular category or because of the operation of the process as a whole.

Target values can be determined in several different ways:

◆ by specification by a regulatory agency or accreditation organization (as in Chapter 11, "Legal and Regulatory Issues in Quality Improvement")
◆ defined by a company executive
◆ defined as expected performance
◆ defined by a customer

One important note: the correct use of a target control chart requires that the different characteristics have the same variability. If the variability is significantly different from one characteristic to the next, then the control limits will be calculated incorrectly. Therefore, characteristics with dissimilar variability should not be placed on a target control chart.

Target Individual X and Moving Range Chart

CRITERION	VALUE
Multiple characteristics to be plotted at the same time?	No
Subgroup size	I
Unique target values for characteristics?	Yes

Target individual X and moving range (IX-MR) charts are, like all variables data control charts, used for evaluating the consistency of variables (measurement) data. The target IX chart is similar to a regular IX-MR chart, with one exception: the plot points on the IX chart are not the individual data values. Instead, the plot points are the difference between an individual data point and its target; so, when a measurement is taken, its target value is subtracted from the actual individual measurement, resulting in the raw difference between the measurement and its target. In other words, the individual data values are "coded" on the target IX chart. There is no subgrouping or calculation of statistics for the target IX chart because each dot on the control chart represents the deviation from its target. The main purpose of the target IX chart is to indicate central tendency (as a deviation from target) for the data set.

As discussed in Chapter 5, the MR chart reflects the variability component of the individual data points. As with every variables data control chart, consistency of central tendency as well as dispersion needs to be evaluated in order to get a true picture of process performance. The MR chart allows for the analysis and evaluation of the consistency of a data set's variability. With target IX-MR charts, the mathematical coding is performed only on the IX values, not the MR values.

Coding data as deviation from target allows similar characteristics to be placed on the same chart, thereby minimizing the number of charts to manage. Typically, hospitals and other health care institutions have many different performance measures to track. With a regular IX-MR control chart, only one characteristic can be evaluated on a single chart. Systems that need to track multiple characteristics would need to use multiple IX-MR charts. The target IX-MR chart eliminates the need for multiple charts by plotting the coded IX values, thus eliminating the differences between means of different characteristics.

Formulas for target IX-MR charts can be found in Exhibit 6-1. Target values can be selected in a number of different ways, as noted previously. The constants A_2, D_3, and D_4 which are used for calculating control limits, are

Exhibit 6-1	Target *IX-MR* Chart Formulas	
	Moving Range	**Individual X**
Plot Point	MR = absolute difference between 2 successive IX values	Coded $IX = IX - $ Target
Average (centerline)	$\overline{MR} = \dfrac{\sum MR}{k-1}$	$Coded\overline{IX} = \dfrac{\sum(IX - Target)}{k}$
UCL	$UCL_{MR} = D_4\,\overline{MR}$	$UCL_{IX} = Coded\overline{IX} + A_2\,\overline{MR}$
LCL	$LCL_{MR} = D_3\,\overline{MR}$	$LCL_{IX} = Coded\overline{IX} - A_2\,\overline{MR}$

k, Number of subgroups used to calculate control limits. MR, moving range.

found in Appendix 5A in Chapter 5. The primary applications of target *IX-MR* charts include

◆ evaluating the consistency of time-ordered variables (measurements) data
◆ tracking the consistency of similar characteristics with different targets on the same chart
◆ reducing the number of charts needed to manage for tracking important measures
◆ tracking the consistency of data that occurs infrequently (such as monthly sales, financial, occupancy, or other infrequently occurring data)
◆ graphing performance measure data as it is collected

The data set used for producing an *IX-MR* chart must meet several requirements for the chart to be valid, including

◆ subgroup size (n) of one
◆ measurements are normally distributed
◆ measurements are independent of one another
◆ similar characteristics are to be placed on the same chart
◆ the unit type from one characteristic to the other is the same

Target *IX-MR* charts are quite useful in producing simple-appearing but comprehensive reports on multiple characteristics and performance measures. The following example illustrates a clinical application of this technique.

Example 6-1

St. Anywhere Hospital is interested in refining the analysis performed in Example 5-5 (see Chapter 5). In that example, an *IX-MR* control chart was generated to better understand how long patients were staying in the hospital after a myocardial infarction. The average length of stay (ALOS) was computed monthly for all patients with a primary diagnosis of myocardial infarction, and an *IX-MR* control chart was created from the data.

Because administrators learned so much from the first study on ALOS after myocardial infarction, they were eager to expand the scope of the evaluation to examine ALOS by service for all other services. Since the end of the last study, data have been gathered to determine the ALOS for all other services (besides treatment of myocardial infarction) provided by the hospital. However, ALOS data have only been gathered for the last 10 months for all other services. Because of this, administrators want to put myocardial infarction ALOS data on the same chart with the "all other services ALOS."

The target ALOS for myocardial infarction is 13 days, and the target for ALOS for all other services is 7 days. The ALOS and targets for myocardial infarction and for all other services can be found in Table 6.2. There has been no case-mix adjustment performed on the data.

Using the data in Table 6.2, and applying the formulas found in Exhibit 6-1, the control limits and centerlines for the *MR* chart portion of the target *IX-MR* control chart are calculated as follows

$$\overline{MR} = \frac{\sum MR}{k-1} = \frac{29}{21} = 1.38$$

$$UCL_{MR} = D_4 \overline{MR} = 3.267(1.38) = 4.51$$

$$LCL_{MR} = D_3 \overline{MR} = 0(1.38) = 0$$

Control limits for the target *IX* chart are as follows

$$Coded\overline{IX} = \frac{\sum IX}{k} = \frac{12.0}{22} = 0.55$$

$$UCL_{IX} = Coded\overline{IX} + A_2 \overline{MR} = 0.55 + 2.660(1.38) = 4.22$$

$$LCL_{IX} = Coded\overline{IX} - A_2 \overline{MR} = 0.55 - 2.660(1.38) = -3.12$$

The deviation from target and *MR* values from Table 6.2 have been plotted together with the centerlines and control limits to form the target *IX-MR* control chart shown in Figure 6.3.

Table 6.2 St. Anywhere ALOS

SUBGROUP	ALOS-MYOCARDIAL INFARCTION	TARGET	DEVIATION FROM TARGET	MOVING RANGES
1	11.2	13	−1.8	—
2	14.8	13	1.8	3.6
3	11.6	13	−1.4	3.2
4	13.1	13	0.1	1.5
5	11.6	13	−1.4	1.5
6	14.8	13	1.8	3.2
7	10.9	13	−2.1	3.9
8	11.6	13	−1.4	0.7
9	12.4	13	−0.6	0.8
	ALOS-ALL OTHER SERVICES			
10	9.1	7	2.1	2.7
11	9.5	7	2.5	0.4
12	7.0	7	0.0	2.5
13	7.3	7	0.3	0.3
14	7.4	7	0.4	0.1
15	8.6	7	1.6	1.2
16	8.2	7	1.2	0.4
17	8.6	7	1.6	0.4
18	8.1	7	1.1	0.5
19	7.8	7	0.8	0.3
20	8.4	7	1.4	0.6
21	8.4	7	1.4	0.0
22	9.6	7	2.6	1.2

Data are for myocardial infarction and all other services. ALOS, average length of stay.

Upon examining the control charts, the administrators noted some useful patterns. Because of the long run below the centerline on the *MR* chart, the variation in ALOS data is unpredictable and out of control according to the runs analysis for control charts. *Subgroups 13 through 22* all have *MR* values below the centerline, indicating either a significant reduction in variation over the time period being evaluated or a significant difference in ALOS variability in myocardial infarction stays vs ALOS for all other services. Assuming that the variation is different between the two different characteristics,

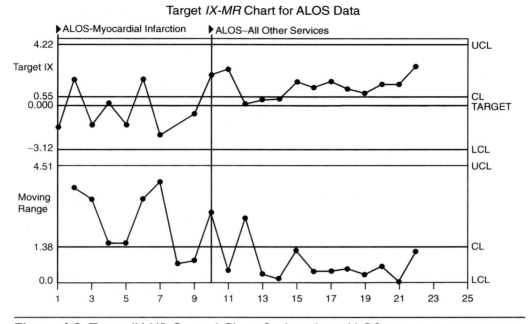

Figure 6.3 Target *IX-MR* Control Chart: St. Anywhere ALOS

the variability of the ALOS for all other services is more consistent and less variable than the ALOS data associated with myocardial infarction visits. In fact, of all the "all other services" ALOS *MR* values, only two fall above the centerline.

Target chart users must realize that, as with any control chart, when the variability chart—in this case an *MR* chart—is out of control, the control limits on the target *IX* chart are not valid because the $\overline{MR}$ value on the *MR* chart is used in the calculation of control limits on the *IX* chart. Because the *MR* chart shows a lack of control, $\overline{MR}$ is not a reliable predictor of variability. Likewise, because $\overline{MR}$ is unreliable for estimating variability, it is also unreliable for accurately calculating the control limits on the target *IX* chart. Therefore, any discussion of special causes on the target *IX* chart should be relegated only to the analysis of how the data points compare to the centerline and to the target.

A great deal of information can be gained from this target *IX* chart. First, there is a shift above the centerline between *subgroups 15* through *22*, indicating that the overall average ALOS has shifted significantly above the average. Specifically, this shift occurs only with the ALOS for all-other-services data. In fact, when looking at the whole chart, the myocardial infarction ALOS data seem to vary randomly about the centerline, but the ALOS for all other services falls above the centerline for all but two of its subgroups. Also, there may possibly be a slight upward trend in the data starting with *subgroup 8* and continuing through *subgroup 22*.

The centerline of 0.55 signifies that, taking into consideration all data on the chart, the data points exceed the target value by an average of 0.55 days for both characteristics. In addition, all of the ALOS all-other-services data fall above target value, which, together with the possible trend upward in overall ALOSs, could indicate a steadily increasing ALOS regardless of the reason for the stay.

As with all target charts, target *IX-MR* charts should be evaluated for several types of patterns:

◆ differences and/or similarities in the variation between characteristics
◆ differences and/or similarities between characteristic averages
◆ shifts, runs, trends, or patterns above and/or below the centerlines
◆ how the individual differences compare to the target values for each separate characteristic
◆ collectively, how the differences across characteristics compare to the overall target line
◆ how the centerline compares to the target line

The target *IX-MR* control chart allows evaluation of more than one characteristic on a single chart because the data are normalized to target values. Not only does the target *IX-MR* control chart allow users to minimize the number of control charts to manage, but it also offers the ability to compare different characteristics and different target values all on the same chart. Additionally, because data are not subgrouped, only one data point is needed before placing a deviation from target value on the chart. Simplicity, power, and ease of use and interpretation make the target *IX-MR* chart a favorite for those with multiple characteristics to evaluate.

In summary, the target *IX-MR* chart is best used in situations

◆ when multiple characteristics must appear on the same chart
◆ to minimize the number of control charts to manage
◆ where data collection opportunities are infrequent
◆ when another point is plotted on the chart after each data collection
◆ when subgrouping of data is either not possible or not economically feasible

The power of the target *IX-MR* chart lies in its ability to separate special cause variation from common cause variation while allowing multiple characteristics to be compared to their target values.

Target $\overline{X}$ and Range Chart

CRITERION	VALUE
Multiple characteristics to be plotted at the same time?	No
Subgroup size	2–9
Unique target values for characteristics?	Yes

Target $\overline{X}$ and range (R) charts are used for evaluating the consistency of variables (measurements) data. Plot points for the target $\overline{X}$ chart are not the subgroup averages like traditional $\overline{X}$ and R charts. Instead, plot points on the target $\overline{X}$ chart are the difference between the average and the unique target value for the characteristic being studied. In this way, the plot points on target $\overline{X}$ charts are very similar to the target IX chart, but the difference is that the target $\overline{X}$ chart uses subgroup sizes of between two and nine, whereas the target IX chart relies on a subgroup size of one. Because the plot points are coded (the difference between the average and its target is plotted, not the actual average), multiple similar characteristics can be displayed on the same target $\overline{X}$ chart. The main purpose of the target $\overline{X}$ chart is to indicate central tendency (as a deviation from target) for the data set.

The R chart, unlike the target $\overline{X}$ chart, specifies no coding or normalization of data. In fact, the construction of the R chart used with the target $\overline{X}$ and R combination is identical to the one discussed in Chapter 5 (traditional $\overline{X}$ and R charts). The R chart reflects the variability component of the subgrouped data points. As with every variables data control chart, consistency of central tendency as well as dispersion needs to be evaluated in order to get a true picture of process performance. The R chart allows for the analysis and evaluation of the consistency of a data set's variability.

By subtracting a target from a subgroup's average, the data are transformed into either plus or minus values around zero (the target). Because all of the values are pluses or minuses, they have the same scale and unit value. Because they are scaled similarly, the characteristics can be compared to each other and can be placed on the same chart. Coding data as deviation from target, therefore, allows similar characteristics to be placed on the same chart, thereby minimizing the number of charts to manage. Reasons for coding data are discussed in more detail in the previous section on target IX-MR charts, but the main reason for performing the transformation for a target chart is to allow multiple characteristics to be tracked on the same chart.

Target $\overline{X}$ and R charts are used in a number of quality improvement applications:

◆   to evaluate the consistency of time-ordered variables (measurement) data

◆ to track the consistency of similar characteristics with different targets on the same chart
◆ to track the consistency of data that occurs frequently enough to allow subgrouping

As with any control chart, the fundamental analysis is based on a few assumptions, primarily to ensure statistical validity.

◆ The subgroup size is between two and nine measurements.
◆ Measurements are normally distributed.
◆ Measurements are independent of one another.
◆ Several characteristics are to be placed on the same chart.
◆ The unit type (dollars, PSI, ALOS, etc.) is the same for all characteristics to be placed on the chart.

Formulas for calculating $\overline{X}$ and R control limits and centerlines are included as Exhibit 6-2. The following example illustrates the use of the target $\overline{X}$ and R chart.

Example 6-2

The office manager at XYZ Clinic (an 11-physician practice) was concerned with cash flow and decided to build on previous work with control charts of weekly receivables (Chapter 5, Example 5-6). Weekly receivables (WR) is defined by the formula

WR = total receivables/weekly sales

Exhibit 6-2 Target $\overline{X}$ and R Chart Formulas

	Range	**Target $\overline{X}$**
Plot Point	R = absolute difference between largest and smallest subgroup value	$Coded\,\overline{X} = (\overline{X} - Target)$
Average (centerline)	$\overline{R} = \dfrac{\sum R}{n}$	$Coded\,\overline{\overline{X}} = \dfrac{\sum(\overline{X} - Target)}{k}$
UCL	$UCL_R = D_4\overline{R}$	$UCL_{\overline{x}} = Coded\,\overline{\overline{X}} + A_2\overline{R}$
LCL	$LCL_R = D_3\overline{R}$	$LCL_{\overline{x}} = Coded\,\overline{\overline{X}} - A_2\overline{R}$

n, Subgroup size; k, number of subgroups over which control limits will be calculated.

and measures the time necessary to collect money owed to the practice for services rendered. The office manager calculated the WR each week or four times per month (n = 4). Then, from the four values taken each month, the subgroup average and range were plotted on an $\overline{X}$ and R chart.

The office manager told many of her colleagues about these analyses and she has attracted the attention of several other office managers who wish to learn what she is doing. Two such managers (one from ABC Clinic and one from DEF Clinic) have called and asked to have their WR data analyzed in the same manner as XYZ. XYZ's office manager has agreed to help with their analyses, but the office managers of each of the other two clinics could only come up with 10 months' worth of data. ABC Clinic had calculated WR from only the first 10 months of last year before giving up. However, DEF Clinic has just recently begun gathering their WR data and currently has 10 months' worth of information. The DEF manager thought this was good for two reasons.

First, to calculate reasonable control limits, between 15 and 25 plot points are needed before control limits can be calculated. Ten months' worth of data is just not enough to calculate fair and representative control limits, but 20 should be. Second, the data on a control chart need to be time ordered. Because the data from ABC Clinic refer to a different time period than those of the DEF Clinic, the two data sets are, in effect, time ordered and can be placed on the same chart.

However, ABC Clinic does a large amount of charitable work, and they also provide services to patients who cannot afford to pay quickly. Therefore, ABC Clinic asks patients to make payment within 10 months. DEF Clinic, however, asks its patients to make payments within 1 month. To analyze data from both clinics on a single chart, the data must be normalized to their respective targets. Therefore, the target $\overline{X}$ and R chart was selected for the analysis. The data that were available for analysis are presented in Table 6.3.

Using the data in Table 6.3 and applying the formulas found in Exhibit 6-2, the control limits and centerlines for the target $\overline{X}$ and R control chart were calculated as follows

$$\overline{R} = \frac{\sum R}{k} = \frac{169.0}{20} = 8.45$$

$$UCL_R = D_4\overline{R} = 2.282(8.45) = 19.28$$

$$LCL_R = D_3\overline{R} = 0(8.45) = 0$$

Calculations for the target $\overline{X}$ chart

$$Coded\,\overline{\overline{X}} = \frac{\sum(\overline{X} - Target)}{k} = \frac{79.4}{20} = 3.97$$

$$UCL_X = Coded\,\overline{\overline{X}} + A_2\overline{R} = 3.97 + 0.729(8.45) = 10.13$$

$$LCL_X = Coded\,\overline{\overline{X}} - A_2\overline{R} = 3.97 - 0.729(8.45) = -2.19$$

Table 6.3 WR Data: ABC and DEF Clinics

								$\overline{X}-$
ABC Clinic								
Month	**Week 1**	**Week 2**	**Week 3**	**Week 4**	**Range**	$\overline{X}$	**Target**	**Target**
1	11.9	6.9	10.9	11.7	5.0	10.35	4	6.35
2	7.2	4.8	7.2	7.1	2.4	6.58	4	2.58
3	15.8	15.4	10.5	3.7	12.1	11.35	4	7.35
4	7.2	6.7	10.3	10.8	4.1	8.75	4	4.75
5	3.4	4.7	7.2	6.4	3.8	5.43	4	1.43
6	12.0	10.7	11.9	1.5	10.5	9.03	4	5.03
7	8.0	6.0	9.7	0.5	9.2	6.05	4	2.05
8	6.3	5.8	14.6	6.8	8.8	8.38	4	4.38
9	10.5	3.6	4.8	8.2	6.9	6.78	4	2.78
10	4.9	7.7	9.8	14.1	9.2	9.13	4	5.13
DEF Clinic								
Month	**Week 1**	**Week 2**	**Week 3**	**Week 4**	**Range**	$\overline{X}$	**Target**	**Target**
11	44.3	38.1	41.1	52	13.9	43.88	40	3.88
12	43.3	53.2	42.7	39.8	13.4	44.75	40	4.75
13	41.5	39.0	44.4	44.2	5.4	42.28	40	2.28
14	46.5	52.3	47.3	40.7	11.6	46.70	40	6.70
15	41.2	44.7	37.3	45	7.7	42.05	40	2.05
16	45.8	41.8	46.2	43.4	4.4	44.30	40	4.30
17	52.2	48.4	35.2	49.4	17.0	46.30	40	6.30
18	42.7	43.1	42.7	44.4	1.7	43.23	40	3.23
19	40.3	44.6	37.4	42.8	7.2	41.28	40	1.28
20	34.3	49.5	47.2	40.4	15.2	42.85	40	2.85

WR, weekly receivables.

The deviation from target and range values from Table 6.3 have been plotted together with the centerlines and control limits to form the target $\overline{X}$ and R control chart found in Figure 6.4.

As always, the range chart must be evaluated first for any sign of a special cause. In this case, there appear to be no indications of special causes. There are no trends, runs, patterns, or points that fall above the upper control limit (*UCL*), indicating that the variability is not significantly different between WR in clinics ABC and DEF. Although the WR numbers do vary at each clinic, there is no indication that one clinic's WR vary significantly more than the other.

The average range value indicates that the variation between WR for any month varies, on average, by 8.45 weeks. The *UCL* on the range chart is a predictor that implies that, for any billing period, the difference between the largest and smallest WR value could be as large as 19.28 weeks. The lower control limit (*LCL*) of 0.0 signifies that there could be no difference between the WR values, i.e., a range of zero. Overall, the variability is consistent from month to month and between ABC Clinic and DEF Clinic.

Because the range chart is consistent, the target $\overline{X}$ chart control limits are reliable predictors of how much the deviation from target

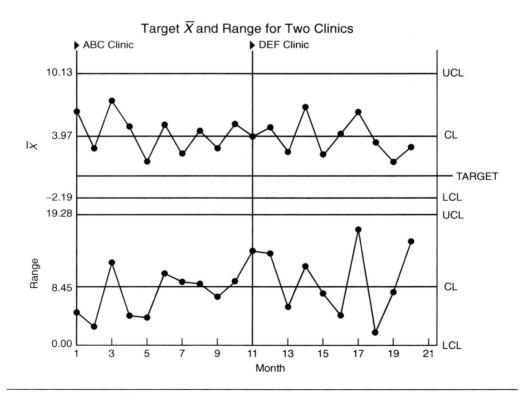

Figure 6.4 Target $\overline{X}$ and R Chart: WR Data

WR, weekly receivables.

values may vary from subgroup to subgroup. The *UCL* on the target chart predicts that there could normally be a WR average that is as much as 10.13 weeks higher than the target, whereas the *LCL* indicates that the average WR for a month could be 2.19 weeks less than the target value. Note that every single average on the target chart fell above the target line, indicating that every single WR average is received later than expected. Because there are no indications of special causes on the target $\overline{X}$ chart, the WR can be expected to consistently vary between 10.13 weeks higher than target, or by as little as 2.19 weeks less than target, regardless of which of the two clinics is being evaluated.

The overall average of 3.97 indicates that over the 20-month period involving both clinics, the WR were, on average, almost 4 weeks longer than the target. Thus, although the clinics each had their own specific payment schedule, patients still took an average of a month longer than required to make full payment, regardless of the clinic. This observation is interesting, because each clinic serves a unique niche in the health care services industry, yet similar results were achieved with a charitable organization and a regular walk-in clinic.

The target $\overline{X}$ and R control chart allows evaluation of the consistency of multiple characteristics on a single chart. By normalizing the data, coded values with a similar scale can be plotted and compared on the same chart with the same vertical axis. Because multiple characteristics can be placed on the same chart, the number of control charts that a team must manage can be minimized.

The target $\overline{X}$ and R chart is best used for

◆ placing similar characteristics on the same control chart
◆ large data sets, for which collection opportunities are plentiful
◆ analyzing subgrouped data when such analysis is preferred and economically feasible
◆ measures for which different characteristics share the same units

Target $\overline{X}$ and R charts are used when sample size is fixed between two and nine. In situations when sample size exceeds nine, the sample standard deviation can be used as a more appropriate measure of variation, as detailed in the next section.

Target $\overline{X}$ and s-Chart

CRITERION	VALUE
Multiple characteristics to be plotted at the same time?	No
Subgroup size	>9
Unique target values for characteristics?	Yes

Target $\overline{X}$ and s-charts are used for evaluating the consistency of variables (measurements) data. Plot points for the target $\overline{X}$ chart are not the subgroup averages like traditional $\overline{X}$ and s-charts or $\overline{X}$ and range charts. Instead, plot points are the difference between the average and the unique target value for the characteristic being studied. These plot points are called "coded" $\overline{X}$ values. The coded $\overline{X}$ plot points on target $\overline{X}$ and s-charts are calculated in identical fashion to the plot points on target $\overline{X}$ and R charts. Target $\overline{X}$ and s-charts are very similar to target $\overline{X}$ and R charts, except for the use of the subgroup standard deviation as the measure of variation. The s-statistic is a better measure of variability than the range when subgroup size (n) is greater than nine.

By subtracting a target from a subgroup's average, the data are transformed into either plus or minus values around zero (the target), i.e., coded. Because all of the values are pluses or minuses, they have the same scale and unit value. Being scaled similarly, data with dissimilar target values can be compared with each other and, given the same scale, can be placed on the same chart. Coding data as deviation from target allows similar characteristics to be placed on the same chart, thereby minimizing the number of charts to manage. Because the plot points are coded (the difference between the average and its target is plotted, not the actual average), similar characteristics can be displayed on the same target $\overline{X}$ chart.

The main purpose of the target $\overline{X}$ chart is to evaluate central tendency (as a deviation from target) for the data set. The s-chart, unlike the target $\overline{X}$ chart, requires no coding of data. In fact, the construction of the s-chart used with the target $\overline{X}$ and s combination is identical to the one discussed in Chapter 5 (traditional $\overline{X}$ and s-charts). The s-chart reflects the variability component of the subgrouped data points in the form of the subgroup standard deviation (s). As with every variables data control chart, consistency of central tendency, as well as dispersion, must be evaluated in order to understand process consistency. The s-chart allows for analysis of the consistency of a data set's variability over time.

Target $\overline{X}$ and s-charts are used in a number of circumstances; including

◆ to track the consistency of similar characteristics with different targets on the same chart
◆ to minimize the number of charts needed to manage important measures
◆ to track the consistency of variables data when a great deal of data can be economically collected and many opportunities exist for data collection
◆ to plot subgroup statistics (an average deviation from target and a standard deviation value) on the control chart each time a new subgroup of data has been gathered

As with other types of control charts, certain conditions must be met for proper application of target $\overline{X}$ and s-charts.

◆ The subgroup size is fixed.

◆ The subgroup size is 10 or more.
◆ Measurements within each subgroup are normally distributed.
◆ Individual measurements within a subgroup are independent of one another.
◆ The unit type (dollars, PSI, ALOS, etc.) is the same for all characteristics to be placed on the chart.

If these conditions are not satisfied, then the control limits or the measurements of dispersion may not be reliable, leading to erroneous interpretations of the charts. Formulas for target $\overline{X}$ and s-charts are found in Exhibit 6-3. The control chart constants in Exhibit 6-3 are based on subgroup size (n) and can be found in Appendix 5A. The following example illustrates the use of the target $\overline{X}$ and s approach.

Example 6-3

In Example 5-9, St. Everywhere Hospital tracked airflow rates in the obstetrics wing of the hospital. The information gained from the analysis was so helpful that the administration wants to expand the analysis to include the infectious disease wing as well. Because of its design, the infectious disease wing requires much higher airflow than the obstetrics ward.

Airflow in the two wings is controlled by two very different air transportation and filtering systems. The target airflow rate for obstetrics is 37 cf/min, whereas the infectious disease wing's target is 78 cf/min. Given the recent interest in evaluating the airflow systems for possible replacement, the administration has asked for an assessment of and comparison between the obstetrics and infectious

Exhibit 6-3 Target $\overline{X}$ and s-Chart Formulas

	s	Target $\overline{X}$
Plot Point	$s = \sqrt{\dfrac{\sum\left(x_i - \overline{X}\right)^2}{n-1}}$	$Coded\,\overline{X} = \left(\overline{X} - Target\right)$
Average (centerline)	$\overline{s} = \dfrac{\sum s}{k}$	$Coded\,\overline{\overline{X}} = \dfrac{\sum\left(\overline{X} - Target\right)}{k}$
UCL	$UCL_s = B_4\overline{s}$	$UCL_{\overline{X}} = Coded\,\overline{\overline{X}} + A_3\overline{s}$
LCL	$LCL_s = B_3\overline{s}$	$LCL_{\overline{X}} = Coded\,\overline{\overline{X}} - A_3\overline{s}$

n, Subgroup size; k, number of subgroups over which control limits will be calculated.

disease airflow systems. For the last 10 days, the infectious disease wing has acquired 10 random samples of airflow measurements each day. Only 10 subgroups of data have been acquired from the infectious disease wing, presenting a bit of a challenge because between 15 and 25 subgroups are needed to calculate representative control limits. Therefore, the last 10 obstetrics wing subgroups will be combined on the chart with the most recent 10 subgroups from the infectious disease wing, providing an opportunity to compare the two wings on the same chart and also provide 20 subgroups for control limit calculations. Because the subgroup size is so large and the wings have different airflow target values, the target $\overline{X}$ and s-chart will be used. The data from the airflow samples are included in Table 6.4.

Using the data in Table 6.4 and applying the formulas found in Exhibit 6-3, control limits and centerlines are calculated for the s-chart portion of the target $\overline{X}$ and s-chart as follows

$$\overline{s} = \frac{\sum s}{k} = \frac{73.7302}{20} = 3.68651$$

$$UCL_s = B_4\overline{s} = 1.716(3.68651) = 6.32605$$

$$LCL_s = B_3\overline{s} = 0.284(3.68651) = 1.04700$$

and control limits for the target $\overline{X}$ chart are calculated as follows

$$Coded\overline{\overline{X}} = \frac{\sum(\overline{X} - Target)}{k} = \frac{-3.31}{20} = -0.17$$

$$UCL_X = Coded\overline{\overline{X}} + A_3\overline{s} = -0.17 + 0.975(3.68651) = 3.42$$

$$LCL_X = Coded\overline{\overline{X}} - A_3\overline{s} = -0.17 - 0.975(3.68651) = -3.76$$

The deviation from target and s-values from Table 6.4 have been plotted together with these centerlines and control limits to create the target $\overline{X}$ and s-chart found in Figure 6.5.

The s-chart shows no trends, runs, patterns, or points that fall outside control limits, indicating that the variability in airflow, as described by the standard deviation (s) is similar between the obstetrics wing and the infectious diseases wing. There seems to be no significant difference in the variability of the airflow. The centerline means that the overall average standard deviation across both

Table 6.4 Airflow Sampling St. Everywhere Hospital

SUBGROUP	OBSTETRICS UNIT				
	1	2	3	4	5
	24.3	35.2	29.2	33.8	30.9
	33.5	36.4	36.6	30.2	35.8
	34.2	40.8	31.5	30.6	31.8
	37.2	31.8	36.3	34.4	35.8
	39.9	33.4	36.1	25.2	36.4
	32.1	26.8	26.2	33.7	28.8
	33.9	33.5	29.1	32.3	34.5
	32.1	28.9	31.0	38.4	30.0
	32.8	30.8	32.0	35.1	36.9
	30.7	27.0	25.8	31.1	32.7
$\overline{X}$	33.07	32.46	31.38	32.48	33.36
Target	37	37	37	37	37
$\overline{X}$ -Target	−3.93	−4.54	−5.62	−4.52	−3.64
S	4.0871	4.3750	3.9749	3.5355	2.9056

SUBGROUP	OBSTETRICS UNIT				
	6	7	8	9	10
	31.4	31.0	34.7	35.0	30.4
	41.0	37.2	40.1	40.4	29.7
	33.1	36.2	34.2	42.0	27.9
	37.0	30.4	29.7	33.6	32.3
	37.9	26.2	37.6	40.6	34.5
	36.1	29.4	37.2	26.5	39.3
	32.3	39.8	33.4	37.4	34.4
	33.6	32.5	35.6	35.0	39.8
	39.5	35.7	37.6	36.2	34.4
	32.0	33.0	40.0	30.8	33.3
$\overline{X}$	35.39	33.14	36.01	35.75	33.60
Target	37	37	37	37	37
$\overline{X}$ -Target	−1.61	−3.86	−0.99	−1.25	−3.40
S	3.3857	4.1018	3.1782	4.7486	3.8404

Table 6.4 *continued*

SUBGROUP	INFECTIOUS DISEASE UNIT				
	11	12	13	14	15
	81.5	73.4	77.2	79.3	79.0
	88.4	81.8	77.2	78.8	79.1
	80.0	82.5	87.8	86.3	80.6
	78.1	83.5	84.1	79.7	86.4
	80.1	76.4	83.0	82.1	81.1
	80.0	81.5	84.0	81.0	76.1
	80.9	74.7	75.2	78.0	78.5
	82.0	80.1	80.7	85.9	87.2
	91.0	79.6	80.1	82.9	83.1
	85.4	82.7	87.7	77.0	74.3
$\overline{X}$	82.74	79.62	81.70	81.10	80.54
Target	78	78	78	78	78
$\overline{X}$ - Target	4.74	1.62	3.70	3.10	2.54
S	4.1677	3.5686	4.3749	3.1840	4.1207

SUBGROUP	INFECTIOUS DISEASE UNIT				
	16	17	18	19	20
	72.9	82.6	79.7	83.2	77.7
	83.6	85.2	80.1	81.0	81.0
	71.9	76.6	79.8	82.9	83.7
	78.9	83.3	81.1	81.9	86.8
	79.2	82.2	80.5	78.8	87.0
	84.5	79.0	77.0	76.8	84.8
	74.1	82.5	84.2	81.2	79.4
	79.7	80.4	85.4	81.0	82.4
	82.8	77.2	77.9	82.0	85.2
	87.4	76.0	81.3	77.8	81.9
$\overline{X}$	79.50	80.50	80.70	80.66	82.99
Target	78	78	78	78	78
$\overline{X}$ - Target	1.50	2.50	2.70	2.66	4.99
S	5.2290	3.1595	2.5517	2.1567	3.0845

Airflow sampling in the obstetrics and infectious disease units at St. Everywhere Hospital.

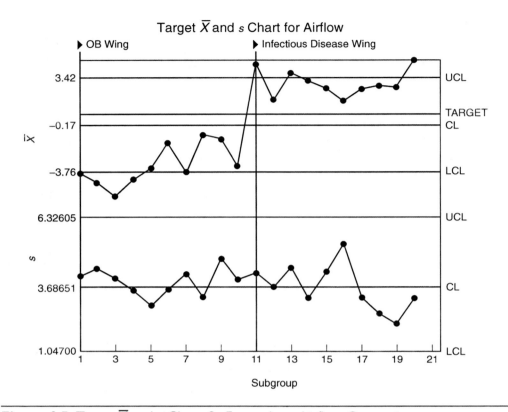

Figure 6.5 Target $\overline{X}$ and s-Chart: St. Everywhere Airflow Comparison

wings is 3.67 cf/min. A day's standard deviation (one subgroup) could normally be as high as 6.33 or as low as 1.05 (the values, respectively, of the UCL and LCL for the s-chart).

Because the s-chart is consistent, the target $\overline{X}$ chart control limits are reliable predictors of normal variation in the subgroup-to-subgroup deviation from target values. The UCL on the target $\overline{X}$ chart indicates that the average airflow could be as much as 3.42 cf/min higher than target. The LCL is a predictor that indicates airflow could normally be as much as 3.76 cf/min lower than the target. All of the first 10 subgroups fall below the centerline of the $\overline{X}$ chart, and all of the last 10 subgroups fall above the centerline. *Subgroups 11, 13,* and *20* fall above the UCL of the target $\overline{X}$ chart, and the first four subgroup values fall below the LCL.

The presence of so many special causes points to a process with an average deviation from target that is unpredictable. Specifically, airflow in the obstetrics unit is significantly lower than the overall average and target line while the infectious disease wing's airflow is significantly higher than both. Highlighted by this chart is the fact that the airflow in the obstetrics unit is much lower than its target requirement, further solidifying the administration's belief that the airflow system in obstetrics is not performing as expected and might possibly need replacement.

Comparatively, airflow in the infectious disease wing is much higher than its target. Maintenance has speculated that it may be because the system in the infectious disease wing has received more complete and thorough maintenance over the years, yielding a stronger, more capable system. Based on this data and other maintenance observations, hospital administration has postponed the acquisition of a new airflow system for the infectious disease wing.

The overall average deviation from target (−0.17) in Figure 6.5 is very close to the target of zero. To compare only these two numbers might lead to an incorrect assumption that the overall average is close to the target value. Of course, this conclusion is erroneous based on the visual display of the data on the target $\overline{X}$ chart. In fact, the reason why the centerline is so close to the target is that the airflow for the obstetrics unit is so much lower than target while the infectious disease wing's airflow is substantially higher.

As with all target charts, several attributes must be carefully examined:

◆ differences and similarities in the variation between characteristics
◆ differences and similarities between characteristic means
◆ shifts, runs, trends, or patterns above or below the centerlines
◆ comparison of individual differences to the target values for each separate characteristic
◆ collectively, how differences across characteristics compare to the overall target line
◆ comparison of the centerline to the target line

The presence of special causes can be determined using the rules for runs analysis of control charts and identification of special causes that were detailed in Chapter 5.

The target $\overline{X}$ and s-chart allows evaluation of the consistency of similar characteristics on a single chart. Target chart techniques create coded data by subtracting target values from subgroup averages. This mathematical calculation results in positive or negative values about a target. In other words, the data are coded to have a similar scale and can therefore be placed on the same chart with the same vertical axis.

The target $\overline{X}$ and s-chart is best used in the following situations:

◆ when similar characteristics are to be placed on the same chart
◆ to minimize the number of control charts to manage
◆ when data collection opportunities are plentiful, and gathering the data is economical and feasible

- ◆ when similar characteristics share the same units, e.g., airflow rates in separate hospital units
- ◆ when data can be subgrouped
- ◆ for larger data sets
- ◆ to achieve greater sensitivity (due to larger subgroup sizes) to process changes than can be achieved with an *IX-MR* or an $\overline{X}$ and R control chart
- ◆ when subgroup size can be fixed from one time period to the next

Like the target $\overline{X}$ and R chart, the target $\overline{X}$ and s-chart was developed to separate special cause variation from common cause variation, thereby allowing a context for problem solving and corrective action. The primary difference between target $\overline{X}$ and R charts and target $\overline{X}$ and s-charts is that the latter is best suited to situations with subgroup sizes of 10 and larger. As mentioned previously, the target $\overline{X}$ and s-chart, because of the large subgroup sizes typically used, results in much higher sensitivity to small changes in the overall process average compared with *IX-MR* charts or $\overline{X}$ and R charts. When a change in the process average could adversely affect important business measures or have dire consequences, greater sensitivity to process average changes is a significant benefit realized by target $\overline{X}$ and s-charts.

Group Charts

Group charts represent a method of plotting multiple characteristics at the same time on the same chart. Traditional and target control charts allow only one characteristic to be placed on each chart at the same time. For example, a subgroup of four ALOS data points might be collected each month at a hospital, with the statistics from that single characteristic plotted on a traditional control chart. One plot point represents the single characteristic (ALOS) placed on the chart for each subgroup. However, suppose that data concerning ALOS are gathered each month for a drug rehabilitation inpatient unit, an intensive care unit, an obstetrics unit, and a pediatric inpatient unit. Four separate traditional control charts would be required for these four groups of data because each of these units has significantly different utilization characteristics. As the number of characteristics increases, so does the number of charts and the necessary work to maintain and analyze the charts.

The target charts described in the previous section allow multiple characteristics to be placed on the same chart but only allow a single characteristic to be plotted at one point in time. Group charts, on the other hand, allow placement of different characteristics on the same chart at the same point in time. Thus, the ALOS data described above could be plotted on the same group chart, with data from each of the patient units representing a single group.

Often institutions try to achieve the same outcome with different methods. For example, different inpatient units may try different techniques for reducing drug administration errors, or different offices in an integrated delivery system may try different methods for improving patient satisfaction. These methods are typically compared against each other using appropriate performance measures to determine which approaches produce better outcomes. Understanding the performance of these different methods allows organizations to optimize allocation of resources to make operational improvements. A "group," then, includes dissimilar data sources that are logically combined together and compared over some specified period of time. Some examples of groups in health care applications could include

- ◆ distinct hospital units with varying patient types and load factors
- ◆ outpatient facilities with separate types of providers, e.g., pediatricians, family physicians, internists
- ◆ home health agencies specializing in different types of patient care, e.g., dialysis, ventilator, pediatric chronic care, and postoperative care
- ◆ several reference laboratories that specialize in particular procedures, e.g., chemistry profiles, hematologic profiles, Pap smears, or cytology exams

Instead of a single line on the graph to represent either averages or ranges (like traditional charts), group charts have two lines: one to highlight maximum group values (MAX) and another for group minimum values (MIN). The MIN line represents the smallest values within groups and the MAX line represents the largest. In order to distinguish among the different characteristics plotted on each MAX and MIN line, each plot point is tagged with a number. The number next to each plot point specifies from which characteristic the MIN or MAX value comes.

No other data except the MIN and MAX values for a group are plotted. This allows only the extreme values within a group to be visible. Even if 20 characteristics were specified for a single group, only two values will appear on the graph—the MAX and the MIN. By specifying groups with a large number of characteristics on a single group chart, important information between the MAX and MIN values could be obscured. Therefore, for group charts to be most effective, the number of dissimilar data sources within a group should preferably be no more than 10 characteristics. This will ensure that important information for one characteristic is not lost between the MIN and MAX lines.

Another characteristic of group charts is that they have centerlines like any other chart, but they do not have control limits. One assumption behind all control charts is that the data with which they are constructed are independent of each other. Usually group charts are employed to track very similar or related data. Often the way in which the data are gathered violates this fundamental assumption of independence. To minimize the impact of violating this assumption, no control limits are placed on group charts.

Group charts, like traditional control charts, are used to track the central tendency of a data set as well as its variability. Thus, group charts have both a central tendency chart (either an IX or $\overline{X}$ chart) and a variability chart (a *MR, R,* or *s*-chart). Each chart should be interpreted separately, but because group charts do not have control limits, different rules are used to identify indications of special cause, based on the following attributes:

◆ runs, as indicated by consecutive, repeating characteristics being displayed on either a MIN or MAX line
◆ patterns, as indicated by collective trends or cycles in the MAX or MIN lines
◆ parallel MAX and MIN plot point lines
◆ the width between MAX and MIN plot point lines either converging or diverging across groups

Group charts should not be used to compare or evaluate data that are unrelated. For example, grouping together hospital admission data with outpatient visit revenues just does not make sense; however, admission data from several different facilities, even with different target values, can be grouped for analysis using these charts. For group charts to be optimally effective, study characteristics should be closely related.

Example 6-4

A managed care organization sought to implement a care management program to improve the care of low back pain. The clinical practice guideline for back pain recommended one of three different outpatient therapies for the condition, but none was clearly proven to be superior to the others in relieving pain. A cohort of 15 patients with low back pain was divided into three groups of five patients each, and each group received one of the three outpatient therapies. Pain scores (on a scale from zero to 50) were recorded for each of the groups daily, with weekly averages maintained over a 6-month time period. Ranges and average scores were then calculated from these data, with results recorded for each treatment method in Table 6.5. MAX (bold) and MIN (bold, italic) values were indicated for the ranges and means for each month's data, leading to creation of the group charts in Figure 6.6. In this case, a group $\overline{X}$ and R chart was used to analyze the data. Each plot point is labeled with the treatment method employed, emphasizing the grouping strategy based on the treatment methods. The upper line on each chart represents the MAX values, while the lower line contains the MIN values. The centerlines on the $\overline{X}$ chart and R chart are obtained from the averages of all the ranges and the mean pain scores, not just MAX and MIN values.

First, the group R chart shows a centerline of 2.2, which is the overall average of all range values for the entire study period. The numbers next to each group on the MIN line (representing the treatment method) demonstrate that of the six groups, four show a *1* next to the

Table 6.5 Pain Scores for Back Pain Therapy Study

	GROUP 1			GROUP 2		
	METHOD 1	METHOD 2	METHOD 3	METHOD 1	METHOD 2	METHOD 3
	25.6	21.5	26.7	25	24.2	26.1
	26.2	21.9	26	25	23.3	24.7
	24.7	21.1	25.9	24.2	21.9	27.5
	24.3	22.9	27.2	26	21.9	27.9
Range	*1.9*	1.8	*1.3*	*1.8*	2.3	**3.2**
$\overline{X}$	25.2	*21.85*	**26.45**	25.05	*22.83*	**26.55**

	GROUP 3			GROUP 4		
	METHOD 1	METHOD 2	METHOD 3	METHOD 1	METHOD 2	METHOD 3
	24.7	22.9	27.1	25.5	22.2	27.4
	25.2	22.4	24.8	25.8	20.6	29.6
	24.7	22.5	25.8	25.3	22.7	28.8
	24.6	18.6	29.9	26	21.9	28.6
Range	*0.6*	4.3	**5.1**	*0.7*	2.1	**2.2**
$\overline{X}$	24.8	*21.6*	**26.9**	25.65	*21.85*	**28.6**

	GROUP 5			GROUP 6		
	METHOD 1	METHOD 2	METHOD 3	METHOD 1	METHOD 2	METHOD 3
	24.2	21.5	27.1	25.8	20.2	26.1
	24.4	23.5	26.5	25.8	23.9	28.9
	25	20.4	26.7	25.6	20.2	28.2
	24.7	20.5	26.9	25.1	20.9	29.1
Range	0.8	**3.1**	*0.6*	*0.7*	**3.7**	3
$\overline{X}$	24.58	*21.48*	**26.8**	25.58	*21.3*	**28.08**

Group $\overline{X}$ and Range for Low Back Pain Study

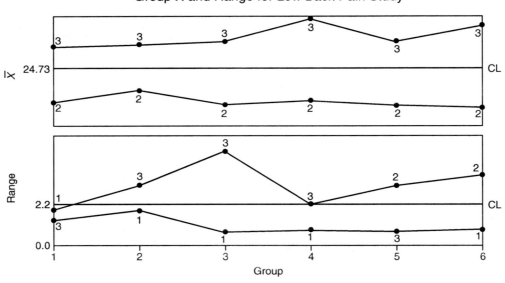

Figure 6.6 Group $\overline{X}$ and R Chart: Low Back Pain Study

plot point. Such a pattern may indicate that treatment *method 1* produces significantly less variation in pain scores than the other methods. The MAX line on the range chart, however, shows that all three treatment methods are approximately equally represented on the line. This indicates that none of the three pain therapies displayed significantly more variation than the others.

The overall average of the group $\overline{X}$ chart is 24.73, meaning that all three methods produced, on average, a pain score of 24.73. The MAX line displays averages from only *method 3*, and the MIN line shows only the number *2* next to all plot points. This chart, then, visually displays a consistent and sustained difference between the average pain scores obtained by the two methods, highlighting the finding that the pain scores produced by *method 3* were significantly higher, whereas *method 2* resulted in significantly lower pain scores. The pain score values for *method 1* fall between the MAX and the MIN lines and therefore are not displayed.

The gap between the MAX and MIN line on the $\overline{X}$ chart represents the largest average difference in pain scores for all three methods. If there were no significant difference in the scores produced between the three methods, the MAX and MIN lines would have converged together, and little (if any) space would exist between them. Also, if the MIN and MAX line numbers alternated between 1 and 3 with no discernible pattern, no method would be recognizably different from the others. In other words, alternating numbers signify the presence of only common cause, random variation between the methods—a signal of no significant difference in pain scores between the methods. In this case, *method 2* clearly produced consistently lower pain scores than the other two methods, and *method 3* returned consistently higher pain scores.

Group charts allow users to plot multiple characteristics at the same time on the same chart. When comparing multiple characteristics with each other, group charts can be used to track all of them on a single chart, thereby simplifying data collection and analysis efforts. The following sections will discuss the types of group charts in more detail.

Group IX-MR Chart

CRITERION	VALUE
Multiple characteristics to be plotted at the same time?	Yes
Subgroup size	1
Unique target values for characteristics?	No

Group *IX-MR* charts are used for evaluating multiple characteristics (sources of data) at the same time and on the same chart. The group *IX* chart is specifically used to track the individual measurements of logically related groups of characteristics through time. MAX and MIN lines are simultaneously displayed on the group *IX* chart. Each line represents the largest and smallest individual values, respectively, across the chart's groups. A number is typically placed next to each plot point to indicate the characteristic that the value represents. Like other *IX* charts, the group *IX* chart's subgroup size (n) is one, and its primary purpose is to indicate central tendency for the data set.

The group *IX* chart indicates central tendency, but the group MR chart reflects the variability component of the individual data points. Like the group *IX* chart, the group MR chart is displayed with two lines: a MAX and a MIN. The MAX line displays the largest values of MRs across the groups, and the MIN line shows the smallest. As with all variables data, central tendency and dispersion need to be evaluated in order to get a true picture of process performance. Knowledge of a data set's average is not sufficient—the underlying variability between the individual data points must also be understood. The group MR chart displays a data set's variability across multiple characteristics on the same chart at the same time.

Neither the group *IX* chart nor the group MR chart has control limits calculated; therefore, group charts are not referred to as control charts.

Group *IX-MR* charts are best employed to

◆ evaluate multiple characteristics on the same chart at the same time

- ◆ evaluate time-ordered variables (measurements) data
- ◆ track data that occurs infrequently (such as monthly sales, financial, occupancy, or other infrequently occurring data)
- ◆ track identical characteristics that occurred at the same time but were generated from different sources

Several assumptions must be satisfied to ensure that the group chart has valid information, including

- ◆ subgroup size of one
- ◆ measurements normally distributed
- ◆ measurements independent of one another
- ◆ identical unit of measure between characteristics

Formulas for group *IX-MR* charts are presented in Exhibit 6-4. An example of the use of the group *IX-MR* chart will illustrate the techniques for analysis and interpretation.

Example 6-5

St. Anywhere Hospital's ALOS study for myocardial infarction was so successful that a managed care organization decided to compare three other hospitals with St. Anywhere. The characteristics or "sources" of data to be grouped together for comparison are the different institutions and their respective ALOS data. The data have been gathered for the last 10 months and can be viewed in Table 6.6.

Exhibit 6-4 Group *IX-MR* Chart Formulas

	Group Moving Range	**Group Individual X**
Plot Point	MAX and MIN *MR* for a group where:	MAX and MIN individual value within a group
	MR = absolute difference between 2 successive *IX* values from the same characteristic	
Average (centerline)	$\overline{MR} = \dfrac{\sum MR}{(k-1)(\# characteristics)}$	$\overline{IX} = \dfrac{\sum IX}{k(\# characteristics)}$
UCL	None	None
LCL	None	None

k, Number of groups; characteristics, the number of sources of data being evaluated within a group.

Bold type highlights MAX values in the table, and values in bold italic represent MIN. To clearly display the differences and similarities among the four hospitals, the data have been placed on the group IX-MR chart shown in Figure 6.7.

Centerline calculations for the group MR chart

$$\overline{MR} = \frac{\sum MR}{(k-1)(\# characteristics)} =$$

$$\overline{MR} = \frac{68.5}{(10-1)(4)} =$$

$$\overline{MR} = \frac{68.5}{36} = 1.90$$

Table 6.6 ALOS for Myocardial Infarction Patients in Four Hospitals

		St. Anywhere	Hospital 2	Hospital 3	Hospital 4
Group 1	IX	**7.4**	3.6	4.2	*2.9*
	Moving Range	—	—	—	—
Group 2	IX	**4.8**	*1.3*	4.6	2.6
	Moving Range	**2.6**	2.3	0.4	*0.3*
Group 3	IX	**8.7**	8.3	5.4	*1.9*
	Moving Range	**3.9**	7	0.8	*0.7*
Group 4	IX	**6.6**	5.4	*2.8*	3
	Moving Range	2.1	**2.9**	2.6	*1.1*
Group 5	IX	5.1	**7.8**	4.9	*1.7*
	Moving Range	1.5	**2.4**	2.1	*1.3*
Group 6	IX	**7.6**	6.1	4.7	*4.4*
	Moving Range	2.5	1.7	*0.2*	**2.7**
Group 7	IX	**6.2**	*1.6*	5.5	3.5
	Moving Range	1.4	**4.5**	*0.8*	0.9
Group 8	IX	7	7	4	*2.9*
	Moving Range	0.8	**5.4**	1.5	*0.6*
Group 9	IX	**6.3**	4.3	4.3	*1.9*
	Moving Range	0.7	**2.7**	*0.3*	1
Group 10	IX	3.7	**7.4**	5.4	*1.9*
	Moving Range	2.6	**3.1**	1.1	*0*

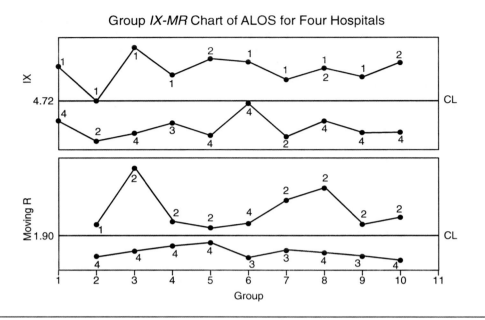

Figure 6.7 Group *IX-MR* Chart: ALOS for Four Hospitals

Centerline calculations for the group *IX* chart

$$\overline{\overline{IX}} = \frac{\sum IX}{k(\#\,characteristics)} =$$

$$\overline{\overline{IX}} = \frac{188.7}{10(4)} =$$

$$\overline{\overline{IX}} = \frac{188.7}{40} = 4.72$$

The data in Table 6.6 are plotted and the centerlines just calculated are used to create the group *IX-MR* chart in Figure 6.7. The group *IX* chart shows the numbers *1* and *2* next to the plot point for *group 8,* signifying that the MAX value is identical for both St. Anywhere and *hospital 2.*

The *MR* chart must be interpreted first to determine the extent of variability across the data set. The overall average ALOS *MR* for all hospitals is 1.90 days, indicating that, on average, the difference between the actual ALOS for any 2 months was about 2 days for all of the hospitals in the study. Of the nine MR values on the chart, seven MAX values come from *hospital 2,* specifying that, compared with the others, *hospital 2* has the largest differences in month to month ALOS; i.e., the variation in ALOS is much greater (more variable) than for any of the remaining three institutions. The MIN line displays the least variation in ALOS from group to group. Note that of the nine *MR* values in the MIN position, six of them are from *hospital 4*. This predominance of *hospital 4* may be an indication that *hospital 4* is more consistent from month to month in its ALOS. The reason for this low degree of variation in that institution cannot be determined from this analysis, but it might be an indication of some difference in the way in which patient stays are handled by *hospital 4*.

Interpretation of the group *IX* chart reveals that the overall ALOS for all hospitals, as indicated by the centerline on the group *IX* chart, was 4.72 days. The centerline for the group *IX* chart shows that for all institutions for the entire length of the study, the ALOS was almost 5 days for a diagnosis of myocardial infarction. The chart also reveals that 8 of the 10 MAX values come from St. Anywhere; i.e., St. Anywhere has a significantly higher ALOS for myocardial infarction than the other three hospitals. *Hospital 4* occupies 7 of the 10 positions on the MIN line, so *hospital 4* not only has the least variation in ALOS but also has the shortest ALOS. With regard to ALOS, the managed care organization chose *hospital 4* to be the benchmark for the region because its overall ALOS is lower and less variable than the other institutions.

Group *IX-MR* charts allow comparison of multiple characteristics at the same time and on the same chart. Like the traditional *IX-MR* chart, the group *IX-MR* chart relies on a subgroup size of one, and the plot points represent individual data values (*IX*) and differences between two consecutive measurements (*MR*). Like all variables data control charts, the *IX-MR* approach uses one chart (the *IX* chart) to depict central tendency and another chart (the *MR* chart) to highlight process variability.

In summary, the group *IX-MR* chart can be particularly useful in grouping data sets with similar characteristics and is best used in situations

◆   to compare identical characteristics with each other
◆   when data collection opportunities are infrequent
◆   when the subgroup size is fixed at one
◆   to minimize calculations and simplify data analysis
◆   to plot multiple characteristics at the same time on a single chart

Group *IX-MR* charts can clearly distinguish performance differences between identical characteristics on one chart. When greater numbers of samples can produce larger subgroup sizes, the group $\bar{X}$ and *R* chart provides a better option for analysis, and that approach is presented in the next section.

Group $\overline{X}$ and R Chart

CRITERION	VALUE
Multiple characteristics to be plotted at the same time?	Yes
Subgroup size	2–9
Unique target values for characteristics?	No

Group $\overline{X}$ and R charts are used for evaluating multiple characteristics or sources of data at the same time and on the same chart. The group $\overline{X}$ and R chart is specifically used to track the average and range of variables data characteristics where groups of logically related data are gathered over some period of time. Like all group charts, the group $\overline{X}$ chart incorporates both a MAX and a MIN line. Each line represents the largest and smallest averages, respectively, from the groups represented on the chart. Each plot point on the graph is labeled with its characteristic number, and those labels provide the basis for analyzing the charts by clearly highlighting patterns or trends of numbers or letters that repeat across MAX and MIN lines. Like other $\overline{X}$ charts, the group $\overline{X}$ chart's subgroup size (n) is fixed between two and nine, and its primary purpose is to indicate central tendency for the data set and the characteristics within its groups.

Although the group $\overline{X}$ chart indicates central tendency, the group R chart characterizes subgroup variation. Like all group charts, the group R chart is displayed with two lines: a MAX and a MIN. The MAX line displays the largest range values across the groups; the MIN line shows the smallest. Each MAX and MIN plot point is tagged with a number that designates the characteristic that is associated with the plot point. Thus, the group R chart displays MAX and MIN range values for all groups across all characteristics at the same time and on the same chart, simplifying comparison of the variability of several identical characteristics against one another without having to maintain separate charts for each measure. Neither the group $\overline{X}$ chart nor the group R chart is configured with control limits. Therefore, group charts are not referred to as "control" charts.

Group $\overline{X}$ and R charts are best employed for comparing multiple characteristics over a period of time. The analytical technique allows for

◆ evaluation of multiple characteristics on the same chart at the same time
◆ evaluation of time-ordered variables (measurements) data
◆ tracking of the consistency of data that occurs frequently and where there exist many opportunities for data collection
◆ tracking of subgroup statistics ($\overline{X}$ and Rs) from identical characteristics that occurred at the same time but were generated from different sources

As with any statistical technique such as the group $\overline{X}$ and R approach, a number of conditions must be satisfied:

◆ subgroup size between two and nine
◆ measurements normally distributed
◆ measurements independent of one another
◆ identical unit of measure between characteristics

The formulas for the group $\overline{X}$ and range approach are included in Exhibit 6-5. The following example illustrates the use of the group $\overline{X}$ and range chart.

Example 6-6

The office manager at XYZ Clinic presented the WR data from her analysis (described in Chapter 5, Example 5-6) at a medical managers' convention. Two managers from similar-sized practices approached her after her presentation with an idea to evaluate the consistency of the WR measure. Each of the three clinics is approximately the same size, with similar billings per month, and the characteristics of interest (WR) are identical. Collectively, they have decided to compare their data with each other by placing their WR data on a group $\overline{X}$ and R chart. The data for the last 10 months are presented in Table 6.7. MIN values for each group are entered in the table in bold italic type; MAX values are simply entered in bold type. To clearly visualize the differences and similarities between the three clinics and their respective WR, the data have been plotted on a group $\overline{X}$ and R chart in Figure 6.8. Calculation of the centerlines

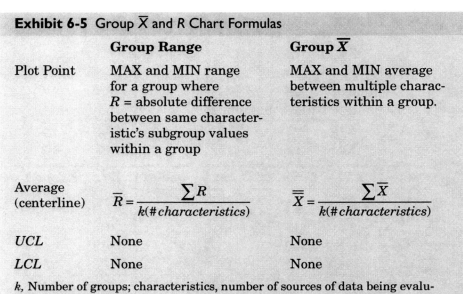

Exhibit 6-5 Group $\overline{X}$ and R Chart Formulas

	Group Range	**Group $\overline{X}$**
Plot Point	MAX and MIN range for a group where R = absolute difference between same characteristic's subgroup values within a group	MAX and MIN average between multiple characteristics within a group.
Average (centerline)	$\overline{R} = \dfrac{\sum R}{k(\# characteristics)}$	$\overline{\overline{X}} = \dfrac{\sum \overline{X}}{k(\# characteristics)}$
UCL	None	None
LCL	None	None

k, Number of groups; characteristics, number of sources of data being evaluated within a group.

for the group $\overline{X}$ and R charts was accomplished according to the formulas in Exhibit 6-5, as follows

$$\overline{\overline{R}} = \frac{\sum R}{k(\#\,characteristics)} =$$

$$\overline{\overline{R}} = \frac{157.9}{10(3)} =$$

$$\overline{\overline{R}} = \frac{157.9}{30} = 5.26$$

$$\overline{\overline{X}} = \frac{\sum \overline{X}}{k(\#\,characteristics)} =$$

$$\overline{\overline{X}} = \frac{328.53}{10(3)} =$$

$$\overline{\overline{X}} = \frac{328.53}{30} = 10.951$$

Table 6.7 Weekly Receivables Data for XYZ Clinic and Two Similar Organizations

GROUP 1	XYZ	CLINIC 2	CLINIC 3	GROUP 2	XYZ	CLINIC 2	CLINIC 3
	8.8	10.6	13		5.4	14.3	12.8
	9.1	5.9	15.4		7.6	10.5	11.5
	8	10.4	10.4		8.5	18.7	11.9
	6.7	12.5	10		9.7	10.9	12.4
$\overline{X}$	8.15	9.85	12.2		7.8	13.6	12.15
Range	2.4	6.6	5.4		4.3	8.2	1.3
GROUP 3	XYZ	CLINIC 2	CLINIC 3	GROUP 4	XYZ	CLINIC 2	CLINIC 3
	4.7	6.4	12.6		7.7	20.2	11.7
	8	13.6	15.3		9.9	14.9	11.5
	8.7	16.8	14		9.2	8.6	14.8
	8.4	11.2	13.5		5.5	9.8	17.2
$\overline{X}$	7.45	12	13.85		8.08	13.38	13.8
Range	4	10.4	2.7		4.4	11.6	5.7

Table 6.7 *continued*

GROUP 5	XYZ	CLINIC 2	CLINIC 3	GROUP 6	XYZ	CLINIC 2	CLINIC 3
	7.6	13.9	14.9		5.9	7.3	13.7
	8.1	7.2	12.5		10.5	10.3	14.4
	11.8	15.6	16.8		7.9	3.4	12
	8	18.5	13		13	7	13.8
X̄	**8.88**	13.8	**14.3**		9.33	**7**	**13.48**
Range	**4.2**	**11.3**	4.3		**7.1**	6.9	**2.4**

GROUP 7	XYZ	CLINIC 2	CLINIC 3	GROUP 8	XYZ	CLINIC 2	CLINIC 3
	10.1	8.8	13.8		3.1	12.2	12.7
	6.1	3.3	12.3		6.8	12.5	15.1
	7.3	10.9	12.1		8.1	12	13.3
	9	14.7	12.4		9.2	16.5	13.8
X̄	**8.13**	9.43	**12.65**		**6.8**	13.3	**13.73**
Range	4	**11.4**	**1.7**		**6.1**	4.5	**2.4**

GROUP 9	XYZ	CLINIC 2	CLINIC 3	GROUP 10	XYZ	CLINIC 2	CLINIC 3
	6.4	13.1	12.8		9.7	10.8	12.4
	6	15.9	12.6		8.7	10.9	17.4
	6.6	9	10.9		10.8	14.8	13.6
	6	8.2	14		8.5	8.9	13.5
X̄	**6.25**	11.55	**12.58**		**9.43**	11.35	**14.23**
Range	**0.6**	**7.7**	3.1		**2.3**	**5.9**	5

The calculated values provide the centerlines for each chart in Figure 6.8, and because the charts are group charts, control limits are not calculated.

From the range chart, the centerline reveals that the overall average WR range across all three clinics is 5.26, indicating that, on average, the difference between the largest and smallest WR for all groups and across all three clinics is more than 5 weeks. For the 10 groups shown, 8 MAX range values come from *clinic 2*, so compared with the others, *clinic 2* has the largest variation in WR. The MIN line on the group *R* chart displays the least variation in WR from group to group. Of all the 10 groups on the chart, half of the MIN ranges come from *clinic 3* and half are from XYZ Clinic (represented by the number *1* next to plot points), indicating that the variability in WR is not significantly different between these two clinics

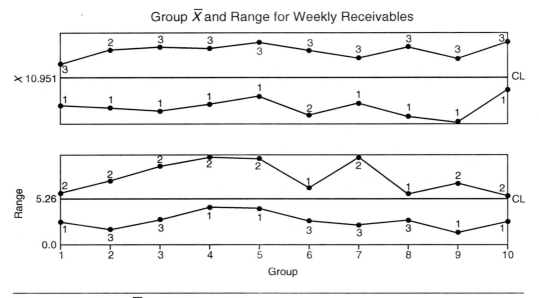

Figure 6.8 Group $\overline{X}$ and R Chart: WR

and that their variability is less, collectively, than the variation displayed by *clinic 2*.

The centerline on the group $\overline{X}$ chart shows that across all groups and for all clinics, the average weekly receivables is 10.95 weeks; that is, all three clinics, collectively, average almost 11 weeks before bills are paid for services rendered. On all group charts, the MAX line shows the largest value within a group and the MIN line displays the smallest. Figure 6.8 reveals that *clinic 3* occupies 9 of the 10 highest average WR (MAX line), whereas XYZ Clinic occupies 9 of 10 plot points on the MIN line. *Clinic 3* thus has a significantly higher WR, XYZ Clinic's WR are lower, and *clinic 2* falls somewhere in the middle.

Overall, *clinic 2* displays the most variability (as seen on the group R chart) compared with the other clinics, but *clinic 3* displays the highest average WR compared with the others. Additionally, XYZ Clinic not only has the lowest overall average WR but also has lower variability compared to *clinic 2*. Therefore, XYZ Clinic may be a good candidate for the other clinics to benchmark, to learn the best ways to minimize WR and thereby maximize cash flow.

Group $\overline{X}$ and R charts allow users to compare multiple characteristics to each other at the same time and on the same chart. Like the traditional $\overline{X}$ and R chart, the group $\overline{X}$ and R chart relies on a fixed subgroup size of between two and nine. Like all group charts, plotted points are the MAX and MIN values of $\overline{X}$ values and range values. The group $\overline{X}$ chart depicts central tendency; the R chart highlights process variability.

Optimum use of the group $\overline{X}$ and R chart can improve evaluation of a process with several parallel streams of data. Ideally, this technique is best used for

◆ comparing identical characteristics
◆ processes in which data collection opportunities are plentiful
◆ subgroup sizes fixed between two and nine
◆ plotting of subgroup statistics (averages and ranges)
◆ plotting of multiple characteristics at the same time on a single chart

Group $\overline{X}$ and R charts are best used with fixed subgroup sizes between two and nine, but as subgroup size grows, another group chart technique becomes applicable, as discussed in the next section.

Group $\overline{X}$ and s-Chart

CRITERION	VALUE
Multiple characteristics to be plotted at the same time?	Yes
Subgroup size	>9
Unique target values for characteristics?	No

Group $\overline{X}$ and s-charts are used for evaluating multiple characteristics or sources of data at the same time and on the same chart. The group $\overline{X}$ and s-chart is used to track the average and standard deviation of variables data characteristics where groups of logically related characteristics are gathered over some period of time. Like all group charts, the group $\overline{X}$ chart incorporates both a MAX and a MIN line, representing the largest and smallest averages, respectively, from the groups represented on the chart. A number is placed next to each MAX or MIN plot point, indicating the source of that value. Group $\overline{X}$ and s-charts clearly highlight patterns or trends of numbers that repeat across MAX and MIN lines. Like other $\overline{X}$ charts, the group $\overline{X}$ chart's subgroup size (n) is fixed and greater than nine. Its primary purpose is to indicate central tendency for the data set and the characteristics within its groups.

The group $\overline{X}$ chart indicates central tendency, but the group s-chart signifies subgroup variation across its groups. Like all group charts, the group s-chart is displayed with two lines: a MAX and a MIN. The MAX line displays the largest subgroup standard deviation values across the groups, and the MIN line shows the smallest. Each MAX and MIN plot point is tagged with a number that designates the group that is associated with the plot point. By doing so, the group s-chart displays MAX and MIN standard deviation values for all groups across all characteristics at the same time and on the same chart, making comparison of the variability of several identical characteristics simpler and eliminating the need to create separate charts for each measure. Neither the group $\overline{X}$ chart nor the group s-chart is configured with control limits. Therefore, group charts are not referred to as control charts.

Group $\overline{X}$ and s-charts are most useful for specific circumstances in health care, particularly for evaluating multiple characteristics simultaneously. The most common applications include

◆ evaluation of multiple characteristics on the same chart at the same time
◆ tracking of the consistency of variables data where large volumes of data can be economically collected and analyzed
◆ plotting of subgroup statistics ($\overline{X}$ and sample standard deviation, s) from identical characteristics that occurred at the same time but were generated from different sources

Group $\overline{X}$ and s-charts are based on a number of statistical principles, and certain conditions must be met for the analysis to be valid.

◆ The subgroup size is greater than nine.
◆ Measurements are normally distributed.
◆ Measurements are independent of one another.
◆ The unit of measure between characteristics is identical.

Formulas for the group $\overline{X}$ and s-charts are listed in Exhibit 6-6. The following example illustrates an application of the group $\overline{X}$ and s-chart technique.

Example 6-7

The administrators of St. Everywhere Hospital have analyzed the air filtering systems of the obstetrics department and the infectious disease unit and determined that some equipment must be replaced (see Example 6-3). Because of these concerns, airflow has been monitored for some time in the hospital, and administrators wish to benchmark their air system against other hospitals. To keep the comparison as fair as possible, only the infectious disease units of three different hospitals have been included in the study. By performing this benchmarking exercise, the administration will be better informed regarding the performance of St. Everywhere's air filtration system compared with some of the other hospitals in the area. For the study, each hospital has sampled airflow rates each day for the last 10 days. Ten airflow measurements ($n = 10$) are gathered at random times during the day from the infectious disease wing of each hospital. Days are treated as subgroups, and an average and a standard deviation statistic have been calculated for each day's airflow data. The other three hospitals are treated as separate sources of in-

Exhibit 6-6 Group $\overline{X}$ and s Chart Formulas

	Group s	**Group $\overline{X}$**
Plot Point	The MAX and MIN s for a group where: $$s = \sqrt{\frac{\sum(x_i - \overline{X})^2}{n-1}}$$	MAX and MIN average between multiple characteristics within a group.
Average (Centerline)	$$\overline{s} = \frac{\sum s}{k(\# characteristics)}$$	$$\overline{\overline{X}} = \frac{\sum \overline{X}}{k(\# characteristics)}$$
UCL	None	None
LCL	None	None

where: k = the number of groups on a chart
characteristics = the number of sources of data being evaluated within a group
n = subgroup size

formation; therefore, the group is defined as a single day's airflow rate for all three hospitals. In this way, the MIN and MAX average and standard deviation for all three hospitals for a single day will be plotted on a group $\overline{X}$ and s-chart. The data for the study can be found in Table 6.8. MIN values in the table are printed in bold italic print, and MAX values are printed in bold print. To clearly visualize the differences and similarities between the three hospitals and their respective airflows, the data have been plotted on the group $\overline{X}$ and s-chart in Figure 6.9. Centerline values were calculated as follows, using the data in Table 6.8 and the formulas in Exhibit 6-6.

$$\overline{s} = \frac{\sum s}{k(\# characteristics)} =$$

$$\overline{s} = \frac{78.2674}{10(3)} =$$

$$\overline{s} = \frac{78.2674}{30} = 2.60891$$

$$\overline{\overline{X}} = \frac{\sum \overline{X}}{k(\# characteristics)} =$$

$$\overline{\overline{X}} = \frac{2682.03}{10(3)} =$$

$$\overline{\overline{X}} = \frac{2682.03}{30} = 89.401$$

When the data in Table 6.8 are plotted with the centerlines from the above calculations, the result is a completed group $\overline{X}$ and s-chart as shown in Figure 6.9.

From the group s-chart, the overall average standard deviation (s) for all three hospitals is 2.61. Comparing the standard deviations of all of the hospitals with that average, it is clear that the variation in airflow from one hospital to the next is different. For the 10 groups shown, all of the MAX standard deviation values come from *hospital 2*, indicating that, compared with the others, *hospital 2* has the largest amount of variation in airflow in the infectious disease unit. On the other hand, *hospital 3* shows the least variation in airflow variability because every one of the group s-chart plot points shows *hospital 3* in the MIN position. Therefore, the air circulation and filtration equipment in *hospital 3* is very consistent in the movement of air each day.

The centerline on the group $\overline{X}$ chart shows that across all groups and for all hospitals the average airflow is 89.40 cf/min. The MAX line on the group $\overline{X}$ chart shows that *hospital 2* consistently has the highest airflow rates of all hospitals in the study. Interestingly, *hospital 2* also displayed the highest variation in air movement, indicating that the airflow equipment is so old or difficult to control that the environmental maintenance staff must increase the overall average airflow to compensate for the difficulty in dealing with its much higher variation. The lowest overall airflow rates are found on the MIN line. *Hospital 3* dominates the MIN line demonstrating the overall lowest airflow rates of all hospitals. *Hospital 3* also displayed the least variation in airflow rates; thus, not only is the equipment handling the airflow more consistently, but *hospital 3* also has a lower overall airflow rate that could possibly mean lower overall utility expenses for the hospital.

In addition to the consistent differences in the standard deviation and average flow rates between all three hospitals, the group $\overline{X}$ chart seems to reveal a gradual increase in the average airflow rates from the beginning to the end of the study. Because the MIN and MAX lines seem to slowly move upward across the group $\overline{X}$ chart, the increase seems to have had an effect on all three hospitals in the study. Some influence has affected all of the hospitals in the study so that the overall average for all 10 days has steadily increased. This finding presents an opportunity for all three hospitals to work

Table 6.8 St. Everywhere Benchmarking Study: Airflow Data

	GROUP 1			GROUP 2		
	HOSPITAL 1	HOSPITAL 2	HOSPITAL 3	HOSPITAL 1	HOSPITAL 2	HOSPITAL 3
	81.2	92.7	81	84	95.6	80
	85.4	92.2	81.1	84.1	94	82.7
	85.7	82.5	83.7	84.8	89	79.7
	86.2	97.8	82.8	87.7	98.9	81.5
	82.7	85.5	82.5	85	88.4	81.5
	85.3	84.8	82.8	82.6	85.5	82.9
	81.9	86.2	80.5	83.7	100.5	80.3
	84.6	88.8	81.9	88.1	91.1	81.7
	84.3	88	81.8	86	85.4	82.5
	85.8	90.8	83.7	81.6	89.1	83.6
$\overline{X}$	84.31	**88.93**	*82.18*	84.76	**91.75**	*81.64*
s	1.7654	**4.5409**	*1.1104*	2.0598	**5.3039**	*1.3159*

	GROUP 3			GROUP 4		
	HOSPITAL 1	HOSPITAL 2	HOSPITAL 3	HOSPITAL 1	HOSPITAL 2	HOSPITAL 3
	84.4	83.1	82.6	84.9	89.6	81.4
	84.5	88.5	82	84.8	94	81.2
	84.4	84.6	82.5	83.8	97.1	82.6
	85.1	95.1	82.2	82	81.2	82.3
	84.8	82.5	81.4	85.6	97.5	82.3
	83	88.2	80.9	86.2	86.9	79.7
	86.6	95.1	82	86	95.3	82.1
	87.2	102.3	82	85.6	95.5	80.6
	83.4	84.7	82.2	81.9	87.8	81.2
	85.2	92	81.2	81.8	93.1	83.9
$\overline{X}$	84.86	**89.61**	*81.9*	84.26	**91.8**	*81.73*
s	1.2834	**6.4325**	*0.5578*	1.7646	**5.2732**	*1.17*

	GROUP 5			GROUP 6		
	HOSPITAL 1	HOSPITAL 2	HOSPITAL 3	HOSPITAL 1	HOSPITAL 2	HOSPITAL 3
	89	101.6	85	89.4	89.1	87.6
	89.1	100	87.7	89.5	94.5	87
	89.8	95	84.7	89.4	90.6	87.5
	92.7	104.9	86.5	90.1	101.1	87.2
	90	94.4	86.5	89.8	88.5	86.4
	87.6	91.5	87.9	88	94.2	85.9

continues

Table 6.8 *continued*

	GROUP 5			GROUP 6		
	HOSPITAL 1	HOSPITAL 2	HOSPITAL 3	HOSPITAL 1	HOSPITAL 2	HOSPITAL 3
	88.7	106.5	85.3	91.6	101.1	87
	93.1	97.1	86.7	92.2	108.3	87
	91	91.4	87.5	88.4	90.7	87.2
	86.6	95.1	88.6	90.2	98	86.2
$\overline{X}$	89.76	**97.75**	*86.64*	89.86	**95.61**	*86.9*
s	2.0598	**5.3039**	*1.3159*	1.2834	**6.4325**	*0.5578*

	GROUP 7			GROUP 8		
	HOSPITAL 1	HOSPITAL 2	HOSPITAL 3	HOSPITAL 1	HOSPITAL 2	HOSPITAL 3
	88.3	97.1	88.1	90.5	96.6	87.3
	90	99.8	87.5	88.4	98.2	88
	91.3	99.4	84.9	89.9	93.8	87.7
	92.9	87	88.9	92.3	90.4	87.5
	93	91.5	85.4	90	97.9	87.8
	91.9	93.3	86.3	93.4	93.1	88.5
	89.2	98.3	87.1	92.6	96.6	87.4
	90.7	99.2	83.7	88.9	98.6	85.9
	92.1	93.7	86.5	85.9	96.8	85.7
	90.4	91.5	86.1	91.5	93.4	85.9
$\overline{X}$	90.98	**95.08**	*86.45*	90.34	**95.54**	*87.17*
s	1.5526	**4.3251**	*1.5443*	2.2495	**2.7044**	*0.9832*

	GROUP 9			GROUP 10		
	HOSPITAL 1	HOSPITAL 2	HOSPITAL 3	HOSPITAL 1	HOSPITAL 2	HOSPITAL 3
	94	97.7	90.6	91.9	97.9	89.9
	92.3	100.9	90	92.1	94.4	90.9
	91.5	102.2	88.6	93.3	96	90.2
	91.4	97.8	89.4	89.8	95.3	90.6
	93.7	92.4	88.5	92.7	100.8	90.4
	93.1	89.1	90.5	94.8	93.7	89
	87.8	105.1	90.4	93.9	102	88.1
	94.7	99.6	90.1	93.7	95.8	91.7
	92.5	94.8	91	92.6	105.8	90.1
	92.2	107	89.8	90.1	105.3	90.7
$\overline{X}$	92.32	**98.66**	*89.89*	92.49	**98.7**	*90.16*
s	1.9147	**5.5438**	*0.8346*	1.5968	**4.4803**	*1.0069*

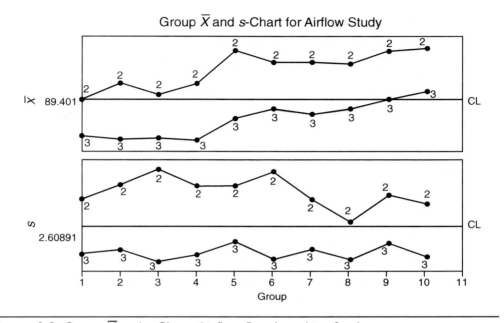

Figure 6.9 Group $\overline{X}$ and s-Chart: Airflow Benchmarking Study

together to determine the cause of the gradual increase, or it could be the result of some unforeseen environmental factor that affected each hospital in the same way, e.g., the sentinel effect of collecting data for analysis.

Group $\overline{X}$ and s-charts allow comparison of multiple characteristics at the same time and on the same chart. Like the traditional $\overline{X}$ and s-chart, the group $\overline{X}$ and s-chart relies on a fixed subgroup size of 10 or greater. Like all group charts, plotted points are the MAX and MIN values of $\overline{X}$ values and s-values that come from logically related groups of data. Like all variables data charts, the group $\overline{X}$ chart depicts central tendency, and the group s-chart delineates process variability.

The group $\overline{X}$ and s-chart provides a powerful means of comparing similar, grouped data when the following conditions are present.

◆ Identical characteristics are to be compared with each other.
◆ Data collection opportunities are frequent, and it is easy and economical to collect the data.
◆ Subgroup size is fixed at 10 or greater.
◆ Subgroup statistics (averages and sample standard deviations) are to be plotted.
◆ Multiple characteristics are to be plotted at the same time on a single chart.

Group Target Charts

Group charts can be used to compare measures that are similar, either from the same organization or from different organizations. Adding the target feature to these techniques expands their use to examine similar characteristics with different expected outcomes. Group target charts are described in the following sections.

Group Target IX-MR Chart

CRITERION	VALUE
Multiple characteristics to be plotted at the same time?	Yes
Subgroup size	I
Unique target values for characteristics?	Yes

Group target IX-MR charts are used for evaluating multiple characteristics or sources of data with unique target values at the same time and on the same chart. Like the target charts, individual data values are subtracted from their targets, and only the differences (deviations from target) are used for plotting purposes. Like all group charts, the group target IX-MR chart is used to track logically related groups of characteristics through time. Both MAX and MIN lines appear on the group target IX chart. Each line represents the largest and smallest deviation from target values, respectively, for all characteristics across the chart's groups. To highlight the characteristic from which the MAX and MIN values came, a number is typically placed next to each plot point identifying the source of the data. Patterns of these numbers on the lines direct the interpretation of the group target IX-MR chart. Like other IX charts, the group target IX chart's subgroup size (n) is one, and its primary purpose is to indicate central tendency for the data set.

Although the group target IX chart indicates central tendency, the group MR chart reflects the variability component of the individual data points. Like the group target IX chart, the group MR chart is displayed with two lines: a MAX and a MIN. The MAX line displays the largest values of MRs across the groups, and the MIN line shows the smallest. The MR chart combined with the group target IX chart is identical to the MR chart used with regular group IX-MR charts. There is no deviation from target calculation with the values found on the group target MR chart. The group MR chart displays the variability of a data set across multiple characteristics on the same chart at the same time. Neither the group target IX chart nor its companion group MR chart has control limits calculated for their respective charts. Therefore, group target charts are not referred to as "control" charts.

Group target IX-MR charts have specific applications in health care, and the technique can best be employed in the following circumstances:

◆ to evaluate multiple characteristics on the same chart at the same time
◆ to compare characteristics that have different target values on the same chart
◆ to evaluate time-ordered variables (measurements) data
◆ to track data that occurs infrequently (such as monthly sales, financial, occupancy, or other infrequently occurring data)
◆ to track identical characteristics that occurred at the same time but were generated from different sources

As with all *IX* charts, several conditions must be met for the analysis of the group target *IX-MR* chart to be valid, including

◆ subgroup size of one
◆ measurements normally distributed
◆ measurements independent of one another
◆ unit of measure between characteristics is identical; target values are different

Formulas for group target *IX-MR* charts can be found in Exhibit 6-7 and notably do not include a provision for control limit calculations because the technique does not produce a traditional control chart. The following example illustrates the use of a group target *IX-MR* chart in a health care setting.

Example 6-8

The managed care organization in Example 6-5 was encouraged by the benchmarking study to begin evaluating hospitals in different regions of the United States where the managed care organization had health plans. The managed care organization staff particularly directed attention to myocardial infarction because previous studies had indicated wide variation in patterns of care among regions. They chose representative hospitals from three different regions of the country and then used the ALOS for all the institutions in each region as the target for these three hospitals. The ALOS target values for myocardial infarction are as follows:

Region 1: 5 days
Region 2: 7 days
Region 3: 9 days

In this example, the characteristics or sources of data to be grouped together for comparison are the three different institutions and their respective ALOS data. A group, therefore, is composed of an ALOS value for each of the three hospitals for a single month. The data have been gathered for each of the last 10 months and can be viewed in Table 6.9. MAX values in the table are printed in bold type,

Exhibit 6-7 Group Target *IX-MR* Chart Formulas

	Group Moving Range	**Group Target IX**
Plot Point	MAX and MIN *MR* for a group where *MR* = absolute difference between 2 successive *IX* values from the same characteristic	MAX and MIN differences between individual values and their targets within a group
Average (centerline)	$\overline{MR} = \dfrac{\sum MR}{(k-1)(\# characteristics)}$	$Coded\overline{IX} = \dfrac{\sum (IX - Target)}{k(\# characteristics)}$
UCL	None	None
LCL	None	None

k, Number of groups; characteristics, the number of sources of data being evaluated within a group.

MIN values in bold italic type. *Hospitals 1* and *2* in *group 9* have the same difference between their ALOS and respective target values; therefore both numbers are in bold italic type, indicating identical MIN plot point values. To clearly display the differences and similarities among the care patterns of the three hospitals, the data in Table 6.9 have been placed on the group target IX-MR chart in Figure 6.10. Calculations for centerlines using the data in Table 6.9 and the formulas in Exhibit 6-7 are as follows:

$$\overline{MR} = \frac{\sum MR}{(k-1)(\# characteristics)} =$$

$$\overline{MR} = \frac{21.0}{(10-1)(3)} =$$

$$\overline{MR} = \frac{21.0}{27} = 0.78$$

$$Coded\overline{IX} = \frac{\sum (IX - Target)}{k(\# characteristics)} =$$

$$Coded\overline{IX} = \frac{25.9}{10(3)} =$$

$$Coded\,\overline{\overline{IX}} = \frac{25.9}{30} = 0.86$$

When the data in Table 6.9 are plotted with the centerlines, the result is a completed group target *IX-MR* chart as shown in Figure 6.10.

From the *MR* chart, the overall average ALOS *MR* for all three hospitals is seen to be 0.78 days; i.e., on average, the difference between the actual ALOS for 2 consecutive months was less than 1 day for all of the hospitals in the study. If any one source of data on a group chart has consistently higher or lower variability, the number related to that source will appear with relatively great frequency

Table 6.9 Group Target *IX-MR* Data for ALOS: Three Hospitals

		HOSPITAL 1	**HOSPITAL 2**	**HOSPITAL 3**
Group 1	ALOS	4.4	8	11.4
	Target	5	7	9
	ALOS - Target	**−0.6**	1	**2.4**
	MR	—	—	—
Group 2	ALOS	5.3	6.6	11.1
	Target	5	7	9
	ALOS - Target	0.3	**−0.4**	**2.1**
	MR	0.9	1.4	**0.3**
Group 3	ALOS	5.2	7.9	11.3
	Target	5	7	9
	ALOS - Target	**0.2**	0.9	**2.3**
	MR	**0.1**	1.3	0.2
Group 4	ALOS	4.1	6.9	10.8
	Target	5	7	9
	ALOS - Target	**−0.9**	−0.1	**1.8**
	MR	**1.1**	1	**0.5**
Group 5	ALOS	5.9	7.5	10.1
	Target	5	7	9
	ALOS - Target	0.9	**0.5**	**1.1**
	MR	**1.8**	**0.6**	0.7
Group 6	ALOS	4.8	7.3	12.3
	Target	5	7	9
	ALOS - Target	**−0.2**	0.3	**3.3**
	MR	1.1	**0.2**	**2.2**

continues

Table 6.9 *continued*

		HOSPITAL 1	HOSPITAL 2	HOSPITAL 3
Group 7	ALOS	5.1	6.3	12.1
	Target	5	7	9
	ALOS - Target	0.1	*−0.7*	*3.1*
	MR	0.3	1	*0.2*
Group 8	ALOS	5.6	7.2	10.6
	Target	5	7	9
	ALOS - Target	0.6	*0.2*	1.6
	MR	*0.5*	0.9	1.5
Group 9	ALOS	4.9	6.9	11.9
	Target	5	7	9
	ALOS - Target	*−0.1*	−0.1	2.9
	MR	0.7	*0.3*	1.3
Group 10	ALOS	4.8	7.7	11.9
	Target	5	7	9
	ALOS - Target	*−0.2*	0.7	2.9
	MR	0.1	*0.8*	*0*

MR, moving range.

next to the plot points on either the MIN or MAX line on the *MR* chart. In this case, however, there appears to be no discernible pattern, indicating that the variation in ALOS seems to be about the same regardless of hospital.

Considering all months, the overall deviation from the target ALOS for all hospitals, as indicated by the centerline on the group target *IX* chart, is +0.86 days. Recall that all of the data plotted on the group target *IX* chart are plotted as the difference between the actual ALOS value and its target. Therefore, the centerline for the group *IX* chart shows that for all institutions for the entire length of the study, the ALOS was almost a day longer than defined by targets.

As with all group charts, the MAX line is plotted with the largest values from a group. All of the MAX values on the group target *IX* chart in Figure 6.10 come from *hospital 3*. Compared with the other institutions, the ALOS at *hospital 3* is not only much higher than its own target, but those differences are much larger than the deviation from target values for the other hospitals. This deviation is especially evident when comparing the MIN line to the target line. The MIN line hovers around the target on the group target *IX* chart, indicating that *hospitals 1* and *2* have ALOS values very close to their expected (target) values. It also indicates that there is a proportion-

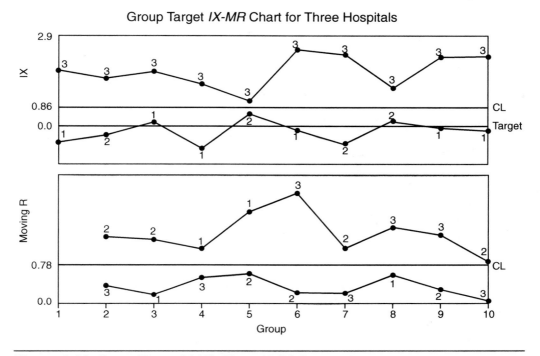

Figure 6.10 Group Target *IX-MR* Chart: ALOS Data

Data for ALOS from three hospitals.

ately larger difference between actual ALOS and the target in *hospital 3*. The managed care organization thus decided to direct its efforts at *hospital 3* because it demonstrated the highest ALOS.

Group target *IX-MR* charts allow comparison of multiple characteristics with different targets to each other at the same time and on the same chart. Like the traditional *IX-MR* chart, the group target *IX-MR* chart relies on a subgroup size of one. The plot points on the group target *IX* chart represent the MAX and MIN differences between individual data values (*IX* values) and their targets. Only the largest (MAX) and smallest (MIN) differences for a group are plotted. On the group target *MR* chart, the MAX and MIN differences between two consecutive values for the same characteristic are plotted per group.

The most useful applications for the group target *IX-MR* chart include those in which

- ◆ identical characteristics with different target values are compared with each other
- ◆ data collection opportunities are infrequent
- ◆ subgroup size is fixed at one
- ◆ calculations are to be minimized and data analysis simplified

◆ multiple characteristics are to be plotted at the same time on a single chart

When subgroup sizes are greater than one, other group target charts should be used, and these charts will be discussed in the following sections.

Group Target $\overline{X}$ and R Chart

CRITERION	VALUE
Multiple characteristics to be plotted at the same time?	Yes
Subgroup size	2–9
Unique target values for characteristics?	Yes

Group target $\overline{X}$ and R charts are used for evaluating multiple characteristics or sources of data with unique target values at the same time and on the same chart. With the exception of subgrouping, these charts are very similar to the group target IX-MR charts. Group target $\overline{X}$ and R charts also share similarities with regular target charts because the plot points are normalized by subtracting target values from subgroup averages. Only the differences (deviations from target) are used for plotting purposes on the group target $\overline{X}$ chart.

Like all group charts, the group target $\overline{X}$ and R chart is used to track logically related groups of characteristics through time. MAX and MIN lines are both displayed on the group target $\overline{X}$ chart. Each line represents the largest and smallest deviation from target values, respectively, for all characteristics across the chart's groups. A number is placed next to each plot point to identify the source of the data, and patterns in the numbers along the MAX and MIN lines direct interpretation of the chart. Like other $\overline{X}$ charts, the group target $\overline{X}$ chart's subgroup size (n) is fixed between two and nine. The primary purpose of the group $\overline{X}$ chart is to indicate central tendency of a data set.

Although the group target $\overline{X}$ chart demonstrates central tendency, the group target R chart reflects the variability component of the individual data points. Like all group charts, the group R chart is displayed with two lines: a MAX and a MIN. The MAX line displays the largest R values across the groups, and the MIN line shows the smallest. The group target R chart is identical to the group R chart that is used in conjunction with regular group $\overline{X}$ and R charts; i.e., unlike its companion group target $\overline{X}$ chart, there is no coding of R values. The group target $\overline{X}$ and R chart does not display control limits and therefore is not referred to as a "control" chart.

The attributes of group target $\overline{X}$ and R charts make them particularly useful under circumstances requiring

◆ evaluation of multiple characteristics on the same chart at the same time

◆ comparison of characteristics that have different expected outcomes
◆ evaluation of time-ordered variables (measurements) data
◆ tracking data that occur frequently enough to allow subgrouping of data
◆ tracking different sources of data that occurred at the same point in time

These techniques require adherence to a few restrictions that validate the analysis. Use of the group target $\overline{X}$ and R chart should be restricted to those data sets for which

◆ subgroup size is between two and nine
◆ measurements are normally distributed
◆ measurements are independent of one another
◆ the unit of measure between characteristics is identical but target values are different

In order to assure that valid conclusions can be made from the analysis, these conditions should be met before the analysis is performed. Formulas for group target $\overline{X}$ and R charts can be found in Exhibit 6-8. The following example demonstrates the use of the group target $\overline{X}$ and R chart.

Example 6-9

After the successful benchmarking analysis depicted in Example 6-6, other office managers became interested in the method of comparing

Exhibit 6-8 Group Target $\overline{X}$ and R Chart Formulas

	Group Range	**Group Target $\overline{X}$**
Plot Point	MAX and MIN range for a group where: R = absolute difference between the same characteristic's subgroup values within a group	MAX and MIN normalized $\overline{X}$ values between all sources of data within a group where $Coded\,\overline{X} = (\overline{X} - Target)$
Average (centerline)	$\overline{R} = \dfrac{\sum R}{k(\#\,characteristics)}$	$Coded\,\overline{\overline{X}} = \dfrac{\sum(\overline{X} - Target)}{k(\#\,characteristics)}$
UCL	None	None
LCL	None	None

k, Number of groups; characteristics, the number of sources of data being evaluated within a group.

WR between clinics. Several managers hoped to produce a report that would help them better understand their collections and compare them with other offices. Because many different offices are now involved, they have significantly different target values for WR, so a group target $\overline{X}$ and R chart was selected for the analysis. Each office manager chose a target value, based on the experience of the office, and a goal for improvement. Three offices were selected for a pilot study, and their target WR are as follows:

Clinic 1: 10 weeks
Clinic 2: 12 weeks
Clinic 3: 15 weeks

In this example, the characteristics or sources of data to be grouped together for comparison are the three different clinics and their WR data for a month. A group, therefore, is composed of the WR coded average and range for each clinic. Grouping the data this way will result in the MAX and MIN coded averages as well as the MAX and MIN R values to be plotted monthly. Table 6.10 lists the data collected over the last 10 months for the three clinics. MIN values are highlighted by bold italic type, and MAX values are emphasized with bold type. *Clinics 1* and *2* in *group 6* have the same coded average and range values; therefore, both the coded averages are in bold type to indicate that they both are maximal. To clearly display the differences and similarities among the WR in the three different clinics, the data in Table 6.10 have been placed on a group target $\overline{X}$ and R chart (Figure 6.11), with centerlines calculated from the data in Table 6.10 and the formulas in Exhibit 6-8.

$$\overline{R} = \frac{\sum R}{k(\# \, characteristics)} =$$

$$\overline{R} = \frac{99.4}{(10)(3)} =$$

$$\overline{R} = \frac{99.4}{30} = 3.31$$

$$Coded\,\overline{\overline{X}} = \frac{\sum (\overline{X} - Target)}{k(\# \, characteristics)} =$$

$$Coded\,\overline{\overline{X}} = \frac{-81.42}{10(3)} =$$

$$Coded\,\overline{\overline{X}} = \frac{-81.42}{30} = -2.714$$

Control limits are not included in group charts and so are neither included in the calculations nor displayed on the chart.

When the data in Table 6.10 are plotted and the centerlines from the above calculations are placed on the charts, the result is a completed group target $\overline{X}$ and R chart as shown in Figure 6.11.

The average range is calculated using all range values in all groups for all sources of variation. The average range of 3.31 indicates the average variation in WR among all three clinics; i.e., that on average, the difference between the lowest and highest WR for any 4-week period is approximately 3.5 weeks. The MAX and MIN lines for the group R chart show no clear runs or trends. Therefore there appears to be no indication of a significant difference in variation among WR at the three clinics.

Table 6.10 WR Data for Three Clinics

	GROUP 1			GROUP 2		
	CLINIC 1	CLINIC 2	CLINIC 3	CLINIC 1	CLINIC 2	CLINIC 3
	8.6	11.5	12.4	6.7	12.3	8.6
	7.9	11.9	12.3	8.7	12.2	8.4
	8.7	15.2	10.7	8.5	9.2	8.9
	8.6	13.2	8.5	9.6	13.8	9.6
$\overline{X}$	8.45	12.95	10.98	8.38	11.88	8.88
Target	10	12	15	10	12	15
$\overline{X}$-*Target*	−1.55	0.95	−4.02	−1.62	−0.12	−6.12
Range	0.8	3.7	3.9	2.9	4.6	1.2

	GROUP 3			GROUP 4		
	CLINIC 1	CLINIC 2	CLINIC 3	CLINIC 1	CLINIC 2	CLINIC 3
	10	9	7.1	7.3	12	9.8
	8.9	13.6	11.5	10.6	13.4	12
	8.3	12.5	9.4	7.9	10.8	10
	9.4	13.7	9.2	8.8	10.8	8.2
$\overline{X}$	9.15	12.2	9.3	8.65	11.75	10
Target	10	12	15	10	12	15
$\overline{X}$-*Target*	−0.85	0.2	−5.7	−1.35	−0.25	−5
Range	1.7	4.7	4.4	3.3	2.6	3.8

continues

Table 6.10 *continued*

| | GROUP 5 | | | GROUP 6 | | |
	CLINIC 1	CLINIC 2	CLINIC 3	CLINIC 1	CLINIC 2	CLINIC 3
	7.6	8.1	7.4	7.4	12.1	10.6
	8.7	10.7	9.5	9.9	11.3	9
	6	10.8	10.7	9.5	10.1	10.8
	10	12.8	12.4	8.3	9.6	11.2
$\overline{X}$	8.08	10.6	10	8.78	10.78	10.4
Target	10	12	15	10	12	15
$\overline{X}$-**Target**	−1.92	−1.4	−5	−1.22	−1.22	−4.6
Range	4	4.7	5	2.5	2.5	2.2

| | GROUP 7 | | | GROUP 8 | | |
	CLINIC 1	CLINIC 2	CLINIC 3	CLINIC 1	CLINIC 2	CLINIC 3
	8.8	12.6	12	9.7	10	8.7
	7.7	10.4	12.5	11.6	10.4	8
	8.5	9.5	7.5	7.1	9.6	7.9
	9.9	10.9	6.4	5.8	11.4	9.2
$\overline{X}$	8.73	10.85	9.6	8.55	10.35	8.45
Target	10	12	15	10	12	15
$\overline{X}$-**Target**	−1.27	−1.15	−5.4	−1.45	−1.65	−6.55
Range	2.2	3.1	6.1	5.8	1.8	1.3

| | GROUP 9 | | | GROUP 10 | | |
	CLINIC 1	CLINIC 2	CLINIC 3	CLINIC 1	CLINIC 2	CLINIC 3
	7.3	7.3	9.2	8.7	10.2	9.5
	6.6	13.3	4.1	8.5	9.1	7.4
	9.6	8	8.3	7.7	9.6	9.9
	8.7	9.4	7.7	5.8	9.4	8
$\overline{X}$	8.05	9.5	7.33	7.68	9.58	8.7
Target	10	12	15	10	12	15
$\overline{X}$-**Target**	−1.95	−2.5	−7.67	−2.32	−2.42	−6.3
Range	3	6	5.1	2.9	1.1	2.5

The overall average WR for all clinics for the entire 10 months is
−2.71, signifying that all clinics averaged almost 3 weeks less than
their targets for WR. There also appears to be a gradual trend downward for the average WR for the entire 10-month period, indicating
that the WR has slowly been reduced over the time period of the en-

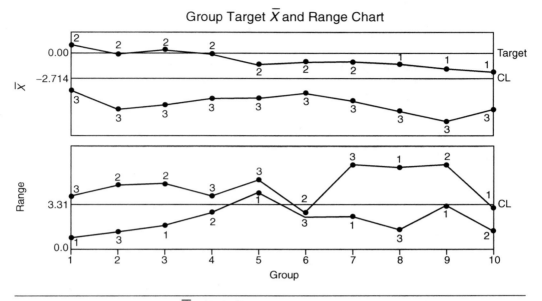

Figure 6.11 Group Target $\overline{X}$ and R Chart: WR Data

tire study. Although this is good news for clinic managers, *clinic 2* shows up on the MAX line for 7 of the 10 months; thus, although WR seem to be decreasing, *clinic 2* still has the highest WR of the three clinics. *Clinic 3* appears to dominate the MIN line, indicating that *clinic 3* has the lowest overall WR compared with the other two clinics. Finally, because almost all of the data for the entire study fall below the target line, WR has performed better than the targets set by the office managers.

Group target $\overline{X}$ and R charts allow comparison of multiple characteristics with different targets at the same time and on the same chart. Like the traditional $\overline{X}$ and R chart, the group target $\overline{X}$ and R chart has a fixed subgroup size of between two and nine. The plot points on the group target $\overline{X}$ chart represent the MAX and MIN differences among different characteristics' group averages and their targets. Only the largest (MAX) and smallest (MIN) differences for a group are plotted on the group target $\overline{X}$ chart. On the group target R chart, range values are calculated for each of the characteristics within a group; then only the MAX and MIN range values for a group are plotted.

Group target $\overline{X}$ and R charts have specific applications in health care, as indicated in the example, and those uses can be summarized as follows:

◆ to compare identical characteristics with different target values to each other
◆ to analyze large amounts of data

◆ to manage fixed subgroup sizes between two and nine
◆ to plot multiple characteristics at the same time on a single chart

When subgroup sizes exceed nine, the group target $\overline{X}$ and s-chart is a more appropriate tool for assessing process data. This technique is described in the next section on group target charts.

Group Target $\overline{X}$ and s-Chart

CRITERION	VALUE
Multiple characteristics to be plotted at the same time?	Yes
Subgroup size	>9
Unique target values for characteristics?	Yes

Group target $\overline{X}$ and s-charts are used for evaluating multiple characteristics or sources of data with unique target values at the same time and on the same chart. These charts are very similar to the group target $\overline{X}$ and R charts except that the subgroup size is 10 or greater, and instead of using the range as an estimate of variability, the sample standard deviation (s) is used. Group target $\overline{X}$ and s-charts share similarities with regular target charts because the plot points on the group target $\overline{X}$ chart are coded by subtracting target values from subgroup averages. Only the differences (the deviations between the average and their targets) are plotted on the group target $\overline{X}$ chart.

Like all group charts, the group target $\overline{X}$ and s-chart is used to track logically related groups of characteristics through time. Displayed on the group target $\overline{X}$ chart are both a MAX and a MIN line. Each line on the group target $\overline{X}$ chart represents the largest and smallest deviation from target values, respectively, for all characteristics within each of the chart's groups. To highlight from which characteristic the MAX and MIN values come, a number is placed next to each plot point. Patterns of these numbers repeating across MAX and MIN lines provide important information regarding the presence of special cause variation, as well as excessive deviation of one characteristic's averages. Like the traditional $\overline{X}$ and s-chart, the subgroup size (n) of the group target $\overline{X}$ and s-chart is fixed and is typically 10 or more. The primary purpose of the group target $\overline{X}$ chart is to indicate central tendency for a data set.

Although the group target $\overline{X}$ chart indicates central tendency, the group s-chart reflects the variability component of the individual data points. Like all group charts, the group s-chart is displayed with two lines: a MAX and a MIN. The MAX line displays the largest s values across the groups, and the MIN line shows the smallest. Unlike its companion group target $\overline{X}$ chart, the group s-chart does not rely on coded s values. The group s-chart displays the variability of a data set across multiple characteristics on the same chart at the same time. Control limits are not used on group target $\overline{X}$ and s-charts, and thus they are not referred to as "control" charts.

Group target $\overline{X}$ and s-charts have a number of applications in health care. The conditions necessary for using these charts include

◆ multiple characteristics on the same chart at the same time
◆ characteristics with different target values
◆ time-ordered variables (measurements) data
◆ data that occur very frequently and can be gathered economically
◆ different sources of data that occurred at the same point in time

Additionally, as with the other charting techniques that have been discussed, group target $\overline{X}$ and s-charts require satisfaction of a few underlying requirements for statistical validity.

◆ The subgroup size is greater than nine.
◆ Measurements are normally distributed.
◆ Measurements are independent of one another.
◆ The unit of measure between characteristics is identical, while their target values are different.

Formulas for group target $\overline{X}$ and s-charts can be found in Exhibit 6-9. The following example illustrates the use of this technique in a health care environment.

Example 6-10

The administration of St. Everywhere Hospital, after reviewing the airflow study results of the obstetrics and infectious disease units, has decided to expand the study to other areas of the hospital. The first targets of the expanded study were radiology, operating rooms, and the medical intensive care unit. Each of the three units uses a different air circulation system for air movement. Because the data are easy to acquire, airflow measurements were gathered for each wing at 10 different times ($n = 10$) randomly throughout the day for 8 days. Because the subgroup size is greater than nine, each wing has a different expected level of airflow (different targets), and the administration wants all of the study data placed on one chart, the group target $\overline{X}$ and s-chart was selected for the analysis. The airflow targets for each wing, in cubic feet per minute, have been acquired from maintenance and are as follows:

intensive care: 85 cf/min
operating rooms: 60 cf/min
x-ray: 45 cf/min

Exhibit 6-9 Target $\overline{X}$ and s-Chart Formulas

	Group s	Group Target $\overline{X}$
Plot Point	MAX and MIN sample standard deviation (s) for a group	MAX and MIN coded $\overline{X}$ values
	s is calculated for each characteristic in a group where $$s = \sqrt{\frac{\sum(x_i - \overline{X})^2}{n-1}}$$	coded $\overline{X}$ values are calculated for each characteristic within a group where $$Coded\,\overline{X} = (\overline{X} - Target)$$
Average (centerline)	$$\overline{s} = \frac{\sum s}{k(\#\,characteristics)}$$	$$Coded\,\overline{\overline{X}} = \frac{\sum(\overline{X} - Target)}{k(\#\,characteristics)}$$
UCL	None	None
LCL	None	None

k, Number of groups; n, subgroup size; characteristics, number of sources of data being evaluated within a group.

In this example, the characteristics or sources of data to be grouped together for comparison are the three different wings and their airflow data each day. A group, therefore, is composed of the daily airflow coded average and s-value for each of the three wings. Grouping the data in this way allows identification of the MAX and MIN coded averages as well as the MAX and MIN s-values for each group. Then, the MAX and MIN values will be plotted for each group each day. The data have been gathered for each of the last 8 days and can be viewed in Table 6.11.

The bold numbers in Table 6.11 highlight the largest group values, and the data in bold italic show the smallest. To clearly display the differences and similarities among the three wings and their airflow rates, the MAX and MIN data in Table 6.11 have been placed on the group target $\overline{X}$ and s-chart in Figure 6.12. Applying the formulas from Exhibit 6-9 to the data in Table 6.11, the centerlines for the group target $\overline{X}$ chart and the group s-chart can be calculated

$$\overline{s} = \frac{\sum s}{k(\#\,characteristics)} =$$

$$\overline{s} = \frac{55.7586}{(8)(3)} =$$

$$\overline{s} = \frac{55.7586}{24} = 2.3233$$

$$Coded\,\overline{\overline{X}} = \frac{\sum(\overline{X} - Target)}{k(\#\,characteristics)} =$$

$$Coded\,\overline{\overline{X}} = \frac{75.82}{8(3)} =$$

$$Coded\,\overline{\overline{X}} = \frac{75.82}{24} = 3.159$$

When the data in Table 6.11 are plotted with the centerlines from these calculations, the result is a completed group target $\overline{X}$ and s-chart, as shown in Figure 6.12. The centerline on the group s-chart

Table 6.11 Airflow Data St. Everywhere Project

	GROUP 1			**GROUP 2**		
	ICU	**OR**	**X-RAY**	**ICU**	**OR**	**X-RAY**
	86.2	61.1	47.1	89	62.2	43.9
	90.4	60.9	47.2	89.1	61.6	52
	90.7	57	55.1	89.8	59.6	43.2
	91.2	63.1	52.3	92.7	63.6	48.5
	87.7	58.2	51.5	90	59.4	48.6
	90.3	57.9	52.3	87.6	58.2	52.6
	86.9	58.5	45.6	88.7	64.2	44.8
	89.6	59.5	49.8	93.1	60.4	49
	89.3	59.2	49.4	91	58.2	51.4
	90.8	60.3	55	86.6	59.7	54.8
$\overline{X}$	89.31	59.57	50.53	89.76	60.71	48.88
Target	85	60	45	85	60	45
$\overline{X}$- Target	4.31	−0.43	**5.53**	**4.76**	0.71	3.88
s	1.7654	1.8154	**3.2836**	2.0598	2.1137	**3.9288**

continues

Table 6.11 *continued*

	GROUP 3			GROUP 4		
	ICU	**OR**	**X-RAY**	**ICU**	**OR**	**X-RAY**
	89.5	59.4	54.6	88.3	60.4	53.3
	90	62	48	90	61.5	51.4
	90.8	57.8	53.7	91.3	61.4	43.6
	84.2	58	51.3	92.9	56.4	55.6
	92.8	60.2	50.7	93	58.2	45.1
	91.2	59.4	53	91.9	58.9	47.8
	86.6	59.6	47.8	89.2	60.9	50.3
	87.8	59.9	50.5	90.7	61.3	40.2
	90.2	59.9	49.4	92.1	59.1	48.6
	88.7	59	54.3	90.4	58.2	47.3
$\overline{X}$	89.18	59.52	51.33	90.98	59.63	48.32
Target	85	60	45	85	60	45
$\overline{X}$- Target	4.18	−0.48	**6.33**	**5.98**	−0.37	3.32
s	2.4769	1.1774	**2.5007**	1.5526	1.7308	**4.6089**

	GROUP 5			GROUP 6		
	ICU	**OR**	**X-RAY**	**ICU**	**OR**	**X-RAY**
	90.5	60.3	50.8	91	59.5	51.8
	88.4	60.9	53.1	89.3	60.8	50.1
	89.9	59.1	52.2	88.5	61.3	45.7
	92.3	57.7	51.4	88.4	59.5	48.3
	90	60.8	52.5	90.7	57.4	45.4
	93.4	58.8	54.5	90.1	56	51.6
	92.6	60.3	51.2	84.8	62.4	51.1
	88.9	61	46.7	91.7	60.2	50.4
	85.9	60.3	46.1	89.5	58.3	52.9
	91.5	59	46.6	89.2	63.2	49.5
$\overline{X}$	90.34	59.82	50.51	89.32	59.86	49.68
Target	85	60	45	85	60	45
$\overline{X}$- Target	5.34	−0.18	**5.51**	4.32	−0.14	**4.68**
s	2.2495	1.1023	**2.9823**	1.9147	2.2192	**2.5245**

Table 6.11 *continued*

	GROUP 7			GROUP 8		
	ICU	**OR**	**X-RAY**	**ICU**	**OR**	**X-RAY**
	88.9	59.5	49.7	89.9	59.4	48.1
	89.1	58.1	52.6	89.8	61.2	47.5
	90.3	58.8	50.7	88.8	62.5	51.8
	86.8	58.5	51.8	87	56.1	50.8
	89.7	60.7	51.2	90.6	62.6	50.9
	91.8	57.9	47	91.2	58.4	43.2
	90.9	61.2	44.4	91	61.7	50.3
	90.7	58.7	55	90.6	61.8	45.7
	89.6	62.7	50.2	86.9	58.7	47.7
	87.1	62.5	52	86.8	60.8	55.8
$\overline{X}$	89.49	59.86	50.46	89.26	60.32	49.18
Target	85	60	45	85	60	45
$\overline{X}$- Target	4.49	−0.14	**5.46**	**4.26**	0.32	4.18
s	1.5968	1.7927	**2.9684**	1.7646	2.1086	**3.521**

ICU, intensive care unit; OR, operating room; X-ray, radiology.

is calculated with all of the *s*-values from all groups and for all data sources (all three wings). Therefore, the *s*-value indicates that the average airflow standard deviation is 2.32 cf/min across all three hospital units. The number *1* on the chart refers to the airflow for the intensive care unit, *2* refers to the operating room, and *3* represents airflow from x-ray. Because the MAX line is tagged only with the number *3*, airflow variation in x-ray is consistently greater than in the other wings, indicating an air regulator problem or some other issue that prevents the system from operating as consistently as the systems in the other units. Additionally, six of the eight MIN *s*-values are tagged with the number *1*, indicating that there is less airflow variation in the intensive care unit. These lower standard deviation numbers suggest that the air circulation unit is either newer, made by a different manufacturer, or in a better state of repair than the others.

The centerline on the group target $\overline{X}$ chart indicates that, on average, all three wings had airflow values that were higher than target by 3.16 cf/min. The MIN line indicates that the lowest airflow consistently came from number 2, the operating room suite. Although the operating room suite shows the lowest airflow when compared with the others, it also falls closest to its intended target airflow rate,

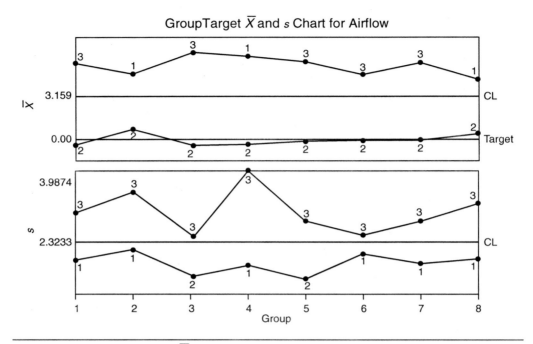

Figure 6.12 Group Target $\overline{X}$ and s-Chart: Airflow at St. Everywhere Hospital

which could translate into lower overall utility costs for the operating room suites while, at the same time, providing airflow which is close to ideal.

Half of the MAX plot points are from x-ray and half are from intensive care, indicating similar, consistently high airflow rates in both wings. The proximity of the target line to the MAX plot point line indicates that these two wings consistently produce airflow levels above their expected target value. This could mean that the air circulation units are being run harder than they need to be, resulting in higher utility costs and potentially shorter useful lives for the equipment.

Group target $\overline{X}$ and s-charts allow comparison of multiple characteristics with different targets to each other at the same time and on the same chart. Like the traditional $\overline{X}$ and s-chart, the group target $\overline{X}$ and s-chart has a fixed subgroup size that is greater than nine. The plot points on the group target $\overline{X}$ chart represent the MAX and MIN differences among different characteristics' group averages and their targets. Only the largest (MAX) and smallest (MIN) differences for a group are plotted on the group target $\overline{X}$ chart. On the group target s-chart, s-values are calculated for each of the characteristics within a group, then only the MAX and MIN s values for a group are plotted.

Ideally, the group target $\overline{X}$ and s-chart can be applied in a number of situations or studies that share the following features.

◆ Identical characteristics with different target values are to be compared with each other.
◆ Data collection opportunities are frequent and inexpensive, allowing large subgroup sizes.
◆ Subgroup size is fixed and greater than nine.
◆ Multiple characteristics will be plotted at the same time on a single chart.

◈ Discussion Points

1. Describe the concept of group control charts. How do they differ from regular control charts? How are they similar?
2. How can target control charts be used in health care organizations?
3. How are targets selected for the control chart?
4. Describe the three types of commonly used group control charts and contrast them with their standard control chart types.
5. How are control limits calculated for each type of control chart?
6. Target charts can also be displayed in group format. Under what circumstances would this approach be useful?
7. What advantages does a group chart have in comparison with a traditional control chart?

Chapter 7

Advanced Statistical Applications in Continuous Quality Improvement

DONALD E. LIGHTER

◆ Introduction

Although control charts provide a powerful way to analyze time-series data, some situations require other statistical approaches to evaluate the information needed by quality improvement teams. When the team is comparing the effects of two or more interventions on a process, they may wish to know which intervention(s) had statistically significant effects on the process. Such situations require more advanced approaches like regression analysis and analysis of variance to determine the degree to which process means vary. Additionally, many statistical techniques require an understanding of distributions, the way that the values of a random variable are distributed as data are collected in an experiment. These empirical distributions (i.e., those that are derived from direct measurements) often conform to theoretical distributions (those that are described by a specific mathematical equation that theoretically would describe the population if a very large number of observations are made), and the type of statistical analysis that can be performed on a data set relates directly to the match between the empirical and theoretical distributions. Although there are hundreds of theoretical distributions, only about a dozen are of practical use for continuous quality improvement purposes, and the most common of these will be discussed briefly in this chapter.

◆ Discrete Distributions

Discrete distributions are applied to variables that have specific outcomes, e.g., heads or tails, success or failure, conforming or nonconforming. Discrete variables often represent counts of events, such as numbers of Caesarean sections (C-sections) or episodes of otitis media (ear infections). These types of data are contrasted with continuous variables that can assume any value within a given interval, such as age or serum sodium values. One of the first tasks in performing advanced statistical studies, as for statistical process control, is to determine what type of data is being collected: discrete or continuous. The data type determines the mathematical approach to analysis, thus ensuring correct inferences from the data. The most useful means of distinguishing between discrete and continuous variables are listed in Table 7.1.

Binomial Distribution

Perhaps the most widely used of the discrete distributions, the binomial distribution applies to situations in which there are just two possible outcomes, often labeled success and failure. The success outcome typically is measured, and probabilities of success are inferred from the data. The designations of success and failure do not connote good and bad, simply two separate outcomes. Outcomes can include variables like heads or tails, dead or alive, improved or not improved. The binomial distribution usually finds application when sample sizes are small, but it may be used for any sample size.

Binomial trials consist of a limited number of experiments, denoted by η, that are independent. The probability of success on any given trial is the same for all the experiments, and the outcome in any trial is not influenced by the outcomes of any of the other experiments. The classic example of a binomial experiment consists of a series of coin tosses with either heads or tails as a result. Calculation of probabilities for these experiments is beyond the scope of this book but can be found in nearly any basic statistics textbook.

The parameters for the binomial distribution are generally represented by π and N, with π representing the proportion of successes and N represent-

Table 7.1 Differentiation: Discrete vs Continuous Variables

	DISCRETE VARIABLE	CONTINUOUS VARIABLE
Characteristics	• Fixed numeric values • No intermediate values between fixed values	• Infinite number of values within an interval • Measurement is usually an estimate of the true value depending on the measurement tool
Examples	• Number of extremities • Episodes of diabetic ketoacidosis • Number of people with hypertension	• Body weight • Systolic blood pressure • Duration of treatment

ing the size of the sample. Using these parameters, the mean of the sampling distribution (μ) is Nπ, and the variance is calculated by

$$(7.1) \quad \sigma^2 = N\pi(1-\pi)$$

When $N\pi \geq 5$ and $N(1-\pi) \geq 5$, the binomial distribution approximates the normal distribution. The parameters define the shape of the binomial curve. The primary application of the binomial distribution in quality improvement (QI) is to evaluate pass and fail outcomes and estimate probabilities of failure.

Poisson Distribution

Primarily directed at populations with rare events, the Poisson distribution is used as the basis for control charts that deal with nonconformities, i.e., relatively rare defects that indicate that a process is not functioning according to specifications. Industrial applications describe the nonconforming unit, which is a unit of production that has enough nonconformities that the unit is rejected. Nonconformities in health care might be nonfatal postoperative infections or episodes of pneumonia that do not respond to appropriate initial antibiotic therapy. There are some basic assumptions that must be met by the data set for the use of the Poisson distribution.

◆ The nonconformities should be independent and random.
◆ The potential number of nonconformities must be quite large (defined in textbooks as infinitely large) and the actual number quite small.

In most applications, the assumptions can only be approximated, so use of the Poisson distribution is generally reserved for those situations where the nonconformity rate is very small. Most notably, the requirement that nonconformities be independent and random often cannot be strictly satisfied because health care decisions are often influenced by factors other than random chance. The Poisson distribution is similar to the binomial distribution and approximates that curve when N is large and π is small.

Hypergeometric Distribution

This discrete distribution is subtly different from the binomial, but it has important applications in the science of QI. The hypergeometric distribution, unlike the binomial, assumes that the sample for measurement is taken from the population without replacement. For example, suppose that a managed care organization knows that the rate of fraud in its network of 1000 providers is 0.014. The hypergeometric distribution would be used to determine the probability that a random sample of 50 providers would include at least one fraudulent provider. Assuming that the fraudulent provider would be removed from the network, the sampling operation would influence the number and the frequency of fraudulent providers remaining in the network. The hypergeometric distribution thus finds application in QI problems in which sampling the population can alter the rate of nonconformity.

◆ Continuous Distributions

In contrast to discrete distributions, continuous distributions represent populations that can have infinitely many values, usually within a finite range. Body heights are often used as an example of a continuous distribution because heights within a population can assume infinitely many values between two finite limits. Although height is measured rather imprecisely, usually only to the closest quarter of an inch or centimeter, the measurement is an approximation for the actual height of each individual in the population, which can have an infinite number of values. This distinction is important when deciding if a data set conforms to a continuous distribution, rather than one that is discrete.

For continuous variables, the most commonly used graphical representation is the probability density function, which can be a histogram but is most often a continuous curve. An example of the Gaussian distribution is included as Figure 7.1. The x-axis represents each value of x, while the y-axis plots the proportion of the population represented by that value of x. These distributions and curves form the statistical foundation of QI.

Normal (Gaussian) Distribution

Probably the most familiar distribution for nearly anyone who has ever received a grade in school, the Gaussian distribution is the basis for what

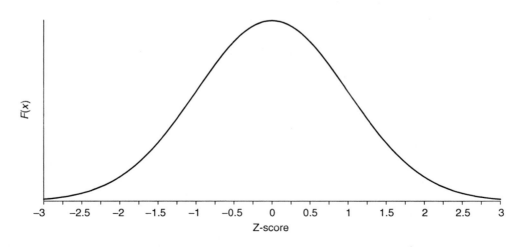

Figure 7.1 Example of Gaussian (Normal) Distribution

$F(x) = y$ term in the standard normal distribution.

many people call grading on the curve. The Gaussian distribution is often termed the "normal" distribution, and it is represented by the equation

(7.2)
$$f(y) = \frac{1}{\sigma\sqrt{2\pi}} e^{-1/2[(y-\mu)/\sigma]^2}$$

where σ is the standard deviation of the population,
μ is the mean of the population,
e is the natural logarithm base = 2.71828 ..., and
π is the geometric constant, π = 3.14159 ...

The limits for the normal distribution are −∞ to +∞. As should be readily apparent, the two parameters μ and σ can vary infinitely, leading to an infinite number of normal distributions. Thus, the normal distribution can be thought of as a family of curves that vary by the population mean and standard deviation. One specific distribution that has broad applicability is the standard normal distribution, obtained by the following transformation

(7.3)
$$Z = \frac{X-\mu}{\sigma}$$

where all terms are the same as defined in equation 7.2, and *Z* is the standard normal distribution score. This transformation can be applied to any normal distribution to obtain a distribution with μ = 0 and σ = 1—i.e., the standard normal distribution. This distribution is particularly useful when discussing populations because *Z*-scores represent the number of standard deviations from the mean. For example, a variable *X* can be transformed via the above equation, and the value of *Z* is the number of standard deviations from the mean that the value of *X* represents. Thus, a *Z*-score of 2.5 indicates that *X* is 2.5 standard deviations from the mean.

Characteristics that must be met for data to be analyzed by a normal distribution are those for any continuous distribution.

◆ The population must be randomly distributed.
◆ Variables can assume any of an infinite number of values along a continuum.
◆ The mean and standard deviation of the population can be measured or calculated.

Although the population mean and standard deviation are not usually known in most practical situations, estimates of these parameters from sample data generally suffice.

Normal distributions underlie nearly all commonly used control charts. Charts such as the $\overline{X}$ and range (*R*) charts, as well as many others that rely on the mean and standard deviation, are based on the assumption that the population is approximately normally distributed and that sample means are also approximately normally distributed. Only in special situations such as rare nonconformities will other types of charts become more appropriate. In spite of the ubiquity of the normal distribution, other types of continuous distributions are used in QI.

t-Distribution

Another of the more famous distributions in statistics is the t-distribution, sometimes called Student's t-distribution after W. S. Gosset, whose pseudonym was "Student." Gosset worked as a beer brewer, and his samples tended to be small, with unknown population means and standard deviations. The t-distribution conforms to the following equality

(7.4)
$$t = \frac{\overline{X} - \mu}{s / \sqrt{n}}$$

where $\overline{X}$ is the mean of the sample,
  μ is mean of the population,
  s is the standard deviation of the sample, and
  n is sample size

The t-distribution generally assumes the shape of a standard normal distribution, but the adjustment for the sample size changes the variability (flatness) of the curve. The sample size defines a parameter called the "degrees of freedom," which is $n - 1$. A comparison of a t-curve with the standard normal distribution can be found in Figure 7.2. A number of calculators for producing t-statistics and curves can now be found on the Internet (Gerdes, 1999). In general, the t-distribution is well approximated by the normal distribution as n becomes larger (>30).

The primary application of the t-distribution in QI occurs in performing hypothesis testing and designing experiments to compare means from different population samples. Specifically designed for situations in which the population standard deviation is unknown, the t-distribution has been generalized to evaluate any parameter via the following equation

(7.5)
$$t = \frac{\hat{\theta} - \theta}{s_{\hat{\theta}}}$$

where $\hat{\theta}$ is the estimate of the parameter based on the data,
  θ is the actual value of the parameter being estimated, and
  $s_{\hat{\theta}}$ is the sample estimator of the standard deviation of the parameter

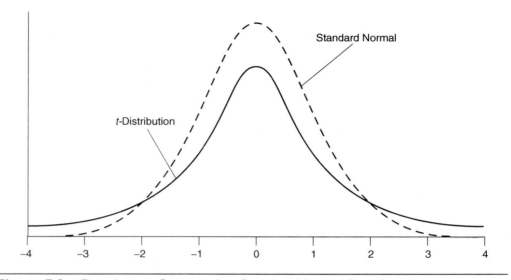

Figure 7.2 *t*-Distribution Compared to Standard Normal Distribution

The *t*-distribution can thus be used to evaluate any parameter that is approximately normally distributed, not just sample means. This property of the distribution makes it very valuable as a statistical tool in QI.

Hypothesis testing will be described in some detail later in this chapter under "Statistical Inference," but a brief description here will demonstrate the value of the *t*-test in evaluating the probability that two means are different. In most cases, an experiment is performed to demonstrate that the means of two populations are different. For example, when testing a new drug, the population of people who received the drug presumably had a better outcome than the population of people who did not receive the drug. However, rather than prove that the results in the two populations are different, statistical tests are designed instead to prove that they are not the same. Although the distinction may seem purely semantic, from a statistical standpoint the difference between the two statements is important because it directly determines the hypothesis that is tested mathematically. In most cases, the experimenter typically states the hypothesis for the trial as the opposite of what is to be proven. This null hypothesis, usually denoted as H_0, postulates that two means are equal, and the goal of the experiment is to demonstrate that the null hypothesis is incorrect, called "rejecting the null hypothesis."

The alternative hypothesis, labeled H_1, states that the two population means are unequal or that one mean is greater (or less) than the other. The *t*-test will provide a *p*-value that represents the probability that the difference between the means of the two randomly selected samples from the population will be as large as or larger than actually observed. A two-tailed *p*-value indicates the probability that the actual difference in the means of the random samples is as large as or larger than the observed difference with either group having the larger mean, whereas a one-tailed *p*-value indicates that same probability but also that one of the two groups (specified before the experiment is performed) has the larger mean. *p*-Values of 0.05 and less are considered for most purposes to be a reasonable level for rejecting the null hypothesis that there is no difference in the means and adopting the alternative hypothesis that the disparity is due to real differences between the population means. It is important to remember that the *p*-value does not provide the probability that the null hypothesis is correct; in fact, it is the probability that the differences in the means could be at least as great as or greater than what was observed in the experiment.

χ^2 Distribution

The χ^2 distribution's probability density function, i.e., the curve, assumes values only between zero and infinity, and the number of degrees of freedom determines the shape of the curve. The advantage of the χ^2 statistic lies in its ability to measure the strength of a relationship, and the statistic depends on the size of the sample used to examine the relationship. The χ^2 statistic finds its most common application in contingency tables, which summarize data between discrete variables with multiple values or categories. A representative 2×2 (read two by two) contingency table is shown in Table 7.2. Comparisons such as that in Table 7.2 are common in QI interventions because in many cases, more than one intervention may be thought to have some benefit. Thus, a QI team may decide to implement two improvements in the system and evaluate each improvement at two different levels to determine which proves most efficacious. For example, an operating room team may test two different types of sterilization for two different lengths of time to determine the effect on bacterial colony counts on instrument packs used in surgical procedures. After gathering data, the team then needs to determine if the differences between the outcomes reaches a sufficient level of statistical significance. For most purposes, researchers adopt a level of significance in which the chance that the results could be due to random error is less than 5%, usually deemed $p < 0.05$.

The χ^2 statistic is used so frequently that computer spreadsheet programs now have built in χ^2 functions that calculate the results of the χ^2 analysis for contingency tables of various sizes. Table 7.2 compares two categories of interventions with two outcomes, but much larger contingency tables are possible. The nature of the relationship between two variables becomes important in the χ^2 analysis because the statistic depends on both the strength of the relationship and the size of the sample in which the comparison is performed. A very weak relationship will require immense sample sizes to become apparent, and a very strong relationship may be unapparent if the sample sizes are too small. Thus, lack of a statistical relationship in the

Table 7.2 2 × 2 Contingency Table

	LEVEL 1	LEVEL 2	TOTAL
Improvement 1	157	293	450
Improvement 2	379	127	506
Total	536	420	956

context of a χ^2 analysis may not imply that one does not exist, only that the relationship was too weak or that the sample size was too small.

F-Distribution

The F-distribution is another family of probability density functions defined by the ratio of two sample estimates for the population variance. The F-statistic compares two sample variances from a given population to determine if the variances are equal; if the sample variances are equal, then the F-ratio is one. The samples are often different in size and composition and may come from the same or different populations. Because the sample sizes are different, the numerator and denominator have different degrees of freedom, usually denoted as m and n. The probability density function of the F-ratio of sample variances defines a family of distributions that are characterized by the two degrees of freedom, as in Figure 7.3.

Most commonly used in analysis of variance (ANOVA) to evaluate the equality of sample means, the F-ratio is defined by the following equality

(7.6)
$$F_{\alpha(m,n)} = \frac{s_m^2}{s_n^2}$$

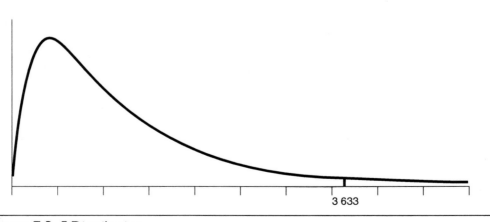

3 633

Figure 7.3 *F*-Distribution

Numerator degrees of freedom = 4; denominator degrees of freedom = 9; p = 0.05; F-critical value = 3.633.

where $F_{\alpha(m, n)}$ is the F ratio for significance level α and degrees of freedom m and n,

s_m^2 is the sample variance of sample m, and

s_n^2 is the sample variance of sample n

The significance level, α (alpha), is generally set at 0.05. The results of ANOVA include a p-value, which represents the probability that the results of the analysis match the assumption of the null hypothesis.

◆ Statistical Inference

In most cases, the distribution of the variable that is being studied is unknown. When sample sizes are large, it is generally safe to assume that the distribution of sample means conforms to the normal distribution, but the size of the sample needed to make the inference of a normal distribution can vary. In some instances, such as when the data assume a χ^2 distribution, a sample size of 15 or 20 may be sufficient. On the other hand, when a population seems to be radically different from the normal distribution, large sample sizes or other mathematical techniques such as logarithmic conversion may be necessary for analysis of the data. The tendency for sample means to approximate a normal distribution as sample size increases is known as the central limit theorem. The important implication of the theorem is the ability to use the normal distribution to make statistical inferences about the mean of a population, even if the variable is not normally distributed. Thus, if sample sizes are sufficiently large, then the samples can be analyzed using statistical principles based on the normal distribution. This fact underlies much of the science of control charting in statistical process control.

The inferences that are made from samples are generally estimates of population parameters, e.g., the population mean, standard deviation, and proportion of the population with a particular characteristic of interest. The corresponding representations are listed in Table 7.3. Once these estimators are known, they can be applied to other useful statistical descriptors, such as the confidence interval. Confidence intervals provide a range of values between which there is a defined probability of finding the population mean. Most frequently used is the 95% confidence interval, which simply means that there is a 95% probability of finding the parameter of interest in the defined interval. For a normal distribution, the 95% confidence interval corresponds closely to 1.96 standard deviations on either side of the mean, so knowing the population standard deviation allows calculation of confidence intervals around the mean. Confidence intervals are usually in the form of the mean ± 1.96 standard deviations for a normally distributed population.

Another important use of distributions in statistical inference includes hypothesis testing. As a QI team is examining the results of an intervention,

Table 7.3 Population Parameters and Their Sample Statistics

PARAMETER	POPULATION	SAMPLE
Mean	μ	$\overline{X}$
Standard deviation (variance)	σ (σ^2)	σ (σ^2)
Proportion	P	$\hat{p}$

the group must frequently determine if an intervention made a significant difference in the outcome of the process. Hypothesis testing provides a way to make this determination. In a typical scenario, the team plans an intervention after performing initial measurements to determine the most likely output from a process. A null hypothesis (H_0) then posits that the intervention will have no effect on the output. The intervention is implemented over a period of time to determine if there is any influence on the process, followed by remeasurement of the output. The results of the new output are then compared to the expected results (no change in output), and the appropriate statistic is calculated to determine if significant differences exist between the output after the intervention and the output that was expected with no intervention. If the differences are determined to be significant, then the null hypothesis is rejected, and the exercise concludes with the fact that the intervention caused a change. The statistic that is used to determine significance will depend on the distribution of the data and on the size of the sample. If the sample size is very large, then the normal distribution may be used to determine significance. If the sample size is limited, then other distributions may be used that match the characteristics of the data.

◆ ANOVA

ANOVA is a statistical technique that deals with variation both within and between groups. Application of ANOVA in health care has always been an important approach to evaluating treatment regimens and analyzing medical data. Many published studies in the medical literature use the ANOVA approach to assess clinical data. The goal of any statistical analysis is to glean the truth about relationships between variables from data that have incumbent errors based on sample variation and process variability. ANOVA is one tool that can be applied to achieve that goal.

Simply stated, ANOVA provides a method of determining whether to affirm or reject the null hypothesis that all population means are equal. For example, a QI team may want to evaluate four different approaches to improving a process before adopting a single procedure. After evaluating the process with each of the four interventions, the degree of improvement of each intercession must be evaluated to determine if the approach was better than the other three. Using ANOVA, the team can determine which of the approaches demonstrated a statistically significant process improvement. In very few cases are the changes different enough to allow ready inference of which treatment is clearly superior, and ANOVA can be used to deduce which of the interventions is preferred.

ANOVA procedures are designed to separate the effects of random error from the effect of an intervention or treatment. Any real-life experiment will have a certain level of variation in the measured effect due to random events not related to the experiment. ANOVA accounts for these random errors while discerning what degree of change in the mean is due to the treatment effect. Essentially, ANOVA separates the total sum of squares (SS) into two parts: one for the differences between groups and the other due to random error. Regression analysis, a topic explored later in this chapter, is another method of performing this type of analysis, and many of the same assumptions and techniques apply to that method as well.

Assumptions for ANOVA

For each treatment group being analyzed, the following relationship applies:

$$(7.7) \quad y = \mu_t + \varepsilon$$

where y is the variable being studied,
$\quad \mu_t$ is the mean of the treatment group t, and
$\quad \varepsilon$ is the normally distributed error

The error term is assumed to be normally distributed, with a population mean of zero and variance defined as σ^2. Defined as a means model, the mean of the tth treatment group, μ_t, is assumed to be the same for all treatment groups because the mean value of the error term is zero. Thus, the following assumptions must be made for ANOVA.

◆ All treatment group observations have the same mean.
◆ Errors are normally distributed and independent.
◆ Errors have a constant variance.

These assumptions can be verified in each ANOVA by creating a graph, such as a histogram, of the observations in each treatment group. If the difference between the means of the treatment groups is large, e.g., if the spread of the observations is different between groups, then the error variance may not be constant. If the graph has outliers, then the assumption of normally distributed error terms may not be correct. Any ANOVA experiment in which samples must be collected sequentially should always be suspected of having error terms that are not independent. In most cases, however, ANOVA experiments can be designed to reduce or eliminate the problem of autocorrelation when results in one time period influence subsequent measurements.

Mathematical Basis for ANOVA

Although this book is not designed as a textbook in statistics, it is useful to understand the basic mathematical underpinnings of ANOVA in order to better understand the output from these programs. SS analyses are designed to determine the closeness with which a mathematical model fits the available data, and this approach provides the basis for many common statistical analyses of data sets. ANOVA uses a property of SS analysis that allows a total SS to be segregated into component parts, as in equation 7.8

$$(7.8) \quad \sum(x - \bar{x})^2 = \sum(x - \hat{x})^2 + n\sum(\hat{x} - \bar{x})^2$$

where x represents each data point,
$\bar{x}$ represents the sample mean,
$\hat{x}$ represents the mean of each subpopulation, and
n represents the size of each subpopulation

The term on the left side of the equality represents the total SS, whereas the terms on the right side of the equation represent the error SS (often called the within-groups SS and the between-groups SS, respectively). Separating these sources of variation is the basis of the ANOVA because the differences in group means caused by random error can be isolated from the differences that are caused by the treatment or intervention. Thus, ANOVA can afford a QI team the ability to determine if differences between treatment groups result from random events that cannot be controlled during the experiment or to the intervention designed by the team.

Computers have made ANOVA much easier. Most computer programs that perform ANOVA have fairly standard output, as shown in Table 7.4, which includes the two types of variation as well as SS and the F-statistic. The columns in the table contain the parameters of interest for the within-groups and between-groups variances and are defined as follows

df = degrees of freedom, calculated as the sample size minus the number of parameters being estimated,
SS = the sum of squares for each variance (equation 7.8)
Mean squares = SS/df
= variance of the sample
F = the ratio of the mean squares

If the between-groups SS is very large, then the difference between the sample means is very large, indicating a large number of groups or a large variation between the groups. The degrees of freedom column provides an

Table 7.4 Output from ANOVA Computer Program

Source of Variation	Degrees of Freedom	Sum of Squares	Mean Square	F
Between Groups	1	0.063	0.063	0.70
Within Groups	18	1.626	0.090	
Total	19	1.689		

estimate of sample sizes so that the reason for a large SS can be quickly determined.

The mean squares represent the variances for each group. Within-group variance values reflect the degree of variation of the means within each group, providing valuable information about the variation due to error. If the variance resulting from between-group variation is small relative to the variance attributable to error, then the means in the samples differ from one another. The F-ratio makes that comparison by dividing the between-groups variance by the within-groups variance. The magnitude of the F-ratio indicates the degree with which the variation resulting from actual differences between groups varies from the variation within groups. A large F-ratio indicates a significant difference between groups, meaning that the alternative hypothesis should be adopted and that the differences are most likely due to the treatment effect. On the other hand, a smaller F-ratio connotes that the differences are not significant, mandating that the null hypothesis should be accepted because there is no difference detectable between the sample means. Stated simply, a large F-value specifies that the differences between groups are statistically significant, whereas a small F-value indicates that the differences are either not statistically significant or attributable to error. Most programs also report a p-value, indicating the level of significance for the difference and validating a decision to accept or reject the null hypothesis.

Applications in QI

ANOVA is an extremely useful statistical tool for QI, as evidenced by the following case study showing how the technique is used in practice.

Example 7-1

St. Anywhere Hospital was having difficulty reducing the waiting time for surgeons between cases in the operating room. After preliminary studies indicated that cleaning the rooms was the major time factor, the surgical support staff implemented a new program of notifying the environmental services department of the need to clean a room approximately 15 minutes before each case had ended. That extra time allowed the environmental services staff enough time to assign a technician to start cleaning the suite almost immediately after the present case ended. The null hypothesis, H_0, posits that the mean times before and after the intervention are not different. The alternative hypothesis, H_1, becomes that the mean times are different. H_1 requires a two-tailed test because the result of the intervention could be either better or worse waiting times. Twenty-five waiting times were randomly selected over a 2-week period before and after the intervention and recorded in Exhibit 7-1. The ANOVA performed by the analysis add-in package in Microsoft Excel is included as Table 7.5. The analysis in Table 7.5 shows that the intervention was deemed effective, with an F-value of 20.134 and a p-value of 0.0000451, which statisticians would report as $p < 0.001$. Thus, the group rejected H_0 and accepted H_1 that the mean times between the before and after groups were different. Because the mean time for

Exhibit 7-1 Surgical Waiting Times Example

ST. ANYWHERE HOSPITAL SURGICAL WAITING TIMES PROJECT	
BEFORE	**AFTER**
15	10
35	15
20	25
45	10
20	10
15	20
25	15
15	20
35	25
25	15
35	10
20	20
30	35
30	15
25	10
35	20
20	10
25	15
45	15
35	20
30	10
15	15
20	10
20	20
25	25

Table 7.5 ANOVA for Surgical Waiting Times

ANOVA: SINGLE FACTOR
SUMMARY

GROUPS	COUNT	SUM	AVERAGE	VARIANCE
Before	25	660	26.4	78.17
After	25	415	16.6	41.08

ANOVA

SOURCE OF VARIATION	SS	DF	MS	F	p-VALUE	F-CRIT
Between Groups	1200.5	1	1200.5	20.13	<0.001	4.04
Within Groups	2862	48	59.625			
Total	4062.5	49				

ANOVA, analysis of variance; SS, sums of squares; df, degrees of freedom; MS, mean square.

the group after the intervention was smaller, the intervention was deemed a success.

The example demonstrates the use of ANOVA to analyze the effect of a single intervention for one variable. Although the sample sizes were the same in this instance because of the symmetric experimental design chosen by the staff, sample sizes do not need to be equal as the next example will show. In that example we will also see how ANOVA can be used for much more complex problems.

Example 7-2

Buoyed by their initial success with the notification of environmental services, the operating room staff decided to tackle the other four problems that they had identified. An intervention was designed for each of the problems, and measurements before and after each intervention were made. Because the staff had a limited amount of time and money to make these changes, they decided to perform each intervention on a single operating room. The rooms were chosen because they were very similar in the types of equipment, staff, volume, and cases performed during the preliminary time study. H_0 for this study hypothesized that the means of the intervention groups did not differ from one another, and H_1 stated that the means differed. Tables 7.6 and 7.7 show the results of the data collection and ANOVA. Another Microsoft Excel add-in called StatPlus was used to perform the analysis, which is reported in Table 7.7.

Notable in Table 7.7 is the addition of a correction factor, termed the Bonferroni correction, in the second matrix (pairwise comparison

Table 7.6 St. Anywhere Waiting Time Experiment

ST. ANYWHERE HOSPITAL

SURGICAL WAITING TIMES PROJECT

BEFORE: ALL ROOMS	AFTER: ROOM 1	AFTER: ROOM 2	AFTER: ROOM 3	AFTER: ROOM 4
15	30	10	35	15
35	10	14	30	10
20	22	15	28	20
45	18	19	24	25
20	20	10	32	10
15	35	14	19	13
25	45	15	25	15
15	20	19	27	15
35	15	24	15	14
25	25	30	19	16
35	10	14	28	17
20	20	18	18	18
30	24	19	29	19
30	20	10	30	10
25	18	13	32	5
35	23	15	38	
20	28	19	20	
25	27	14	17	
45		18	19	
35		22		
30				
15				
20				
20				
25				

probabilities: Bonferroni correction). Because multiple comparisons are being performed, the probability of rejecting at least one true null hypothesis increases; thus, some statisticians impose a correction factor to the *p*-values, multiplying each *p*-value by the number of tests in order to reduce the probability of making this type of error. Any time multiple comparisons are made, the Bonferroni correction provides some assurance against inappropriate rejection of a true null hypothesis.

Table 7.7 Between-Groups ANOVA: St. Anywhere Waiting Time Experiment

PAIRWISE MEAN DIFFERENCE (ROW–COLUMN)

	AFTER: ROOM 1	AFTER: ROOM 2	AFTER: ROOM 3	AFTER: ROOM 4
After: Room 1	0	6.178	−2.749	7.98
After: Room 2		0	−8.926	1.8
After: Room 3			0	10.73
After: Room 4				0
MSE = 41.339				

PAIRWISE COMPARISON PROBABILITIES (BONFERRONI CORRECTION)

	AFTER: ROOM 1	AFTER: ROOM 2	AFTER: ROOM 3	AFTER: ROOM 4
After: Room 1	1.000	**0.026**	1.000	**0.004**
After: Room 2		1.000	**0.000**	1.000
After: Room 3			1.000	**0.000**
After: Room 4				1.000

Using the SS in each of the matrices for the four interventions, an overall F-statistic is calculated by summing the mean SS for between-group variation and dividing that value by the sum of the mean SS for within-group variation as follows

$$F = \frac{137.307 + 1067.11 + 8.24 + 1261.5}{75.295 + 19.57 + 63.637 + 58.17} = \frac{2474.157}{216.672} = 11.419$$

The F-value of 11.419 is significant at $p < 0.001$, indicating that further analysis of each factor can be performed. As can be seen from the first matrix in Table 7.7 (pairwise mean differences: row–column), differences existed between nearly all of the measured mean waiting times, ranging from as little as 1.8 minutes to as much as 10.7 minutes. The second matrix (pairwise comparison probabilities: Bonferroni correction) reduces the relationships to p-values, and significant p-values are noted in bold type. Thus, the experiment demonstrated that differences existed between the interventions. Because a difference exists, the group needs to know which of the interventions contributed to the difference. A similar analysis is performed to test the individual hypotheses for each of the interventions or H_0. No difference exists between the mean waiting times before and after the intervention. A one-way ANOVA was performed for the four interventions, using the baseline data, with the results presented in Table 7.8. The results of the analysis indicate that *interventions 2* and *4* were effective, but *interventions 1* and *3* were not. Thus, H_0 would be accepted for *interventions 1* and *3*, but rejected for *interventions 2* and *4*.

Although these analyses may seem rather complicated, even more complex evaluations can be performed with ANOVA and the concept of factorial experiments. Many situations in medical organizations call for interventions in very different environments, adding more factors for analysis by ANOVA. For example, the St. Anywhere experiment with four different interventions could have been complicated by differences in the operating rooms in which

Table 7.8 Comparison of Interventions with Baseline Waiting Times

ANOVA: SINGLE FACTOR—INTERVENTION 1
SUMMARY

GROUPS	COUNT	SUM	AVERAGE	VARIANCE
Before: All Rooms	25	660	26.4	78.167
After: Room 1	18	410	22.8	71.242

ANOVA

SOURCE OF VARIATION	SS	DF	MS	F	*p*-VALUE	F CRIT
Between Groups	137.307	1	137.307	1.824	0.18	4.08
Within Groups	3087.111	41	75.295			
Total	3224.419	42				

ANOVA: SINGLE FACTOR—INTERVENTION 2
SUMMARY

GROUPS	COUNT	SUM	AVERAGE	VARIANCE
Before: All Rooms	25	660	26.4	78.167
After: Room 2	20	332	16.6	24.674

ANOVA

SOURCE OF VARIATION	SS	DF	MS	F	*p*-VALUE	F CRIT
Between Groups	1067.111	1	1067.11	19.57	**<0.001**	4.07
Within Groups	2344.8	43	54.53			
Total	3411.911	44				

continues

Table 7.8 *continued*

ANOVA: Single Factor—Intervention 3
SUMMARY

Groups	Count	Sum	Average	Variance
Before: All Rooms	25	660	26.4	78.167
After: Room 3	19	485	25.526	44.263

ANOVA

Source of Variation	SS	DF	MS	F	*p*-value	F crit
Between Groups	8.240	1	8.240	0.13	0.72	4.07
Within Groups	2672.737	42	63.637			
Total	2680.977	43				

ANOVA: Single Factor—Intervention 4
SUMMARY

Groups	Count	Sum	Average	Variance
Before: All Rooms	25	660	26.4	78.167
After: Room 4	15	222	14.8	23.886

ANOVA

Source of Variation	SS	DF	MS	F	*p*-value	F crit
Between Groups	1261.5	1	1261.5	21.69	**<0.001**	4.10
Within Groups	2210.4	38	58.17			
Total	3471.9	39				

St. Anywhere operating room waiting times experiment.

the interventions were made. Suppose that two of the operating rooms had automated anesthesia equipment and the other two had older equipment, which changed the rate at which patients could be induced and recover from anesthesia. The differences in the rooms would add another factor to the experiment—anesthesia equipment with two levels, automated and manual. The intervention experiment would become a two-way analysis of variance, with two factors: one with two levels and the other with four levels. The mean waiting time between cases would then be defined by the following equality

mean waiting time = overall mean + intervention effect + anesthesia equipment effect + interaction + error

The two-way ANOVA models can also be expressed as a means model, just like the one-way models.

$$(7.9) \quad y_{ijk} = \mu_{ij} + \varepsilon_{ijk}$$

where y_{ijk} is the outcome variable for the ith level of one factor and the jth level of the other factor for the kth replicate,

μ_{ij} is the mean for the ith level of one factor and the jth level of the other factor, and

ε_{ijk} is the error for the ith level of one factor and the jth level of the other factor, for the kth replicate

Replicates occur when there are multiple observations for each combination. The error term accounts for replicates, assuming a normal distribution of the error terms with mean 0 and variance σ^2.

Graphs are useful tools to visually evaluate the distribution of the data (assumed to be independent and normally distributed) and the relative equality of the variances (assumed to be virtually equal). Frequency histograms are useful for assessing the distribution, and box plots provide more information about variance. These charts were performed for the data in the two-way ANOVA experiment and are included as Figure 7.4 and Figure 7.5.

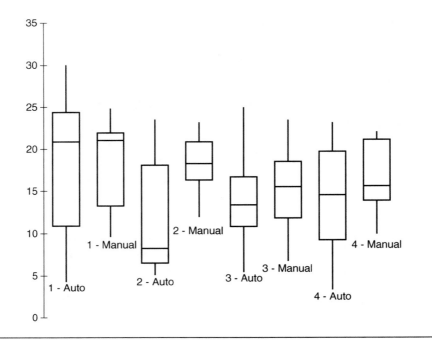

Figure 7.4 Box Plot for Surgical Waiting Time Data

Numbers, intervention type; Manual/Auto, anesthesia equipment type.

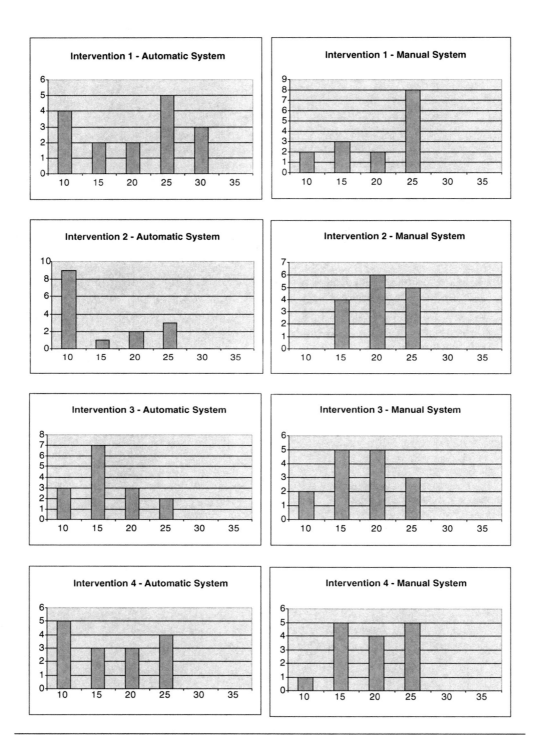

Figure 7.5 Histograms for Surgical Waiting Time Data

The box plot in Figure 7.4 displays the data distribution by quartiles. The line inside the box represents the median of the data, and the top and bottom edges of the box are plotted by the third and first quartiles, respectively. The lines emanating from each end of the plot indicate the upper and lower range of the data. The length of the lines, called whiskers by statisticians, can be no greater than 1.5 times the interquartile range defined by the upper and lower limits of the box (defined as the inner fences of the plot). Although no outliers appear on this plot, any points that fall outside the inner fences are plotted individually and appear as points on the graph.

Histograms, shown in Figure 7.5, also provide information regarding distribution of the data. The graphs shown in the figure are known as frequency histograms because they reflect the frequency of sample values at each interval. For this analysis, intervals of 5 minutes were chosen: 5 minutes, 10 minutes, 15 minutes, etc. The number of values within each of these ranges was then plotted to produce the histogram for each interval. The histograms indicate only moderate conformity with the assumption of a normal distribution of the data, but with samples of this size, such distributions are not unusual.

A two-way ANOVA for the mean waiting time influenced by the four interventions and the anesthesia equipment is presented in Table 7.9. The output from the ANOVA program includes three effects, in contrast to the one-way analysis, which had only one effect. A great deal of information about the relative importance of each of the factors can be gleaned from the mean SS data. Each of the SS contributes to the total, and the relative contribution of each can be ascertained by observing the relative values of each mean SS. The rows represent each factor, as follows

sample (row) effect ....intervention type (4 levels)
columns effect....................anesthesia equipment type (2 levels)
interaction effect...............effect produced by combining factors
within groups ....effect of variation within each group (error)

The within-groups mean SS appears to be the smallest and thus is the least contributor to the total SS. The other effects are substantially smaller, and the significance of the relatively small differences between the factors cannot be appreciated until the SS values are corrected for degrees of freedom, leading to mean square (MS) values. Because they are adjusted for degrees of freedom, the MS values convey the relative importance of the variance of each factor. F-values, noted before to be ratios of variances, are calculated by dividing each MS by the MS for the within-groups MS, to provide the relative importance of each factor relative to random error. A large F-value indicates that the factor MS is very important in producing the variation between samples, thus indicating a statistically significant factor effect. The table includes the p-value for each F-statistic, as well as the critical F-value for a significance level of 0.05.

Table 7.9 Two-Way ANOVA for St. Anywhere Surgical Waiting Times

ANOVA

Source of Variation	SS	DF	MS	F	p-value	F crit
Sample	251.72	3	83.91	2.47	0.07	2.68
Columns	207.95	1	207.95	6.12	0.01	3.92
Interaction	157.61	3	52.54	1.55	0.21	2.68
Within	4074.84	120	33.96			
Total	4692.12	127				

In the mean surgical waiting time example, the results of the ANOVA are presented in Table 7.9. The sample effect, which reflects the influence of the first factor (intervention type), has an F-value of 2.47, which is very close to the F-critical ($p = 0.05$) value of 2.68; this proximity is reflected by the p-value of 0.06, which is only slightly greater than the desired level of 0.05. On the other hand, the columns (anesthesia equipment type) effect is significant, with an F-value greater than the F-critical value and a p-value of 0.01. The interaction effect relates the intervention type and anesthesia equipment type to determine if an interaction between the two factors has a significant effect on the mean waiting times. The relatively small F-value and a p-value of 0.20 indicate that little or no interaction factor exists in this experiment.

Although based on relatively complex statistical constructs, ANOVA provides a powerful tool in QI. Performance of these analyses can help identify the best interventions to achieve the goals of the QI team, and use of ANOVA in validating the results of interventions can help QI managers better justify corporate efforts at improvement.

◆ Regression Analysis

Perhaps one of the most versatile of statistical tools, regression analysis has been applied to a huge variety of situations in which possible relationships must be investigated. The simplest case, linear regression, relates a variable, termed a dependent variable, to a second variable, the independent variable, by the following equality

(7.10) $\quad y = \alpha + \beta x + \varepsilon$

where y is the dependent variable,
$\quad\quad\alpha$ is the y intercept term (can connote the value of y when x is zero, if applicable),
$\quad\quad\beta$ is regression coefficient, which is the slope parameter in the simple linear model,

x is the independent variable, and
ε is the error term

This equation defines the relationship between a dependent and an independent variable in a simple linear regression. The actual relationships should conform to a linear equation, such as $y = \alpha + \beta x$, and the coefficients in the linear regression above provide information on the strength and direction of the effect of the independent variable on the dependent variable. The sources of error in the equation usually include problems with variation in the sample data.

Multiple regression expands the utility of this technique to situations in which many independent variables are related to a dependent variable. Because most real-life conditions involve more than one independent variable influencing a dependent variable, multiple regression usually proves much more useful than simple linear regression.

The power of regression surpasses mere correlations between dependent and independent variables, however. If the model seems to adequately reflect the relationship between the variables, then regression equations can be used to predict the dependent variable from the independent variables. For QI applications, that feature of regression provides the ability to evaluate the potential outcomes of interventions in the future, particularly as conditions in the work environment change. For example, if a QI team has performed a regression analysis and determined that five factors are related to a particular outcome, then changing each of the factors in the regression equation should provide insight into changes in the outcome. Regression equations can thus be used to perform "what if?" analyses as QI teams are designing interventions to improve quality.

Assumptions for Regression

As with any statistical procedure, regression techniques require that data sets meet a few criteria before the procedure can be applied. Although almost the same, the assumptions for linear regression and multiple regression differ slightly, as detailed in Table 7.10. Unfortunately, these assumptions are rarely met perfectly in practice, but the regression technique is robust enough to tolerate some deviation from the requirements. The most important of these assumptions, however, is that of linearity. The relationships between independent and dependent variables must be nearly linear for regression to produce valid results.

Mathematical Basis for Regression

All regression methods are based on the concept of least squares, which finds a mathematical fit to the data that minimizes the variance of the data from the model estimated from the regression analysis. The method calculates residuals, which are the differences between the expected value for each

Table 7.10 Assumptions for Linear and Multiple Regression

TYPE	DATA SET REQUIREMENTS
Linear	• Data fit a straight line model
	• Errors are normally distributed with mean 0
	• Errors are independent
	• Errors have constant variance
Multiple	• Independent variables are linearly related to the dependent variable
	• Errors are normally distributed with mean 0
	• Errors are independent
	• Errors have constant variance

dependent variable data point and the actual value of the dependent variable obtained by collecting data. The residuals are then used in the following equation

$$(7.11) \quad \hat{\beta} = \frac{\sum (x_i - \bar{x})(y_i - \bar{y})}{\sum (x_i - \bar{x})^2}$$

where $\hat{\beta}$ is the regression coefficient or the slope parameter for a linear equation,

x_i is the ith observation of the independent variable x, and

y_i is the ith observation of the dependent variable y

The $\bar{x}$ and $\bar{y}$ terms are the means for the independent and dependent variables, respectively. Once the estimate for the slope is determined, the intercept term can be found by substituting the means for the independent and dependent variables and then solving the linear equation for $\hat{\alpha}$

$$(7.12) \quad \hat{\alpha} = \bar{y} - \hat{\beta}\bar{x}$$

The calculated values provide the basic parameter estimates for the regression model.

Although knowing the intercept and regression coefficient is the goal of the regression process, a number of other important issues must be addressed. In computerized regression analyses, a number of other statistics are reported that further define the relationship between dependent and independent variables. The first, called the coefficient of determination or R^2, relates the degree of variation in the dependent variable that can be assigned to the independent variable. This statistic is used to define the degree with which changes in y are related to changes in x, rather than just random error. R^2 values are reported as proportions (decimals), e.g., 0.556, but are usually thought of in terms of percentages, e.g., "55.6% of the variation in y is explained by x." Because R^2 is always positive, it provides no information on whether the effect is positive or negative. Because the direction of the effect is important, another statistic is often calculated, the correlation coefficient. Usually denoted by r, the correlation coefficient can be the square root of R^2 or can be calculated by the following

$$(7.13) \qquad r = \frac{\sum (x_i - \bar{x})(y_i - \bar{y})}{\sqrt{\sum (x_i - \bar{x})^2} \sqrt{\sum (y_i - \bar{y})^2}}$$

x_i is the ith observation of the independent variable x,
$\bar{x}$ is the mean of the ith set of independent variables,
y_i is the ith observation of the dependent variable y, and
$\bar{y}$ is the mean of the ith set of dependent variables

The numerator can be positive, negative, or even zero, so the value of r can indicate the direction of the effect of the independent variable on the dependent variable. It is important to note, however, that the correlation coefficient is different from the regression coefficient (compare equations 7.11 and 7.13). Where the regression coefficient can assume the value of any real number, the correlation coefficient will always be between –1 and +1.

For multiple regression, these statistics have a somewhat different interpretation. R^2, the coefficient of determination, now represents the relationship between all of the independent variables and the dependent variable. Other statistics that are usually reported include the multiple R or multiple correlation, which is the square root of R^2. The multiple correlation is the maximum correlation between the dependent variable and a combination of all of the independent variables.

An adjusted R^2 is often calculated for multiple regression analyses that account for degrees of freedom, providing more information about the relationship as new independent variables are added. In many cases, as new independent variables (sometimes called predictors) are added to the analysis, the value of R^2 will continue to increase and approach one. The adjusted R^2 calculates the effect of increasing the number of variables and reducing the degrees of freedom and helps determine if adding more variables will improve the model.

Standard errors are reported for all of the regression coefficients, in addition to t-statistics and p-values. These values come from a null hypothesis stated as H_0: all regression coefficients are equal to zero. Some programs also include upper and lower 95% confidence limit bounds for the coefficients. The t-statistic is calculated as the ratio between the coefficient and the standard error. These statistics are useful in determining which variables can be dropped from the model.

Table 7.11 Example ANOVA for Regression Analysis

ANOVA

	DF	SS	MS	F	p-VALUE
Regression	7	4138.253	591.179	2.495	0.083
Residual	29	6873.219	237.008		
Total	36	11,011.472			

Every multiple regression analysis also includes an ANOVA as part of its output. The ANOVA arises from the null hypothesis above, and it usually reports data in the format shown in Table 7.11. The now familiar format of the ANOVA report indicates the SS for the regression variables and the residuals (error terms), along with the F-value and p-value for the indicated degrees of freedom. Because the F-statistic is the ratio of the regression variance (MS) to the residual variance, a large F-value indicates that the variation due to the regression variables is statistically significant.

Many multiple regression programs will also provide a number of graphs that can be used to determine if the assumptions necessary for a valid analysis are met. These plots include

◆ observed dependent values vs predicted values
◆ residuals vs predicted values
◆ residuals vs independent variable values
◆ normal probability plot of residuals

These graphs help determine how closely the regression assumptions are met and should be evaluated before the results of the regression analysis are accepted.

The first graph, observed vs predicted values of dependent variables, confirms the fit between the data and the regression equation. An example scatterplot of observed vs predicted values is included as Figure 7.6. The goal of this analysis is not only to reduce the variation for each score to a minimal level but also to determine if the variation in predicted values is uniform throughout the range. In Figure 7.6, the variance of observed values seems fairly uniform throughout the range of the data, although the points seem to be less dispersed at higher values. However, the variance appears to be uniform enough to satisfy the regression assumption that the variance should be constant across all values.

Figure 7.7 presents the residual vs predicted values for the same data. This graph helps determine if the regression assumptions of linearity are satisfied. Because the residuals determine the degree of variation in the data, plotting the residuals against the predicted values provides a visual means for checking linearity. If a curved pattern appears in this plot, then

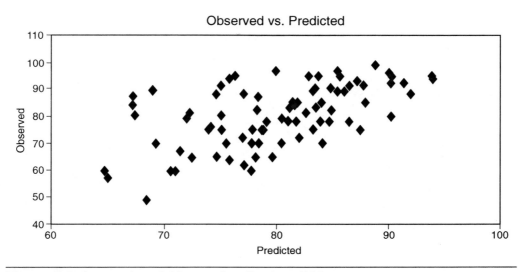

Figure 7.6 Scatterplot of Observed vs. Predicted Values

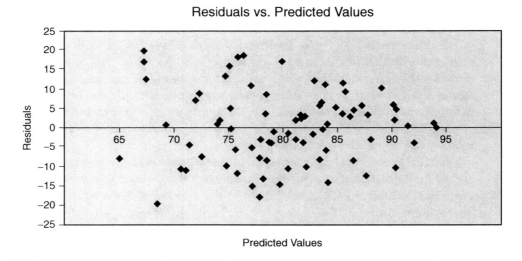

Figure 7.7 Scatterplot of Residuals vs. Predicted Values

the assumption of linearity may not be fulfilled. Additionally, if points on the plot appear to be clustered in one or more areas, then the variance may not be constant across the population, leading to errors in the regression. The plot in Figure 7.7 seems to demonstrate just such a pattern, because the width of the plot seems to decrease as the values approach 100. In these cases, mathematical transformations are sometimes necessary to obtain a valid analysis. Outliers are also significant in this plot because they may indicate that the error terms may not fit a normal distribution. A normal

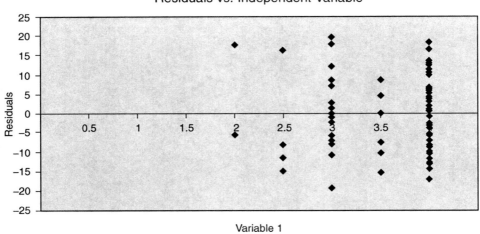

Figure 7.8 Scatterplot of Residuals vs. Independent Variable I

probability plot usually provides the best examination for normality in the residual terms.

Another useful analysis compares the residuals vs independent variables. An example of this analysis is found in Figure 7.8. This analysis provides another check on the variance across the samples, and as shown in the figure, the variance, represented by the residuals, should be relatively consistent across all levels of the independent variables. If the variance appears to be different at each level, then the regression assumption of constant variance for the error terms may be violated.

Finally, the normal probability plot of residuals is the best way of verifying normally distributed error terms. Figure 7.9 demonstrates normally distributed residuals, which essentially plot the N-score of the residuals against the residual values. If the values are normally distributed, then the graph is linear, as in Figure 7.9. If the normality assumption is violated, then outliers may appear or the graph may be curved rather than linear.

Applications in QI

The breadth of applications for regression make it a tool for nearly any situation in which relationships must be defined or when future outcomes can reasonably be predicted from historic data. Defining relationships prior to designing and implementing QI interventions can prevent costly projects that have little effect on quality. Without a demonstrated relationship between an intervention (independent variable) and an outcome (dependent variable), a QI team could create a project that would do nothing more than consume resources and generate costs. Thus, if there is any doubt about a relationship between an outcome and contemplated interventions, a regression

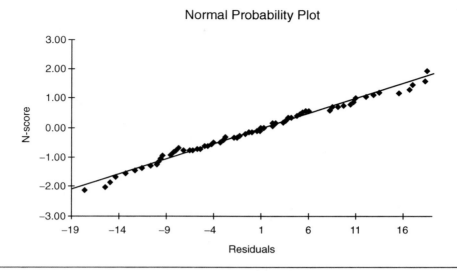

Figure 7.9 Normal Probability Plot of Residuals vs. Dependent Variable

analysis could help better define the relationship and even help determine which interventions are of greatest potential benefit.

Simple linear regression is used extensively to define a relationship between two variables. An example of this application follows.

Example 7-3

The office manager of XYZ Clinic was trying to determine if new patient waiting times were related to patient satisfaction, with the goal of determining whether the staff needed to work on improving the time it took new patients to see the doctor. The practice collected patient satisfaction information after each new patient visit, and after a period of 2 months had collected 100 surveys. During that same time, the staff recorded waiting times for patients to see the doctor, and they then decided to compare the waiting times with the patient satisfaction scores. The satisfaction scores comprised an average of five different questions patients answered about their experience at the clinic, none of which specifically addressed waiting time. Thus, a direct relationship could not be inferred, and linear regression was chosen as the method for establishing the correlation. The results of the regression analysis are provided in Table 7.12.

According to the regression output, the equation describing the estimated regression relationship between waiting time and satisfaction scores was as follows

(7.14) estimated patient satisfaction score $= -0.01 \times (\text{waiting time}) + 3.88$

Table 7.12 XYZ Clinic Results of Linear Regression

REGRESSION STATISTICS

Multiple R	0.439
R^2	0.192
Adjusted R^2	0.183
Standard Error	0.775
Observations	100

ANOVA

	DF	SS	MS	F	SIGNIFICANCE F
Regression	1	14.02	14.02	23.33	<0.001
Residual	98	58.90	0.60		
Total	99	72.93			

	COEFFICIENTS	STANDARD ERROR	t-STAT	p-VALUE	LOWER 95%	UPPER 95%
Intercept	3.88	0.17	22.84	<0.001	3.54	4.21
Wait Time	−0.01	0.002	−4.83	<0.001	−0.015	−0.006

Multiple R, multiple correlation; R^2, coefficient of determination.

The analysis demonstrates that the score is negatively affected by a long waiting time because the regression coefficient is −0.01. The ANOVA demonstrates that the regression effect is highly significant, with an F-value of 23.328 and a p-value substantially less than 0.05. The waiting time graphs of residuals and the regression line are presented in Figure 7.10. The regression appears significant because the line appears to fit the data and the residuals appear to be distributed uniformly over the range of values. The R^2 value in Table 7.12 indicates that 19.2% of the variation in satisfaction scores is predicted by waiting times. Thus, the clinic manager concluded that waiting time for new patients was a significant predictor of patient satisfaction.

The example demonstrates the value of linear regression analysis in identifying relationships of importance to QI teams. A factor that accounts for nearly 20% of patient satisfaction seems important enough for a QI team to consider.

Multiple regression can be used for more complex situations, when several factors may be affecting a specific outcome. A typical use of multiple regression can be seen in the following example.

Example 7-4

The XYZ Clinic staff was heartened to know that new patient waiting time was a significant factor because it provides several opportu-

Wait Time Residual Plot

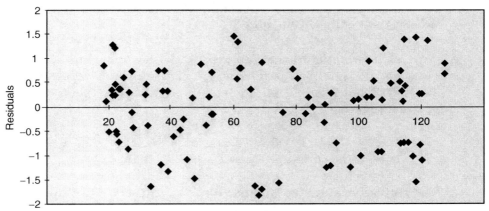

Wait Time Line Fit Plot

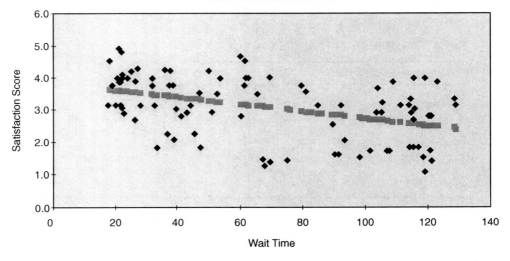

Figure 7.10 Residual Plots: XYZ Clinic Waiting Times

nities for change and improvement. The staff wanted to evaluate other potential predictors of patient satisfaction, so they checked the information available for the 100 new patients that they used in the initial evaluation of satisfaction scores. The following information was obtained from the chart audits:

◆ time spent with the physician (minutes)

◆ blood tests performed (binary variable, i.e., zero if a blood test was not performed and 1 if a blood test was performed)
◆ total cost of the visit (dollars)

This information was added to the database and a multiple regression analysis was performed, with the results reported in Table 7.13 and Figure 7.11. The results provided the following regression equation

(7.15) score = 1.843 − 0.006 × (waiting time) + 0.079 × (time with MD) + 0.140 × (blood test performed) + 0.000 × (total cost)

The regression statistics are also reported in Table 7.13. The R^2 value indicates that 49% of the satisfaction score can be attributed to the independent variables, and the adjusted R^2 is in the same range at 46%. The multiple R is important in this example, since it represents the correlation between the satisfaction score and a linear combination of the independent variables; in this instance, the multiple correlation (multiple R) value of 0.70

Table 7.13 Results of Multiple R for XYZ Clinic

REGRESSION STATISTICS

Multiple R	0.70
R^2	0.49
Adjusted R^2	0.47
Standard Error	0.63
Observations	100

ANOVA

	DF	SS	MS	F	SIGNIFICANCE F
Regression	4	35.78	8.95	22.88	**<0.001**
Residual	95	37.14	0.39		
Total	99	72.93			

	COEFFICIENTS	STANDARD ERROR	t STAT	p-VALUE	LOWER 95%	UPPER 95%
Intercept	1.843	0.332	5.56	<0.001	1.185	2.501
Wait Time	−0.006	0.002	−3.2	<0.002	−0.010	−0.002
Time with MD	0.079	0.011	7.41	<0.001	0.058	0.100
Blood Test	0.140	0.126	1.11	0.27	−0.110	0.389
Total Cost	0.000	0.001	0.83	0.41	−0.001	0.001

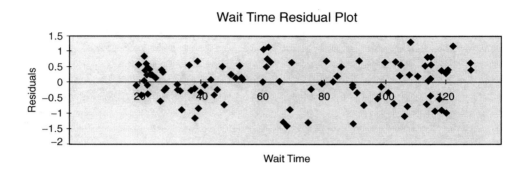

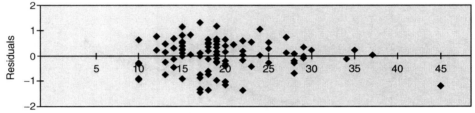

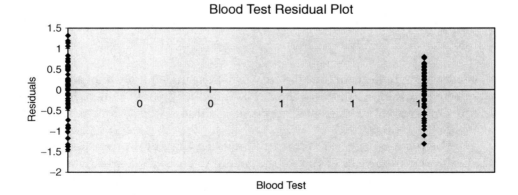

Figure 7.11 XYZ Clinic Multiple Regression Plots

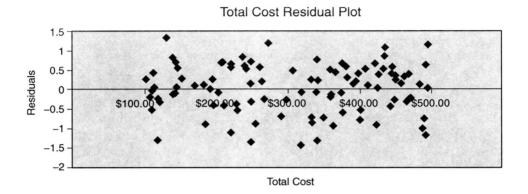

Figure 7.11 *continued*

is very high, indicating that the satisfaction score is highly dependent on the selected variables. Similarly, the ANOVA demonstrates the high level of significance for this regression, with an *F*-value of 22.88 and a significant *p*-value of $p < 0.001$.

The residual analysis plots in Figure 7.11 are of interest because they specify the adherence of the regression analysis to the underlying assumptions. All of the residual plots appear to have random patterns of distribution, except for the variable *time with MD,* which demonstrates gradually decreasing variation as the time increased. Because most of the points are clustered near the mean, part of the reason for the differing variances could be smaller sample sizes at longer times. In any event, the regression must be tempered with the idea that the variance in *time with MD* may not be constant. Finally, the residual probability plot demonstrates that the residuals follow a nearly normal distribution.

Returning to the regression equation in equation 7.15, the effects of each of the independent variables on the satisfaction score appear to be quite disparate. The coefficient for *waiting time* in the regression equation is −0.005, which indicates that as waiting time increases by 20 minutes, the satisfaction score will decrease by 0.1 points. Thus, if targets are set using patient satisfaction scores, then reducing waiting time by 20 minutes can be expected to add 0.1 to the average satisfaction score. Similarly, *time with MD* has a substantial effect on the satisfaction score. Each additional 10 minutes spent with the physician will add 0.8 to the satisfaction score. If the goal of the team is to improve the patient satisfaction score, then the most useful intervention would be to increase the time that the patient spends with the physician.

The other two variables, *blood test performed* and *total cost of visit*, are not significant in the analysis, as indicated by low *t*-statistics and high *p*-values. In fact, the regression can be performed again, first by eliminating the least significant variable (*total cost of visit*), and then reevaluating the output to see if the *blood test performed* variable becomes significant. Often, when insignificant variables are eliminated, the predictive power of the regression equation improves.

These examples are relatively simple, but they exemplify the utility of regression in QI. Because regression is so widely used in nearly every sector of the business world, many variations of the basic technique have been developed (Piegorsch 1998).

◆ Analysis of Means

Analysis of means (ANOM) provides another method of performing a statistical evaluation on a data set, but this technique is not time-series related. Thus, it is not a control chart per se, but rather is a method of comparing individual performance to that of the system in which the individual functions. Additionally, the ANOM procedure described here is designed for ratios of attribute ("count") data and will not be statistically valid for continuous variables or ratios of continuous variables. Some examples of the types of ratios that are designed for ANOM include Caesarean section rates (number of Caesarean sections divided by the total number of live births) and beta blocker prescription rates (number of patients with myocardial infarction treated with beta blockers divided by the total number of patients with myocardial infarction). The analysis of variance techniques discussed previously provide information on whether at least one mean differs from all the others. ANOM, however, provides information regarding whether one or more means differ from the average of all the means.

Many organizations are measuring the performance of physicians, hospitals, and other health care professionals as a way to determine adherence to diagnostic or treatment recommendations. In most cases, these comparisons involve gathering count data, such as the number of Caesarean section (c-section) procedures, and then producing a bar graph comparing a provider to peers. If the provider deviates more than, say, two or three standard deviations from the mean number of procedures performed by the peer group, then that provider is usually labeled an outlier and targeted for intervention. The fallacy of this approach lies in the lack of consideration of provider characteristics in the analysis. Although a managed care organization may compare all the providers within a state or group of states with one another, those providers may be practicing in facilities ranging from sophisticated university medical centers to small community hospitals with limited resources. For example, a comparison of c-section rates for all of the obstetricians in a state usually does not account for the fact that referral centers generally have higher rates than community hospitals. Thus, the perinatologist at the university center would be expected to have a higher c-section rate than an obstetrician in a rural community. Failure to account for these different expected rates could lead to erroneous targeting of the university perinatologist, ignoring a community obstetrician with an excessive rate for that practice setting, or, just as bad, ignoring a practitioner with an excessively low c-section rate that causes significant quality problems. Many organizations perform severity adjustment, as discussed in Chapter 10, "Making Continuous Quality Improvement Work: Care Management," but even the severity adjustments may not adequately take the work environment into account.

The performance improvement paradigm discussed in Chapter 9, "Strategies for Implementing Quality Improvement," suggests that problems with quality are most often related to the process and not the people. ANOM presents a method of evaluating individual performance within the context of the process in which the performance occurs, such as the rate of use of a certain medication relative to the usage rate of peers. Using an approach that accounts for common cause variation, ANOM creates output that includes upper and lower control limits (usually termed "common cause limits"), based on each individual unit of measurement (in this case, a provider doing c-sections). A vertical band of common cause limits is placed around each individual in the analysis to determine the presence of common cause, or attributable cause, variation.

ANOM can be considered a stratification technique, which divides a large group of individuals into smaller subgroups according to specific characteristics. For example, a stratification technique for a population of diabetics may divide the group into subgroups based on their glycohemoglobin (hemoglobin A1c) levels. ANOM provides a more sophisticated method of stratifying a population, based on the performance of each individual relative to that which would be expected based on the environment in which the individual functions. The ANOM procedure produces stratification of individuals within a group based on expected performance within a particular work environment, identifying whether the variation in the individual's performance is a result of common cause or if it can be attributed to some other factor.

ANOM requires a stable process, i.e., one in which the mean and variation are not continually changing. Thus, an ANOM may start with a control chart analysis to establish stability of the process. Once stability has been ensured, the data are reanalyzed by an individual data component, rather than as a time series. Physician prescription patterns provide an example of this technique. A QI team may want to evaluate physician prescription patterns for a particular agent such as selective serotonin reuptake inhibitors (SSRIs) relative to all agents in that class. The team would first determine the overall rate of SSRI usage over a period of time using a control chart, and if the mean of that process appears to be stable for the study group, then the team would reevaluate the data to determine individual prescription rates, followed by ANOM to determine if each individual physician is using SSRIs as expected. Without ANOM, raw rates of usage would be calculated and compared, and the "high utilizers" would be targeted for intervention. Of course, that group would include psychiatrists, who normally would have higher rates of utilization, leading to unnecessary expense and irritating network physicians who are performing according to expected patterns of care. ANOM eliminates this problem by identifying those physicians who fall outside common cause limits, making the intervention much more effective and economical.

The formulas for ANOM are included as Table 7.14. These equations account for the differences between each individual measurement unit's opportunities to demonstrate the target behavior by adjusting the control limits with the number of possible events for each individual. These formulas are approximations to the actual formula for calculating upper and lower "decision lines," as they are termed in ANOM. The precise formula can be found in standard statistical process control references, and the number of standard deviations used to calculate the upper and lower limits (the "3" in the formulas in Table 7.14) varies according to the number of degrees of freedom, the probability of incorrectly rejecting the test hypothesis, and the number of means being tested. More detail can be obtained from Ryan (Ryan, 1989). For samples of means involving 30 or more individuals, the estimate of three standard deviations will provide approximately a 0.3% risk of incorrectly identifying individuals outside of decision limits. An example will provide further insight into this approach.

Example 7-5

St. Anywhere Hospital's Pharmacy and Therapeutics Committee is trying to determine if some physicians on the staff are overusing the new fourth-generation cephalosporin antibiotic, CefdeY2K, since it came out nearly 3 years ago. They have data from the past 12 months on ordering patterns by physician, and they have performed a simple analysis analyzing usage patterns for the five physicians in the in-

Table 7.14 Formulas for Analysis of Means

CHART PARAMETERS AND LIMITS

Plot Point

$$P_i = \frac{ObservedEvents(i)}{PossibleEvents(i)}$$

Average (centerline)

$$Mean = \frac{\sum ObservedEvents}{\sum PossibleEvents}$$

Individual Upper
Common Cause Limit

$$UCL_i = Mean + 3 \bullet \sqrt{\frac{Mean(1 - Mean)}{PossibleEvents(i)}}$$

Individual Lower
Common Cause Limit

$$LCL_i = Mean - 3 \bullet \sqrt{\frac{Mean(1 - Mean)}{PossibleEvents(i)}}$$

Where

P_i is the proportion of target events for each individual in the analysis

Observed Events (i) is the count of target events that occurred for the individual unit

Possible Events (i) is the total number of events which could have occurred or actually did occur

Observed Events is the total of all target events observed in the population

Possible Events is the total of all events that could have occurred or did occur in the population

ternal medicine department. The data from the past 12 months are presented in Table 7.15. A control chart was constructed to determine if the process was in control, and the resulting *p*-chart is included as Figure 7.12. The *p*-chart revealed no special causes, and the committee decided to examine each physician's prescribing behavior and elected to proceed with the ANOM.

The committee decided to first evaluate a histogram with each physician's utilization rates. The graph in Figure 7.13 was produced, revealing relatively high rates for *physicians 3* and *4,* but otherwise unremarkable findings. The other three physicians had relatively low usage but nothing that appeared notable to the committee.

The ANOM chart in Figure 7.14 produced an interesting pattern, however. Common cause limits were calculated using the formulas in Table 7.14 and the data in Table 7.15. Particularly notable are the variable upper and lower common cause limits, because each limit calculation includes a factor that reflects the individual physician's total number of chances to prescribe the drug. When the actual proportions of CefdeY2K were placed on the chart with the common

Table 7.15 CefdeY2K Utilization Rates

CefdeY2K

Physician	Month 1	Month 2	Month 3	Month 4	Month 5	Month 6	Month 7	Month 8	Month 9	Month 10	Month 11	Month 12	Total
1	1	2	1	2	1	1	1	1	1	2	1	1	15
2	3	4	1	3	5	3	5	2	2	1	3	3	35
3	5	7	5	4	6	4	5	6	6	6	4	7	65
4	3	3	5	5	6	4	2	4	5	3	5	5	50
5	1	2	1	1	1	0	3	0	0	1	2	0	12

All Cephalosporins

Physician	Month 1	Month 2	Month 3	Month 4	Month 5	Month 6	Month 7	Month 8	Month 9	Month 10	Month 11	Month 12	Total
1	29	21	14	23	21	18	19	23	12	14	10	14	218
2	45	31	29	34	19	32	40	21	38	46	42	17	394
3	41	42	48	39	42	35	29	42	35	26	19	20	418
4	16	18	14	15	22	12	10	20	14	12	16	17	186
5	24	20	17	21	26	17	19	16	12	26	29	32	259

Proportion

Physician	Month 1	Month 2	Month 3	Month 4	Month 5	Month 6	Month 7	Month 8	Month 9	Month 10	Month 11	Month 12
1	0.034	0.095	0.071	0.087	0.048	0.056	0.053	0.043	0.083	0.143	0.100	0.071
2	0.067	0.129	0.034	0.088	0.263	0.094	0.125	0.095	0.053	0.022	0.071	0.176
3	0.122	0.167	0.104	0.103	0.143	0.114	0.172	0.143	0.171	0.231	0.211	0.350
4	0.188	0.167	0.357	0.333	0.273	0.333	0.200	0.200	0.357	0.250	0.313	0.294
5	0.042	0.100	0.059	0.048	0.038	0.000	0.158	0.000	0.000	0.038	0.069	0.000

CefdeY2K use among physicians in the internal medicine department at St. Anywhere Hospital.

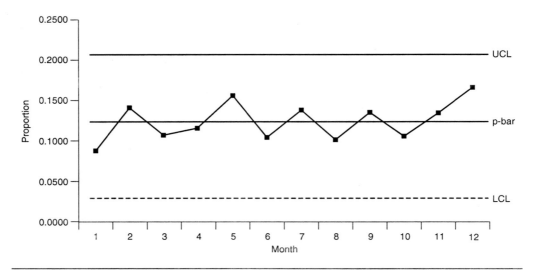

Figure 7.12 *p*-Chart of Physician Ordering Habits for CefdeY2K

Data are from Example 7-5.

Histogram of CefdeY2K Usage

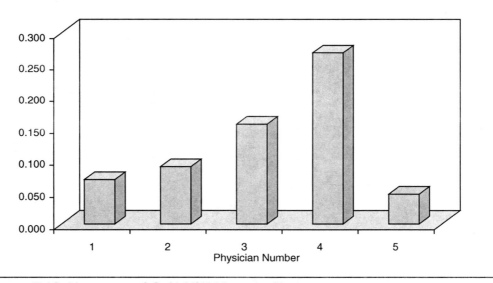

Figure 7.13 Histogram of CefdeY2K Usage by Physician

cause limits, *physician 4*'s proportion of CefdeY2K was demonstrably above the upper common cause limit, *physician 5*'s level was below the lower common cause limit, and the other three practitioners were within these limits. Although *physician 4* attracted a great deal of attention because of the cost of the drug, *physician 5* also gained the

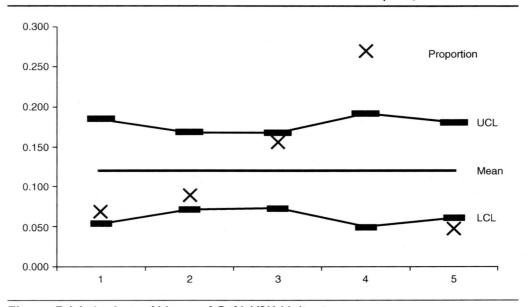

Figure 7.14 Analysis of Means of CefdeY2K Utilization

committee's interest because of relatively low levels of utilization, indicating a potential quality of care issue. More thorough examination of the charts of these two practitioners was warranted by the findings of the ANOM.

This analysis demonstrates a fairly typical outcome of an ANOM procedure. Attributable causes are identified above and below common cause limits, with the majority of subjects falling within these limits. As with other types of statistical analysis, attributable causes must be investigated to determine the underlying problem before specific interventions are designed to eliminate the obstacle to quality.

The usefulness of ANOM in stratifying populations is also demonstrated by the example. Three subgroups were identified by the analysis: overprescribers, underprescribers, and those who prescribed the drug according to expectations. Stratifying populations is a valuable method for targeting interventions based on underlying problems, rather than blanketing the population with less effective educational material or ill-advised QI projects. Not only will the interventions be more successful in producing a desired outcome, but they will also be more economical because they can be much more specific and direct.

ANOM is a technique that determines if a subgroup or individual mean is different from the population mean. By tailoring control limits to specific subgroups or individuals, values outside common cause limits can be identified to stratify a population and better direct QI interventions to optimize success. The technique provides substantial power for evaluating individuals or subgroups within a population for a specific characteristic that is not time dependent. ANOM can augment traditional control charts to provide more detailed information about a population and improve the opportunities for QI projects to achieve successful outcomes.

◆ Design of Experiments

Although not intuitively obvious, all of the approaches described in this chapter require an appropriately designed model for analysis. The concepts of experimental design underlie these issues, and the use of these models can provide a much more robust analysis. The design of an experiment, or intervention in QI terms, determines the type of analytical tools that will be used in analyzing the results for statistical significance. The use of design of experiments (DOE) concepts assists in optimizing experiments or in determining the best ways to analyze data from an experiment.

The first and most important concept in designing interventions is to anticipate possible sources of variation. Virtually all of the tools discussed in this chapter have statistics that estimate actual values of parameters in a model, such as regression coefficients, correlation coefficients, and standard errors. Included in all of these analyses is some correction for error, otherwise known as random variation, that results from other influences on the data. In the XYZ Clinic example, the R^2 value of 0.49 signifies not only that 49% of the variation is due to the regression variables, but also that 51% of the variation is due to other factors that are not identified in the regression equation. The goal of any experiment is to identify as many variables as possible that influence the outcome of the experiment. However, because that goal is seldom achievable, as many variables as possible are selected and either varied or held constant so that the effects of the experimental intervention can be properly assessed.

Another important concept of the DOE approach involves varying several factors at the same time. Most research applications try to control the experimental environment and vary only one element at a time so that the effect of that element can be studied precisely. Examples abound in the medical literature, and such an approach has been instrumental in creating a scientific medical system. On the other hand, rarely do these experimental environments reflect reality. These experiments are often deemed "controlled" studies because all factors but one are held constant; in real-life situations, however, everything seems to change at the same time. Altering one factor usually sets off a chain reaction of modifications that involve several factors at once. Additionally, QI interventions are nearly always implemented in the real world, not a laboratory, necessitating analysis of many factors simultaneously to determine which have noteworthy effects on a process. Techniques such as ANOVA and regression help dissect out the individual contributions of many factors in an intervention, providing important information about the factors that are important in a process. After these factors are identified, the tools of statistical process control can determine the statistical state of control of a system so that the effects of change can be properly assessed.

Another key feature of DOE involves rational subgrouping. This concept has particular relevance when multiple factors are involved in an experiment because preconceived notions of variable grouping may prove erroneous. Although most experiments involve designing groups and subgroups to maximize the information obtained from the trials, the results may require further analysis to evaluate the efficacy of the grouping strategy. Analysis after the fact sometimes reveals patterns that would have remained undiscovered if the data were not reexamined.

A common experimental configuration for health care QI teams is termed the 2^3 (read 2 by 3) design, which connotes three factors with two levels each. This model allows for eight combinations of factors, and can be represented by a cube like the one in Figure 7.15. The cube in the figure represents an experimental combination of the three factors, *a, b,* and *c,* each of which has two levels that can be denoted by +1 and −1. Each numbered corner of the cube represents an experimental run in which one of the factor levels is varied. Table 7.16 lists all the combinations of factors and levels for a 2^3 full factorial design, which means that all factors and identifiable interactions are included in the analysis. Larger experimental models, which have large numbers of variables and multiple levels for each factor, create even larger tables. In those situations, the number of factors is often reduced by a number of techniques to produce fractional factorial designs, a topic which is beyond the scope of this book. A number of books and Web sites are noted in

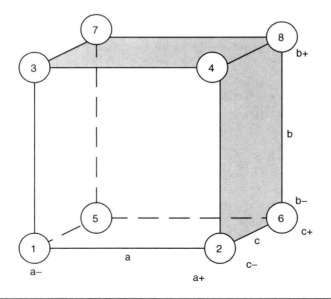

Figure 7.15 2^3 Full Factorial Experimental Design

Table 7.16 Combinations for a 2^3 Full Factorial Experiment

TRIAL NUMBER	FACTOR A	FACTOR B	FACTOR C	RESULTS	VARIABLE NAME
1	−1	−1	−1	Result -a-b-c	m
2	+1	−1	−1	Result a-b-c	n
3	−1	+1	−1	Result −a + b-c	o
4	+1	+1	−1	Result a + b-c	p
5	−1	−1	+1	Result -a-b + c	q
6	+1	−1	+1	Result a-b + c	r
7	−1	+1	+1	Result −a + b + c	s
8	+1	+1	+1	Result a + b + c	t
	0	0	0		

the Additional Reading section that provide more information on creating fractional factorial designs.

The goal of analyzing data from a multifactorial experiment is to determine the effect of each factor and any interactions between factors. The usual method for determining the effect of each factor individually, known as the main effect of that factor, is as follows.

1. Calculate the mean for all results for which the factor is at level +1.
2. Calculate the mean for all results for which the factor is at level −1.
3. Subtract the mean of the results for which the results were negative from the mean of the results for which the factor was positive.
4. Each factor's main effect can be calculated in turn using the above procedure.

An example calculation for the variable a in Table 7.16 would conform to the following equation

(7.16)
$$\text{main effect of } a = \frac{n + p + r + s}{4} - \frac{m + o + q + t}{4}$$

$$\text{main effect of } b = \frac{o + p + s + t}{4} - \frac{m + n + q + r}{4}$$

$$\text{main effect of } c = \frac{q + r + s + t}{4} - \frac{m + n + o + p}{4}$$

Interaction effects result from the interactions of two, or even all three, factors to change the results of the response variable. Although these effects are more complex, they can be similarly understood. Two factor interactions are calculated as follows.

1. For each two-factor interaction, find the mean of all the results in which the two factors are the same sign (either both +1 or both –1).
2. Find the mean of all the results in which the two factors are oppositely signed (one factor is +1 and the other is –1).
3. Subtract the mean for the oppositely signed factors from the mean for the same signed factors. The result is the estimated interaction effect.

Using the variable names in Table 7.16 again, the interaction effect between variables a and b can be calculated according to the following

(7.17)
$$\text{interaction effect } a \times b = \frac{m+p+s+t}{4} - \frac{n+o+q+r}{4}$$

$$\text{interaction effect } a \times c = \frac{m+o+r+t}{4} - \frac{n+p+q+s}{4}$$

$$\text{interaction effect } b \times c = \frac{m+n+s+t}{4} - \frac{o+p+q+r}{4}$$

The interaction of all three variables simultaneously may be accounted for, as well, and this calculation is somewhat more complex. The method of calculating the three-factor interaction is as follows

(7.18)
$$\text{interaction effect}(a \times b \times c) = \frac{n+o+q+t}{4} - \frac{m+p+r+s}{4}$$

The net effect of these interactions can be important to the results of the experiment and emphasize the reasons for performing studies that include multiple factors.

The existence of interaction effects also amplifies the need for randomization during experimental design. If factor combinations are not randomly assigned to each of the experimental runs, then experimental bias may lead to spurious conclusions. Most health care workers are familiar with this concept from reading medical literature. When testing new drugs or therapies in human or animal models, most study designers attempt to randomize the subjects in the trials to ensure that characteristics of the subjects do not alter the outcomes of the experiments. For example, an experimental design would not examine all males before all females, but would instead alternate subjects by gender to avoid a spurious effect caused by the order in which subjects were evaluated. Similarly, if QI trials are being performed, the factor levels used in the trials must be randomized as much as possible. Of course, randomization is not always possible; for example, if a study is to be performed evaluating patient satisfaction during a particularly busy time of year in an emergency department, the effect of that time of year cannot be eliminated. However, the study design team should recognize these types of problems and try to randomize factor levels in the study to the greatest extent possible.

The following example can better illustrate the effect of a designed experiment approach to a management problem in health care.

Example 7-6

Returning to the XYZ Clinic, the staff has decided to further explore some of the interventions that they attempted in the earlier example. Because they have identified some of the more important interventions that improve patient satisfaction scores, they have decided to try to improve those scores using a designed experiment. They found in their multiple regression analysis that the significant variables were *waiting time* and *time with MD*, and the insignificant variables were *blood test performed* and *total cost of visit*. They were not really convinced that the *total cost of visit* was insignificant (in real life!), so they designed an experiment that involved the next 50 new patients enrolling in the clinic. Using *waiting time, total cost of visit,* and *time with MD,* they created an experiment that separated the patients into one of eight different groups, as found in Table 7.17. The *waiting time* variable was tested at two levels, the usual time (−1) and a reduced time (+1) obtained by expediting the check-in process; the *time with MD* variable levels were obtained by having physicians spend extra time with patients designated by the staff as "special needs" patients (+1) according to the experimental design; and the *total cost*

Table 7.17 Design for Patient Satisfaction Experiment at XYZ Clinic

TRIAL NUMBER	WAITING TIME	TIME WITH MD	TOTAL COST OF VISIT	SCORE	SD OF SCORE
1	−1	−1	−1	2.5	0.8
2	+1	−1	−1	3.2	0.7
3	−1	+1	−1	3.6	0.9
4	+1	+1	−1	4.1	1.0
5	−1	−1	+1	3.2	0.7
6	+1	−1	+1	3.8	0.9
7	−1	+1	+1	4.2	1.1
8	+1	+1	+1	4.8	0.8

SD, standard deviation.

Table 7.18 Results of Factor Analysis for XYZ Clinic Experimental Design

FACTOR 1	FACTOR 2	FACTOR 3	EFFECT
waiting time			0.30
	time with MD		1.00
		total cost of visit	0.65
waiting time	time with MD		0.45
waiting time		total cost of visit	0.00
	time with MD	total cost of visit	0.25
waiting time	time with MD	total cost of visit	0.05

of visit variable was altered by providing patients with a 50% reduction in their bill (+1) based on the experimental design. The scores and sample standard deviations are shown in Table 7.17.

Main and interaction effects were calculated with the use of equations 7.16 through 7.18 and are reported in Table 7.18. Confirming the results of the multiple regression analysis, *time with MD* exerts a significant main effect, but not surprisingly, the *total cost of visit* variable has attained importance in the experiment. A significant interaction effect can be readily identified as that between *waiting time* and *time with MD*.

The staff then produced a number of graphs that are illustrated in Figure 7.16. The interactions are most significant when the lines approach perpendicularity and least significant when the lines are parallel. The staff noted that the most significant interactions seem to be those involving *time with MD*. Thus, the time spent with the doctor remains the most important factor for the staff to improve, but the data in Table 7.18 indicate that the staff may also see notable improvements by lowering costs also.

The fact that the QI team gleaned more information from the experiment, specifically that cost was a factor when it was varied experimentally, is an important lesson to remember, because any variable that has been deemed insignificant based on analyses using historic data can readily assume new importance when studied prospectively.

◆ ## Sources of Data for QI

One of the most important tenets of QI can be distilled down to an aphorism: "In God we trust; all others bring data." Nearly every QI intervention relies on data for determining where to intervene and how successful an intervention has been. Unfortunately, data in health care are often difficult to obtain,

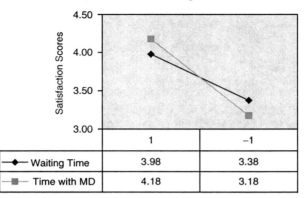

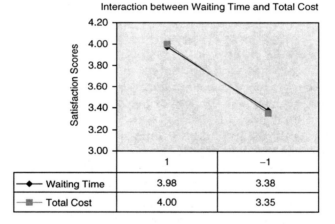

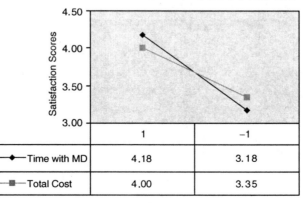

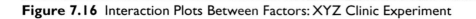

Figure 7.16 Interaction Plots Between Factors: XYZ Clinic Experiment

especially if they relate to patient care. In general, two types of data are required in health care studies: clinical data and administrative data. This section will detail the advantages and disadvantages of sources for each of these data classes.

Administrative Data

The health care system has extensively automated the collection and analysis of administrative data over the past few decades. The resulting data analyses are routinely used for a number of decisions, from resource allocation in hospitals and other institutions to insurance benefit coverage by employers and insurers. In most cases, use of administrative data can provide the information necessary to make important business decisions, but it is often problematic to extend those decisions to clinical environments, as has been demonstrated by some of the major problems that have arisen in the managed care delivery systems around the country.

Administrative data sets are typically obtained from insurance claims data. Providers of various types—physicians, hospitals, home health agencies, rehabilitation centers, etc.—send information about patient encounters to insurance companies or third-party payers so that the payer can determine the amount to reimburse the provider. The data that are submitted generally include the following information:

◆ patient name and demographic information
◆ diagnosis code(s) relating to the patient visit
◆ procedure code(s) for services provided the patient during the visit
◆ provider name and demographic information
◆ place where the services were rendered
◆ dates and times of the services
◆ authorization information, when required
◆ other information, such as reason for the services, whether the services were related to pregnancy or an accident, etc.

The coding scheme used in the United States provides only cryptic information about the services rendered, and often the paucity of clinical information causes the payer to refuse to pay a claim for lack of information. In spite of this lack of information, many insurers and other payers try to infer information about the quality of clinical services from these databases. Measures such as the Health Plan Employer Data and Information Set (HEDIS), used by the National Committee for Quality Assurance (NCQA) to evaluate managed care plans, are plagued with problems caused by inability to confirm data sources without expensive and time-consuming data collection programs.

Many insurers and employers are now creating data warehouses that contain massive numbers of medical claims in order to analyze population health and costs. Data warehouses are huge databases that accumulate data from several sources and then create records for individual transactions that are more complete than typical medical claims. For example, an insurer may place information into one of these warehouses from its claims management system, its pharmacy management system (often a subcontractor's data), surveys performed by staff, telephone logs maintained online, physician and nurse reviewer notes, medical management databases of interventions with patients and providers, and other disparate sources. Such databases require a tremendous effort to create and maintain, as well as highly sophisticated programming to match data sets by some code, e.g., the patient (or member) code, so that all of a patient's data are maintained in a coherent record. Validating data in the data warehouse can prove daunting, even for the most advanced management information systems. Thus, analyses based on these databases must be suspect until the validity of the underlying data can be ascertained.

Claims data inevitably originate with providers. Hospitals, on the whole, tend to have fairly accurate data capture systems that are implemented at the site of care and automate the collection and reporting of transaction data. Physicians, however, tend to collect and report data manually, with numerous opportunities for error between the physician and the final bill submitted for payment. Capitation, a method of prepaying physicians for services instead of paying for each service after it has been rendered, has become a complicating factor in contemporary health care data management. Because physicians are no longer paid for submitting a claim and because submission of claims entails time and cost for the physician, many doctors do not submit claims for services covered by capitation arrangements. Thus, payer databases often lack important information about services provided to their beneficiaries, leading to more errors in analysis and interpretation. Although medical claims data are intended to represent the essential information about the services provided to a patient during a medical encounter, the information remains inadequate in most situations.

Other sources of administrative data include physician and hospital computers because the raw data for health care claims are contained in those systems. In some cases, obtaining provider data from their systems can prove more helpful than obtaining data from an insurer's data system. As data are received in the insurance company computer, special programs called filters analyze the data for any obvious errors, such as the 100-year-old man with a diagnosis of term pregnancy. Although these filters are generally very reliable, in some instances the programs have errors that eliminate valid data or add information to a record that invalidates the data. These types of errors are often insidious and difficult to find and often remain unrecognized until serious errors finally become evident during data analysis.

Financial data management has reached a high degree of sophistication among both payers and providers. Accounting programs are available for nearly any size organization, and those data have generally been reliable for analysis. In health care systems, however, the financial information provides only limited utility for making decisions regarding QI interventions because most projects will have an impact on patient care. Thus, financial systems can provide only a portion of the information needed for QI teams in health care.

As medical billing systems have become more automated, the types of errors that occur in claims data have become limited to the human interactions with the systems, such as during data entry in the provider's office or as claims processors transfer data from insurance forms to the insurer's claims management computer system. Electronic data capture and transfer will gradually eliminate these errors, leading to more robust systems for QI analysis. Analytic tools for end users are also becoming much easier to use, and even user-friendly spreadsheet programs now have sophisticated data analysis capabilities for QI programs. As the validity of administrative databases improves and the tools for analysis become even more usable, a new era of QI activity will become possible.

Clinical Data

At the present time, sources of clinical data are limited. Relatively few providers have automated clinical data collection and storage systems, and the use of electronic medical records is gaining acceptance in the health care delivery system very slowly. Typical clinical data sources are provider medical records, predominantly maintained by physicians and nurses. A number of other potential sources must be considered as well. Pharmacy data often are quite robust because pharmacies have highly developed data management systems to optimize reimbursement. The sophistication of those systems often ensures a more accurate data set than can be obtained from medical charts. Patients themselves can sometimes serve as a source of clinical data through questionnaires about their clinical condition.

Medical charts have remained the gold standard for clinical data, and many performance measures required by the NCQA in the HEDIS data set require medical chart reviews to obtain data for calculating the measures. Chart reviews are tedious, expensive endeavors that require trained chart extractors, usually registered nurses, who must pore over paper charts that are often unorganized, with handwriting that is difficult to read. In preparation for chart reviews, qualified personnel must prepare chart extraction survey forms or computer programs that direct the chart reviewers to specific data items that are needed for the analysis. Even with substantial preparation, chart reviews often fail to achieve their purpose because of difficulty finding information or problems reading the information that is in the chart. In spite of all of these difficulties, chart reviews often are the sole source of certain types of clinical data.

Other potential sources of clinical data include laboratory vendors, who may be sole source contractors for some health plans. Because clinical laboratories are nearly all automated, patient laboratory values are available in computerized format, and if appropriate programming support is accessible, the patient lab data can be matched to records with diagnoses and other procedures so that specific lab values can be tracked as part of a disease-management program.

Direct data collection from physicians is usually a difficult method of obtaining clinical data, but a well-designed study can gain physician support and cooperation in collection of information. Specific projects that do not intrude on a physician's patient-care time can be accomplished by having simple, rapidly completed forms that the provider can fill out as part of the patient encounter. In most cases, physicians should be involved in designing the study and the data collection forms to improve compliance by participating providers.

As computerized patient records are used by more providers, a wealth of clinical data will become available for studies of clinical quality. Computerization of the medical chart will allow direct entry of information about patient care by the provider, allowing rapid analysis of the data and more targeted interventions. Quality improvement projects will include computerized reminders and "just-in-time" educational systems that can help enhance the quality of care as it is occurring, rather than after the fact as is currently done. Because information management will continue to improve, the future of quality in the health care delivery system is particularly bright.

◆ Discussion Points

1. Discuss the difference between discrete distributions and continuous distributions. What kinds of variables are involved in the analysis of each type of distribution?
2. What is the function of the null hypothesis in evaluating a quality improvement intervention? What types of statistical inference tests are applicable in testing a null hypothesis?
3. Discuss the use of analysis of variance (ANOVA) in quality improvement. How can ANOVA be used to evaluate quality improvement projects?
4. Regression analysis consists of simple linear and multiple regression. Discuss the difference between the two and provide sample applications that use each technique.
5. How can planned experiments assist in quality improvement efforts? Provide an example from your experience in which a designed experiment could be of use.
6. Discuss sources of clinical and administrative data. What are the difficulties in obtaining data from each of these sources for quality improvement studies?

◆ # Notes

Gerdes G. (1999). *Student's t-distribution*. Retrieved September 2003, from *http://jevons.sscnet.ucla.edu/gerdes/java/Graphics2D/tDist.html*

Piegorsch W. (1998). An introduction to binary response regression and associated trend analyses. *Journal of Quality Technology, 30*(3), 269–281.

◆ # Additional Reading

Berk K., and Carey P. (1998). *Data analysis with Microsoft Excel*. Pacific Grove, CA: Duxbury Press.

Box G. E. P., and Draper N. R. (1987). *Empirical model-building and response surfaces*. New York: John Wiley & Sons.

Lane D. (1999). *Hyperstat online*. Retrieved September 2003, from *http://www.ruf.rice.edu/~lane/hyperstat/index.html*

Ryan T. P. (1989). *Statistical methods for quality improvement*. New York: John Wiley & Sons. *StatSoft electronic statistics textbook*. Retrieved September 2003, from *http://www.statsoft.com/textbook/stathome.html*

Younger M. S. (1979). *Handbook for linear regression*. Belmont, CA: Duxbury Press.

Chapter 8

Clinical Processes: Clinical Practice Guidelines

DONALD E. LIGHTER
NEDA LEWIS

Introduction

Over the past two decades, the private and public sectors have dramatically changed methods of financing health care. In a move away from relatively unstructured, open-ended payment mechanisms, payers have instituted systems for capping costs. These new payment arrangements have encouraged providers and insurers to develop systems for ensuring that care is appropriate, but many problems have arisen regarding questions of quality of care. The public has begun to ask critical questions regarding the health care system.

◆ Is quality care being delivered?
◆ How is quality measured?
◆ What kind of quality information should be available to the public?

Over the last 50 years, medical progress has typically been measured by the development of innovative technical information about diseases, diagnostic techniques, and treatment modalities. There has not been a great deal of attention paid to developing systematic information about the methods of the delivery of health care to individuals or to populations. Studies of these issues have concentrated on the high degree of variation in clinical practices for basic conditions (Agency for Healthcare Research and Quality, AHRQ, formerly known as the Agency for Health Care Policy and Research, AHCPR, 1995).

History of Clinical Practice Guidelines in Health Care

Nearly all stakeholders in the system need information to improve the quality of care. Health planners need to know which interventions actually improve the health of populations so that they can create budgets that enhance the health of the greatest number of people. Patients and medical professionals need to know which quality interventions produce improvements in overall health in order to decide which to apply to individual health care regimens. Health administrators must justify the allocation of increasingly limited resources to these new modalities. Organizations that pay for health care need to realize value for their health care dollars, and outcomes data will provide that reassurance.

All of these considerations led Congress to establish the Agency for Healthcare Research and Quality (AHRQ), formerly known as the Agency for Health Care Policy and Research (AHCPR), as a result of Public Law 101-239, the Omnibus Budget Reconciliation Act of 1989. The AHRQ is a part of the U.S. Department of Health and Human Services and replaces the National Center for Health Services Research and Health Care Technology Assessment. The agency was created in part to respond to concerns about the variability in health care practices and concern about the efficacy of health care services. The mission of the AHRQ is to improve the quality, appropriateness, and effectiveness of health care by supporting research and improving access to health care. Since the publication of the Institute of Medicine's seminal book, *Crossing the Quality Chasm*, in 2001, the AHRQ has also focused on the issue of medical errors in an effort to reduce harm to patients through better quality improvement (QI) efforts. The AHRQ was also charged with the development and continuous updating of clinical practice guidelines (CPGs). The AHRQ conceptualized CPGs to be clinically relevant and useful to a variety of health professionals to assist them in determining how diseases and other health conditions can most effectively and appropriately be prevented, diagnosed, treated, and managed. Additionally, the guidelines are to be used by the health care industry in judging the provision of health care and improving quality.

Soon after its creation, the AHRQ solicited the help of the Institute of Medicine (IOM), a branch of the National Institutes of Health, regarding the development of CPGs. The IOM provides information and advice concerning health policy to government, the corporate sector, the medical professions, and the public. After being asked for help by the AHRQ, the IOM immediately convened an expert committee to define key terms, identify attributes of good guidelines, and provide technical assistance for other aspects of guideline development. Through this process, the IOM fashioned a definition of CPGs as "systematically developed statements to assist practitioner and patient decisions about appropriate health care for specific clinical circumstances" (Field and Lohn, 1990). Two important points follow from this definition. First, the methodology defined in CPGs must be systematic, rigorous, and explicit; and second, CPGs must be based on the best medical evidence available.

In addition to establishing the AHRQ, Congress created the Forum for Quality and Effectiveness in Health Care to develop and review "clinically relevant guidelines that may be used by physicians, educators, and health practitioners to assist in determining how diseases, disorders, and other health conditions can most effectively and appropriately be prevented, diagnosed, treated and managed clinically." The law establishing this function (the Omnibus Budget Reconciliation Act of 1989) requires that CPGs conform to the following principles.

◆ Guidelines must be based on the best available research and professional judgment.

◆ Guidelines must be presented in formats appropriate for use not only by physicians, but also by other health care practitioners, providers, medical educators, medical review organizations, and consumers.

◆ Guidelines must include treatment-specific information or contain specific recommendations for clinical treatments and conditions in forms appropriate for use in clinical practice, educational programs, and quality and appropriateness review.

Through these legislative efforts, Congress established mandates to create CPGs to assist in the delivery of health care and measure outcomes of care. Sources of CPGs have proliferated very rapidly over the past few years in response to these legislative initiatives. The AHRQ has developed several guidelines over its relatively short life, and other sources for guidelines now include specialty societies, managed care organizations, and health research organizations. The number and variety of guidelines grew so rapidly that the AHRQ created a National Guideline Clearinghouse on the World Wide Web (Agency for Healthcare Research and Quality, AHRQ, formerly known as the Agency for Health Care Policy and Research, AHCPR 1999).

◆ Use of CPGs in Health Care

CPGs have been recognized as one method of defining, measuring, and evaluating the cost and quality of care (Thomas, et al., 1998; McCulloch, et al., 1998; Collins, 1998; Shrake, et al., 1994). Purchasers of health care services view practice guidelines as a positive step in improving the quality of care, allowing them to finally place a value on their health care expenditures. The Health Plan Employer Data and Information Set (HEDIS), created by the National Committee for Quality Assurance (NCQA), uses medical review criteria derived from practice guidelines to measure health plan performance and produce provider report cards. Managed care organizations use CPGs to measure variation in patterns of care in their networks of providers for a number of clinical conditions. Importantly, though, CPGs should not be construed as algorithms for health care practice or legal standards of care. Rather, they fit into the Shewhart plan-do-study-act cycle (Agency for Healthcare Research and Quality, AHRQ, formerly known as the Agency for Health Care Policy and Research, AHCPR 1995), and as such they are continually works in progress. Thus, CPGs have a salient role in the QI process and are expected to improve the quality of care by reducing variation and providing continuous oversight into the process of care. By using the QI techniques described in previous chapters, CPGs become the nidus of the efforts to optimize care of disease and improve the health of the population. Used in this manner, CPGs become tools to create standards of quality and medical policy. Figure 8.1 demonstrates the use of CPGs in the medical policy development process.

Once guidelines have been developed, they are used to expand QI efforts by producing medical review criteria and performance measures, as indicated in Figure 8.1. Medical review criteria define the issues within the guideline that require attention for potential quality problems, e.g., obtaining quarterly hemoglobin A1c (HgbA1c) levels in diabetics. Sources for the criteria include administrative data analysis, chart audits, and input from experienced clinicians and patients with a specific condition. Some examples of medical review criteria include

◆ annual professional eye examinations for people with diabetes
◆ use of steroid inhalers in asthmatics
◆ prenatal screening for nutritional adequacy in pregnant women
◆ completion of immunization schedules by 2 years of age
◆ initiation of beta blocker therapy after a myocardial infarction

Once these possible problem areas are identified, the QI team spends time with clinicians and data analysts to determine which performance measures can adequately assess the issue. For the criteria above, a list of possible performance measures could include

◆ rate of eye examinations by an ophthalmologist or optometrist in diabetics
◆ rate of use of steroid inhalers in asthmatics
◆ rate of use of steroid inhalers or the number of inhalers per asthmatic per year if nearly all asthmatics were found to use the inhalers
◆ rate of nutritional screens documented in prenatal charts
◆ immunization rates for 2-year-old children
◆ rate of beta blocker use after a myocardial infarction

These and other similar measures have been used nationally for several years to assess health care organizations on quality of care, and some of these measures have been part of the HEDIS data set in the past, as well as currently.

Returning to Figure 8.1, once the performance measures have been defined and actual data analysis completed, QI teams design interventions to improve care. For example, a program may be initiated to educate asthmatic patients and their physicians about the benefits and low risk of steroid inhalers, with the aim of increasing the number of asthmatics who use these

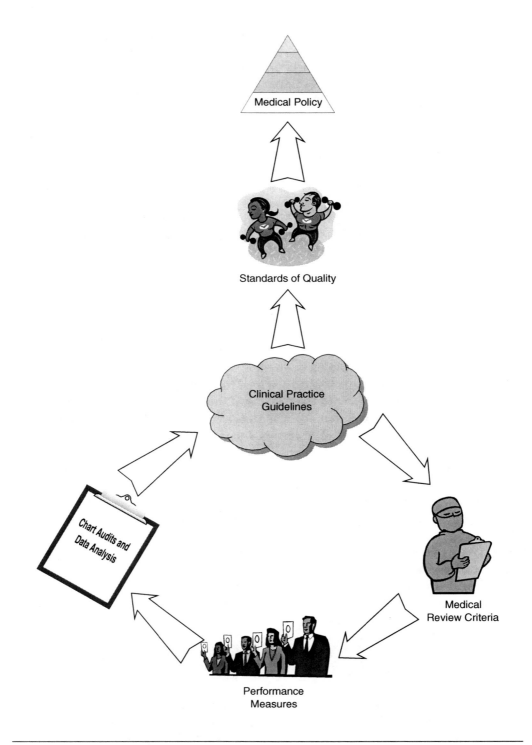

Figure 8.1 Medical Policy Development Cycle

medications for maintenance therapy. Once the program has had enough time to demonstrate an effect, the follow-up analysis is performed to compare pre- and postintervention rates and evaluate the effect of the intervention. In some cases, the effects of the intervention may be measured with control charts, as in any industrial QI project; however, many interventions in health care involve only pre- and poststudy analysis.

If the interventions have been successful in effecting change, then the QI program becomes incorporated into the CPG. At this point, most quality assurance programs would consider this project a success and move on to another problem area. The QI approach, however, involves continued monitoring of the improvement to ensure that progress and gains are maintained and that the intervention continues to be productive. Additionally, once the intervention has been incorporated into the guideline, the QI team should begin concentrating on identifying other potential changes that could enhance the process. Using the example of steroid inhaler use in asthma, once the educational program has been successfully implemented and can be sustained, the team may begin working on other types of interventions, such as having pharmacists provide physicians with feedback from encounters with patients during prescription refills. Because prescription refills occur more frequently than office visits, the physician can use this information to optimize the patient's therapeutic regimen between regular encounters. Other areas of the CPG should be examined at each review to unearth any other potential improvement interventions. The goal should be to bring care patterns into compliance with the CPG, or, if the current patterns of care appear to produce superior outcomes when compared with the CPG, to revise the CPG to reflect these better practices. In either circumstance, the emphasis is on continually improving the quality of care.

The major problem encountered when trying to initiate QI projects using CPGs is the difficulty in measuring health care quality, because physicians and analysts rarely agreed on valid metrics. CPGs can serve as a model for understanding and measuring health care by providing a framework that will promote the development of measures that can be validated statistically. One of the tenets of QI is particularly germane: "You can't manage what you can't measure." Organizations that use CPGs are able to define measures that help them better manage patient care.

Another impediment faced in QI implementation in health care is the expectation of decreased costs through QI. Historically, QI interventions in industry have been associated with decreased costs (Anassi, et al., 1994; Natsch, et al., 1998; Citrome, 1998). Payers, i.e., industrial and business people, are accustomed to seeing an immediate return on investment when improvements are made in a manufacturing process, but some health interventions may only manifest improvement over a period of years. For instance, when women have better prenatal care, their babies are healthier, and the deliveries are less likely to be fraught with complications. The cost of caring for compromised babies—those who are premature or have infections or other preventable complications—far exceeds the cost of prenatal care, but the cost of caring for the severely affected infant is spread over a period of years. The financial impact of the lack of prenatal care extends far into the future, and some payers may posit that the upfront expenditure for prenatal care will not be regained if the family switches to another health insurance plan or finds employment elsewhere. However, if all payers invested in these cost-saving enhancements, then all would benefit from the savings, lowering the overall cost of care.

An example of the shortsighted approach to health care finance occurred when payers embarked on health care cost reduction programs, pushing providers and insurers into cost containment initiatives that limited stays in the hospital or shunted patients to other modes of care. To a certain extent, these measures reduced the slack in health care utilization; however, as with any business practice, most of these programs reached a level at which further reductions in expenditures were associated with increasing administrative costs and lower net cost reduction, thus decreasing the marginal rate of return. Some providers and insurers then tried to reduce essential services, leading to a vocal public backlash (Associated Press, 1999) and increasing costs in the health care delivery system. In response to these public outcries, the health care industry has begun to examine QI strategies as a means of reducing costs. Concurrently, these QI approaches are expected to improve the health of the population, adding value to health expenditures. Although there are still few data indicating cost savings, some studies have demonstrated salient effects on costs as QI programs become implemented more widely (Khoury, 1998).

As the quality of care improves, patient satisfaction with care should also increase. Patient surveys are assuming greater importance in evaluating health care because the patient's perception of the outcome of care is as important as the provider's interpretation of the patient's clinical results. Payers, employers, and providers are all coming to recognize the importance of patient perceptions in determining the value of health care interventions because these attitudes determine the patient's willingness to adhere to treatment regimens and follow-up care that will allow continuous improvement in outcomes (Bassetti, et al., 1999; Hershberger, et al., 1999; Apter, et al., 1998).

Finally, CPGs can decrease complication rates by reducing unnecessary variation in care. A number of studies using disease management programs that include CPGs have indicated such improvements as reduced rates of Caesarean sections and neonatal morbidity (Burton and Joffe, 1998), improved outcomes for congestive heart failure (Tilney, et al., 1998), and decreased rates of hospital utilization for acute exacerbations of asthma (Buchner, et al., 1998; McDowell, et al., 1998). Most care management programs use CPGs as the focus for analysis and interventions. Payer organizations as diverse as the federal government and small employers are beginning to recognize that without some mechanism to continually improve quality, the long-term return on health care investment will not be realized.

◆ Creation of CPGs

Presently, the process for creating CPGs varies substantially among organizations. Because of this variation, the quality of guidelines is not uniform, requiring some effort on the part of QI teams to modify any existing guidelines to ensure adequate evidence for any recommendations made, as well as adapting the CPG to local practice variations. The process described in this book outlines the ideal method for creating CPGs and provides input from local patients and professionals.

Several steps are required to ensure the creation of optimal clinical guidelines.

- selection of an appropriate disease process or clinical problem for the guideline
- creation or adoption of the CPG
- validation of the CPG through literature review and expert consensus
- finalization of the CPG by an inclusive implementation task force
- dissemination of the guideline
- follow-up studies to determine the efficacy of the guideline and implementation process

These steps are represented in the flowchart in Figure 8.2.

Selection of a Clinical Condition for Guideline Development

As the universe of medical conditions is surveyed, the task of finding just one condition for guideline creation may seem daunting. A screening process must be applied to find the health condition that will benefit most from the organization's efforts. The type and goals of the organization will weigh heavily in the decision, and financial factors will always be involved. Some pertinent goals of various stakeholders are listed in Table 8.1. In a consumer-driven health care delivery system, consumer needs and desires must be considered the ultimate goal, but the goals of all the stakeholders in the system will factor into how medical conditions are selected for intervention.

Taking into account all of the objectives listed in Table 8.1, the list of criteria for selecting a clinical condition for CPG development would include diseases or conditions in which

- improvement is possible
- outcomes are suboptimal
- costs of care are high
- improvements can be expected to produce cost savings
- the condition afflicts a large number of people
- people with the condition can be readily identified
- the pathophysiology of the condition is well understood
- interventions are relatively easy and inexpensive to implement

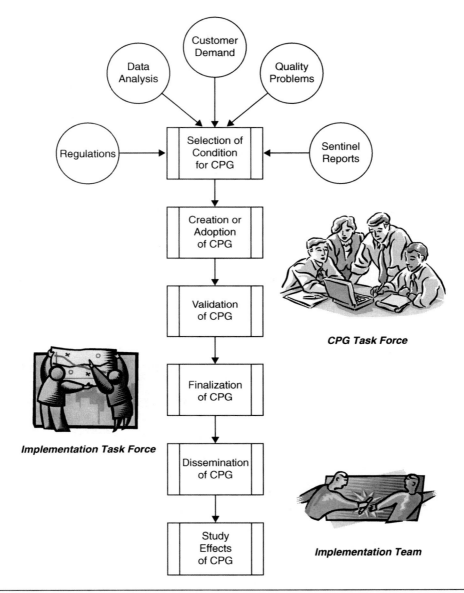

Figure 8.2 CPG Development Process

CPG, clinical practice guideline.

- ◆ consumers value change for the condition
- ◆ regulatory bodies value change for the condition
- ◆ data can be collected relatively easily
- ◆ validated performance measures already exist

Obviously, no condition meets all of these criteria, but any condition that is selected should address as many of these issues as possible. Also, note that

Table 8.1 Stakeholder Goals for CPGs

STAKEHOLDER	GOALS
Patients/Consumers	✓ access to the best medical care possible ✓ protection from untenable financial burdens ✓ pain and complication control and management ✓ limited disruption of lifestyle ✓ maintenance or improvement of quality of life
Physicians	✓ minimal limitations on resources to perform patient care ✓ professional autonomy in decision making ✓ compensation appropriate to the level of care provided ✓ respect for professional abilities
Hospitals	✓ financial resources to provide the infrastructure for patient care ✓ freedom to manage resources according to local standards ✓ minimal oversight by outside agencies and accrediting bodies ✓ community support of health care system
Allied Health Professionals	✓ few or no limitations on resources to provide care for patients ✓ collegial working relationships with physicians and other health professionals ✓ limited oversight by regulatory bodies ✓ respect for skills and professionalism
Employers	✓ good medical care for employees ✓ lowest cost possible ✓ high return on investment ✓ documentation of quality
Insurance Companies	✓ high internal rate of return and shareholder value ✓ cooperative relationships with providers ✓ high quality services, both administrative and medical ✓ competitive position in the marketplace ✓ minimal regulation from government agencies and accrediting organizations
Special Interest Groups	✓ maximum resources allocated for people with a specific condition ✓ open access to care ✓ high quality services and medical treatments
Society	✓ high value services for resources dedicated to health care ✓ continual improvement in the health of the population ✓ research and development in the health care system to enhance medical diagnosis and treatments

CPG, clinical practice guideline.

the criteria are not listed in order of importance because they may vary in significance in different organizations. For example, consumer advocacy organizations will tend to be less concerned about the potential for cost savings or success of interventions than the potential for the CPG to produce improvements in the target condition. Conversely, payers will probably conduct a cost–benefit analysis that will include issues regarding data collection, expected cost savings as a result of the interventions, the cost of diagnostic and therapeutic modalities, and other financial issues. Providers will be less concerned with the cost than with the efficacy of any interventions in making medical practice easier and improving the health of patients. Thus, the type of organization and its goals constitute critical factors in the approach to CPG development.

Creation or Adoption of the CPG

Once a condition has been identified, a comprehensive, expert CPG task force should be assembled to profile the process of diagnosis and treatment. The task force should include any potential contributors to the guideline from the health care field, payers, and even consumers, if possible. Teams should have sufficient expertise to be able to consider scientific evidence regarding patterns of care, but they also should be devised to address the effects on consumers who must deal with the system. Often, one or more consumers who have the condition can provide a perspective to the task force that a purely scientific approach may ignore. An example of a CPG task force for childhood immunizations could include the following team members:

◆ pediatricians and family physicians
◆ parents
◆ school nurses
◆ nurse practitioners
◆ state health officials
◆ county health officials
◆ teachers
◆ school principals
◆ insurers
◆ infectious disease specialists

Team composition must be customized for each clinical condition, as well as for the nature of the organization and the local environment. Medical professionals can include any allied health professionals, and it is incumbent on the organization that convenes the team to evaluate the clinical condition and ensure that all affected professionals are represented.

As detailed in earlier chapters, the continuous quality improvement (CQI) approach suggests that early steps in the analysis should include a flowchart and methods of documenting the course of the clinical problem from exposure to risk factors through initial encounters with providers, diagnosis, treatment, and ultimate outcomes. Because flowcharts can become especially complex in some disease processes, it is often helpful to break the entire process into more manageable subprocesses termed "episodes of care." These episodes describe specific exacerbations or events in the disease process. For example, an episode of care in diabetes could be the onset, diagnosis, and management of diabetic ketoacidosis. The concept of episodes of care is especially useful in evaluating processes for potential areas of intervention and in performing the analyses involved in disease management.

Many disease processes have already been characterized in this manner by organizations such as the AHRQ, specialty societies, universities, and some insurers; but the proliferation of CPGs has also created a somewhat confusing degree of redundancy and contradiction. Some conditions, such as congestive heart failure, may have several CPGs available, and the practice patterns suggested by these disparate guidelines can sometimes conflict with one another. Many published CPGs assume the availability of certain resources such as cardiac catheterization, which may not be accessible where a guideline is to be implemented. Thus, when CPGs are already available, the job of the CPG task force becomes adapting one or more guidelines for local use. A number of Internet-based sources for CPGs are listed in Table 8.2.

If a CPG has not been previously published, then the task force must undertake the arduous mission of creating a CPG from scratch. Rather than

Table 8.2 Internet Sources for CPGs

ORGANIZATION	WEB SITE
AHRQ (formerly AHCPR)	http://www.ahcpr.gov/clinic http://www.guideline.gov
Evidence-Based Medicine Resource Center	http://www.ebmny.org/cpg.html
American Association of Clinical Endocrinologists	http://www.aace.com/clin/guidelines
American College of Radiology	http://www.acr.org/dyna/?doc=departments/stand_accred/standards/standards.html
American Association of Respiratory Care	http://www.aarc.org/resources/cpgs_guidelines_statements
American College of Cardiology	http://www.acc.org/clinical/statements.htm
American College of Rheumatology	http://www.rheumatology.org/research/guidelines/index.asp
American Society of Anesthesiologists	http://www.asahq.org/publicationsAndServices/sgstoc.htm
CDC Prevention Guidelines	http://www.phppo.cdc.gov/cdcRecommends/AdvSearchV.asp

Table 8.2 *continued*

ORGANIZATION	WEB SITE
Canadian Medical Association	*http://www.cma.ca/cpgs/index.html (requires membership in CMA)*
	http://mdm.ca/cpgsnew/cpgs/index.asp (does not require membership in CMA)
University of Washington	*http://www.stat.washington.edu/TALARIA/TALARIA.html*
University of Iowa	*http://www.vh.org/adult/provider/familymedicine/ FPHandbook/FPContents.html*
Emory University	*http://www.medweb.emory.edu/MedWeb*
AMA	*http://www.ama-assn.org/ama/pub/category/4837.html*
NIH	*http://www.nlm.nih.gov/databases/alerts/clinical_alerts.html*
NHLBI	*http://www.nhlbi.nih.gov/guidelines/index.htm*
University of California, San Francisco	*http://medicine.ucsf.edu/resources/guidelines*
NSW Public Health Division, Australia	*http://www.health.nsw.gov.au/public-health/clinprac/ clinprac.html*
Cancer Care—Ontario	*http://www.cancercare.on.ca/access_PEBC.htm*
McMaster University, Canada	*http://hiru.mcmaster.ca/COCHRANE/DEFAULT.HTM*
American Academy of Allergy, Asthma, and Immunology	*http://www.jcaai.org/Param*
University of Dusseldorf	*http://www.uni-duesseldorf.de/WWW/AWMF/ll/ll_list.htm (German)*
American Psychiatric Association	*http://www.psych.org/clin_res/prac_guide.cfm*
Institute for Clinical Systems Integration	*http://www.icsi.org*
American Academy of Pediatrics	*http://www.aap.org/policy/paramtoc.html*
Ontario Medical Association	*http://www.gacguidelines.ca*
American Association for Respiratory Care	*http://www.hsc.missouri.edu/~shrp/rtwww/rcweb/aarc*
	http://www.rcjournal.com/online_resources/cpgs/ cpg_index.asp
American College of Physicians	*http://www.acponline.org/sci-policy/guidelines*
Alberta Medical Association	*http://www.albertadoctors.org/resources/guideline.html*
US Army	*http://www.qmo.amedd.army.mil/pguide.htm*
Veterans Health Administration	*http://www.oqp.med.va.gov/cpg/cpg.htm*

AHCPR, Agency for Health Care Policy and Research; CDC, Centers for Disease Control; AMA, American Medical Association; NIH, National Institutes of Health; NHLBI, National Heart, Lung and Blood Institute; NSW, New South Wales.

searching the medical literature to validate an existing CPG that has been adapted for local use, ad hoc creation of a CPG requires a thorough literature review as an initial step. Searches of the medical literature and Internet resources can be expedited with the use of automated search tools, and experts on the CPG task force usually contribute valuable references for the group to evaluate. The group then pores over the information to identify those sources with the greatest scientific validity, which will be used as the basis for the guideline. The task force drafts the CPG in a format that conveys important information concisely, usually in a flowchart. Samples of an exemplary format can be found on the AHRQ Web site (Agency for Healthcare Research and Quality, 1999. Documentation of each step in the flowchart generally resembles a review article in the medical literature, but the AHRQ has pioneered guides for clinicians and consumers that are more concise and focused on the information that these two groups of stakeholders need. Examples of these guides can be found on the Web site noted.

Validation of the CPG

No guideline will withstand the rigors of professional scrutiny without scientific evidence or expert consensus to support its recommendations. If the CPG task force adopts an existing guideline, the guideline should already include a literature search; however, a subsequent search should be done before the CPG proceeds to implementation because the published CPG may be a year or two old. New evidence may have appeared in the literature that can either confirm the validity of the existing guideline or show that changes are required. For those steps in the CPG that cannot be documented in the medical literature, consensus among the experts on the task force serves to validate the recommendation; however, those areas should be clearly indicated in the CPG so that practitioners can assess the soundness of the guideline. For the CPG to be credible with health care professionals, it must reflect the most recent evidence available or consensus among recognized authorities.

If the task force creates a new CPG, then the literature search should have been performed as part of the initial development activity. Each step in the diagnosis and treatment schema should be documented, either by a valid literature source or by consensus among the panel of experts on the CPG task force. Only rarely will the practice patterns of a CPG be fully supported in the medical literature, so agreement among the experts on the task force will be necessary in nearly all CPGs. One method of indicating the strength of literature or expert support is to use a rating system such as the one described in Table 8.3. Such a rating system provides health care professionals with important information about the nature of the recommendations in the CPG.

Although consensus statements are considered an adequate interim step, the CPG task force should make every effort to cite literature sources whenever possible. As CQI techniques become more widespread in health care,

Table 8.3 Rating System for Evidence in a CPG

CLASS	DESCRIPTION
1	Strong support in the medical literature; judged to be sound medical practice
2	Moderate support in the medical literature; probably sound medical practice, but further research should help clarify the recommendation
3	Little or no support in the medical literature; strong consensus among the experts on the task force that this recommendation represents sound medical practice according to current practice standards
4	Little or no support in the medical literature and marginal consensus among task force experts; the recommendation represents the majority opinion of the task force but not unanimous consent

studies using statistical process control will be able to add information for use in creating CPGs. In the meantime, however, literature sources and expert consensus are the best tools available.

Implementation of the Guideline

If budgets are limited, the work groups that create and validate CPGs may also be required to finalize the product for distribution and follow-up. If organizational structure and financing permit, however, a separate task force for implementation and long-term evaluation of the guideline will provide a new set of eyes to assess the validity and practicality of the CPG. The CPG implementation task force should consist of representatives from as many affected stakeholders as possible, including providers, payers, and consumers. Composition of the CPG implementation task force will depend on the type of organization that is developing the guideline. For example, a provider organization will want to include patients, hospital representatives, local employers, and insurers. Hospitals need to include their physicians and other health professionals involved in the care rendered via the CPG, community leaders, patients, and payers (insurers and employers that directly contract with the hospital). State organizations and agencies like Medicaid bureaus will invariably need to include special interest groups in any task forces. Although the composition of task forces may vary, the function is the same: to ensure that the content and implementation of the guideline will meet the needs of all concerned stakeholders. Ensuring that the guideline meets these needs is often very difficult, and compromises may be necessary; however, the scientific underpinnings of the CPG should be preserved.

The implementation task force should be convened with the goal of soliciting input from pertinent representatives. The task force leader must set the tone of meetings to encourage constructive input and discourage hidden agendas. Task force members should understand that the recommendations of the experts who created the CPG are well founded and that only further credible scientific evidence can alter the CPG. The goals of the implementation task force include

◆ design of the final draft of the CPG
◆ formulation of a plan for disseminating the guideline
◆ promoting patient and provider education in use of the guideline
◆ measuring results of guideline use and interventions
◆ update of the CPG at regular intervals

These essential steps take the CPG from the drawing board to the community, and the task force should be constituted to achieve this goal.

A complete CPG should be written much like a scientific review article but with a few important differences. Scientific reviews generally present the results of a comprehensive literature search and comparison of similar articles. The CPG must contain a similar review, but several other features must be included, among them

◆ a description of the patient population for whom the CPG was developed
◆ a listing of the panel or task force involved in developing the CPG, often with brief biographies to document qualifications
◆ a critical pathway that details the practice recommendations in a graphic format
◆ a step-by-step description of the proposed diagnostic and treatment interventions for patient care

These voluminous reports promote a scientific approach to each CPG, but they usually are not useful to practitioners charged with treating many patients daily, each with a different clinical condition.

Patient care occupies the majority of a busy clinician's time, and practice aids like CPGs must be concise if they are to be usable. Formats such as those created by the AHRQ and the Institute for Clinical Systems Integration (ICSI) (Institute for Clinical Systems Integration, 1999) have found acceptance among practitioners because they summarize guidelines effectively. Generally, the format consists of the following elements: (1) a qualification section that defines patient characteristics for the guideline, (2) a flowchart of the clinical pathway so that the clinician can rapidly assess where the patient falls in the clinical schema, (3) footnotes amplifying certain steps of the pathway to provide further information or to quickly explain the rationale for the recommendation, and (4) appendices with any necessary forms or tables. Guides for clinicians, such as those created by the AHRQ and ICSI, are summaries of CPGs that concisely summarize the salient parts of a CPG for busy practitioners.

The first section of the guideline must succinctly detail the patient attributes that qualify them for the guideline. Depending on the CPG, this information could be a list of symptoms, diagnosis codes, procedure codes, or a specific procedure. The evaluation by the clinician determines the patient's suitability for the guideline, so this section must be very precise. The AHRQ guideline for unstable angina provides a good example. The qualification section presents a list of presenting symptoms and uses the Canadian Cardiovascular Society classification for angina as a resource for categorizing patients who would possibly benefit from the clinical recommendations in the guideline.

The second section of the CPG, the flowchart, provides a rapid overview of the entire process for the practitioner. Because most providers have little time to devote to perusing long textual documents during a busy day, the flowchart performs a useful function by having information presented graphically for rapid assimilation. The physician can place a patient within the clinical pathway quickly and then determine the next steps for the patient's care according to the practice recommendations.

Next in the CPG are footnotes that refer to specific steps in the guideline. These notes serve a number of purposes, such as further explaining a specific recommendation, describing the rationale underlying a step in the process, or referencing specific local issues such as resource availability. Although the notes may provide a fair amount of detail, the clinicians' guides usually limit the footnotes to specific, critically important issues.

Finally, the "short-form CPG" should contain tables, graphs, and forms that expedite the clinician's use of the guideline. Tables and graphs are usually geared toward presenting diagnostic and treatment criteria succinctly. For example, the four-step diagnosis and treatment schema for asthma would be presented in tabular format in a CPG for asthma. Forms are often added as a means of collecting data or submitting information to payers for reimbursement, but this section can also include patient education information such as brochures and tracking sheets for important clinical data.

Dissemination of the guideline can be a monumental task. Organizations such as insurers, who have several thousand network providers, will have much different logistical problems than group practices with only a few practitioners. Getting this information to all possible users can be a daunting and expensive job, especially because each of the guidelines must be updated periodically, necessitating the sending of revisions. Posting guidelines on the Internet can attenuate the cost and effort of distribution. The Internet offers myriad advantages over typical paper distribution methods.

◆ Updates can be disseminated immediately.
◆ Specific users can be notified of updates immediately using Internet-based "push" technology that allows users to request updates from the Web site as soon as they occur.
◆ CPGs can be interactive; i.e., when a practitioner wishes to view a footnote, the Web browser can go to that footnote and then back to the flowchart with minimal effort.

◆ CPGs are available from nearly everywhere.
◆ Information is stored centrally, rather than in libraries in practitioners' offices.
◆ The cost of maintaining a Web site is far lower than printing and mailing to thousands of users.

The list in Table 8.2 details some of the major sites for clinical guidelines on the Internet and provides some direction in effective ways of using the Internet for guideline dissemination.

Providers and consumers must be educated about the purpose and nature of the guidelines. Many physicians might perceive these instruments as "cookbook" medicine, a phrase that is anathema to physicians. The approach to educating providers will depend on the type of organization that is supporting the guideline. Organizations usually can design incentives that improve practitioner adherence to guidelines. A provider organization will often have some influence over the clinician, either through an employment relationship, membership in the provider organization, peer contacts, or credentialing. Insurers control reimbursement, and hospitals often can produce incentives through privileging and specialty facilities. In some circumstances, barriers to implementation can limit the effectiveness of the CPG (e.g., time constraints or poor design of the CPG package). A Barriers Analysis, which is a process that helps identify obstacles to implementation, should help uncover underlying reasons for noncompliance, provide a means for changing the implementation approach, and eliminate the obstacles.

Consumers have a stake in the CPG implementation process, also. If CPGs are appropriately applied, consumers should benefit from higher quality medical care. However, many consumers balk at CPGs because of a lack of understanding of the nature and use of the tools and because their physicians have a poor opinion of the CPG process. Patients must understand that their physicians still manage their medical care and that a CPG simply provides the latest information on the clinical condition, as well as some methods of measuring the effectiveness of care. Patient education must be geared toward the educational level of the population and requires insight into the target group. Many organizations establish an eighth-grade reading level for published materials, but analysis of a particular population's educational level proves useful for customizing patient information.

The organization must also be prepared to implement the CPG. If practitioners are expected to follow certain procedures or collect data while using the CPG, the organization must ensure that the processes for these steps in the CPG are made as straightforward and foolproof as possible. For example, if the clinician is required to report a certain finding to a central database for tracking, then the reporting process should be as simple and expeditious as possible. CPGs that add to a physician's workload are doomed to fail.

Data collection tools must be easy to use and geared toward collecting information at the site of care, rather than relying on recall. Many physicians quickly forget details of patient encounters, so concurrent data collection optimizes accuracy. Forms should be short, simple, and quickly completed. If an automated data-gathering tool is selected, then the system must be responsive and user friendly. After the information is collected, form handling should be limited to putting the form in an envelope for delivery to data analysts. As with all other implementation steps, providers should be involved in planning and implementing these procedures. Most barriers to implementation can be circumvented if providers assist in the planning phase.

As the implementation plan is being developed and executed, the providers on the task force should also direct attention to medical review criteria. As stated previously, medical review criteria identify issues within the CPG that are expected to produce variation or lapses in quality. The medical professionals who will be using the CPG are in the best position to establish which steps in the guideline are likely targets for measurement and intervention. After the medical review criteria are selected, then the task force can determine the best performance measures for evaluating patterns of care as the CPG is introduced into the medical community.

An important part of selecting performance measures is establishing operational definitions that specify the data elements needed to measure the parameters selected in the medical review criteria. If certain data elements are not available or are difficult to obtain, then the task force may reconsider the medical review criteria to find criteria that can be measured economically. A number of sources of well-documented performance measures with solid operational definitions are listed with their Web sites in Table 8.4.

Table 8.4 Sources for Performance Measures

RESOURCE	WEB SITE
NCQA	http://www.ncqa.org/Programs/HEDIS/index.htm
Foundation for Accountability	http://www.facct.org/facct/site/facct/facct/Measures
JCAHO	http://www.jcaho.org
National Quality Measures Clearinghouse	http://www.qualitymeasures.ahrq.gov
Malcolm Baldrige Award Criteria	http://www.baldrige.gov
Leapfrog Group	http://www.leapfroggroup.org/consumer_intro2.htm
CMS: End-Stage Renal Disease Indicators	http://www.cms.gov/esrd/1.asp
HIV Guidelines: HRSA	http://www.hivguidelines.org/public_html/center/quality-of-care/perform_guide/perform_guide.pdf

NCQA, National Committee for Quality Assurance; JCAHO, Joint Commission on Accreditation of Healthcare Organizations; CMS, Centers for Medicare and Medicaid Services; HIV, human immunodeficiency virus; HRSA, Health Resources and Services Administration.

A frequently used source for the health care industry is HEDIS, designed by the NCQA, but numerous organizations are working industriously to create and validate even more measures.

Performance measures represent one of the important products of CPGs. Not only do they assess process efficiency and effectiveness, they can be designed to evaluate outcomes of the process of care defined by the CPG. Medical professionals must be involved in defining the medical review criteria from CPGs, but consumers often become involved in determining which measures are of importance for evaluating processes of care. Only after the criteria are selected and performance measures defined is the CPG ready for implementation.

Users of CPGs

Once these instruments are in the marketplace, one may question who will actually use the CPGs. Obviously, the target groups are providers and consumers, but many others will also find use for the information gleaned from CPG QI studies, including managed care organizations, policy makers in the public and private sectors, provider organizations, governing boards of health care institutions, researchers, consumers, and attorneys and the legal system. All of these potential users must be aware of the limitations of guidelines and their usefulness. Table 8.5 lists some of the uses that each of these groups might find for CPGs.

Managed care organizations adopt CPGs to assist with medical management. Much of the impetus for this use of guidelines is the need for saving money and for satisfying regulatory and certification organizations. The goal of using CPGs should always be to improve the quality of care, which will not always be consistent with the need of managed care organizations to cut costs. Effective managed care organizations reconcile these two goals and create a mix of QI and utilization management that optimizes value. Several important benefits can accrue to managed care organizations using CPGs, not the least of which is standardization of medical utilization criteria that are developed in conjunction with their provider networks. Many managed care organizations use national guidelines that provide only a bare framework for utilization management decision making, and conflicts frequently arise when local practice variations differ from the national guidelines. Having local provider input on the guidelines is one way of defusing those disagreements. Additionally, CPGs serve as the core of an effective care management program (see Chapter 10, "Making Continuous Quality Improvement Work: Care Management"), and a CPG that has been adapted for local use by network physicians and providers is more likely to promote a successful program.

Guidelines also form the basis for analyses of the patterns of care provided to the members of the managed care organization. Performance mea-

Table 8.5 Uses for CPGs

User Group	Potential Uses
Managed Care Organizations	✓ care management programs ✓ utilization management criteria ✓ identification of cost management opportunities ✓ evaluation of quality management opportunities ✓ provider credentialing and recredentialing
Public Policy Makers	✓ resource allocation for populations ✓ development of systemwide medical policy ✓ evaluation of providers, institutions, and health care organizations
Provider Organizations	✓ improve efficiency and effectiveness of care ✓ evaluation of practitioners ✓ enhance consumer satisfaction
Governing Boards of health care institutions	✓ measurement of efficacy of care ✓ benchmark institution with others locally and nationally ✓ implement quality improvement system for clinical services
Researchers	✓ produce findings and comparisons of clinical interventions ✓ benchmarking
Consumers	✓ evaluate health care providers and organizations in terms of quality ✓ compare providers regarding issues of interest ✓ better understand the process of care and individual responsibility
Attorneys and the Legal System	✓ develop standards of quality and medical policy
Providers	✓ better definition of expectations of payers and public ✓ ready source for current practice patterns ✓ method of comparing performance with other providers

sures can have a financial component, as well as a quality component, and that information can be used to analyze areas for intervention to contain costs. Approaching cost containment in this way is more likely to garner the support of network providers because they have had input into the decision-making process. Using similar information, managed care organizations can evaluate the performance of network providers and institutions with the goal of promoting quality and identifying targets for QI and cost-containment efforts. This type of analysis can lead to decisions regarding a provider's continuation in the network of a managed care organization.

Public policy makers have long sought methods of making objective decisions regarding medical policy and provider evaluation. Many areas in the country are publishing report cards with comparisons of providers and payers based on poorly defined criteria, often relating more to cost than to quality. Use of the performance measures from CPGs could alleviate much of that problem. The NCQA and the Foundation for Accountability continually work to improve the measurement systems for managed care organizations, but nationally recognized CPGs could add a dimension of measurement that has heretofore been unavailable.

Organizations of providers are similarly concerned with operational efficiency and cost containment. Medical directors in these groups frequently encounter situations in which they have no means of discussing a practitioner's patterns of care objectively, and CPGs could provide a scientific basis for evaluating the quality of the practice patterns of each group member. The group could measure the performance of each clinician against a cohort of peers and determine what areas of improvement are needed, both at a group level and for each individual practitioner. Objective criteria for such analyses are currently unavailable, but CPGs promise to create the framework for unbiased evaluations.

Similarly, governing boards of health care institutions can seek opportunities for increasing organizational efficiency and improving quality by using CPGs to evaluate care. Frequently, these boards consist of lay people who must follow the guidance of providers at the institution, and, as with any group of professionals, opinions of quality issues can differ. CPGs are adopted by the institution and its providers and thus can be used to gauge the effectiveness of the institution using impartial measures that have been accepted by the entire institution. As more health care organizations compete for contracts, the ability to objectively measure and improve performance becomes even more critical. CPGs provide one tool to assist institutional boards in guiding their organizations in a more rational direction.

Researchers in health care policy also can benefit from broader dissemination of CPGs. As defined patterns of care are corroborated by scientific measurement and tracking, more data will be available to make comparisons between different providers, institutions, and patterns of care. The data will allow analyses that provide information on factors contributing to better outcomes and help direct research efforts into promoting improved care and population health. When CPGs are uniform across study groups, researchers can use CPGs as experimental protocols that serve as the basis for their studies.

Consumers should also be able to enjoy great benefit from CPGs. At the present time, consumers who want to understand the recommendations of their practitioner for care almost need the same knowledge base as the doctor. CPGs help consumers become involved in their care, because the expectations for both patients and providers are clearly outlined in good guidelines. As the consumer movement that began in the late 20th century matures, more people will want to take control of their medical care, and

CPGs present one way that they can have a greater understanding of a disease process and how they need to be involved.

Attorneys are beginning to use CPGs as standards of care, which, unfortunately, subverts the nature of guidelines. Guidelines are not standards of care, but guidelines for quality, and medical policy can emanate from the guidelines once the information has been validated by implementation and study. Using CPGs as standards of care in a legal sense is erroneous and should be discouraged. However, as CPGs mature and as medical policy and standards of quality become codified by the evidence that accumulates through QI studies, the legal system can begin to rely on the resulting standards and policies.

Although listed last in Table 8.5, providers should receive very important benefits from CPGs. In the early stages of managed care, providers rarely knew what these organizations' expectations were regarding care for specific illnesses. Most provider manuals contained lists of procedures that required permission from the payer before they could be ordered for patients, and seldom would the rationale for the list be included. Physicians, especially, have grown increasingly frustrated with the disruption in patient care that such an approach causes. CPGs can offer an alternative approach, because physicians who adhere to CPGs will automatically know when procedures are allowed and what criteria are needed for the payer to approve the tests. The ultimate goal, of course, is to relieve the system of the prior authorization process that is most onerous to physicians. In addition to this benefit, providers can also use CPGs and their attendant performance measures to evaluate their own performance with that of their peers. Provider performance should cluster about a mean, just as with any group measurement, and the performance measures associated with CPGs can provide the information that providers need to make these comparisons among themselves.

Although they have been defined for over a decade, the potential for CPGs is just now being recognized. As health care organizations move further into QI efforts, CPGs provide one means for coordinating efforts to improve care. Properly constituted, CPGs have all of the elements of a QI blueprint for success, and nearly every stakeholder in the health care delivery system will benefit as these useful tools become more prevalent.

◆ Discussion Points

1. Describe the evolution of clinical practice guidelines in health care from their original inception to present implementation.
2. How are clinical practice guidelines used in the health care delivery system? What are the advantages of using clinical practice guidelines? The disadvantages and caveats?
3. Describe the process of creating a clinical practice guideline in a provider organization. How are health professionals involved? What other stakeholders should be involved in the process?

4. Follow the Web links in Table 8.2 to examine the sources for guidelines. Do all of the sites have clinical practice guidelines in the same format? Which format is most effective at conveying the necessary information?

5. Discuss methods of gaining provider cooperation in creating and using clinical practice guidelines. Include in your discussion possible barriers to provider cooperation and barriers to implementation.

6. Choose a disease with which you are familiar and create a clinical practice guideline using the format described in this chapter. If this disease is particularly complex, you may want to choose an episode of care for your analysis.

7. Describe how various stakeholders in society use clinical practice guidelines. Discuss the advantages and disadvantages of these uses.

◆ **Notes**

Agency for Healthcare Research and Quality, (AHRQ), formerly known as the Agency for Health Care Policy and Research (AHCPR). (1999). *National guideline clearinghouse.* Retrieved September 2003, from *http://www.guideline.gov/index.asp*

Agency for Health Care Research and Quality. (1999). *Clinical information.* Retrieved September 2003, from *http://www.ahcpr.gov/clinic*

Agency for Healthcare Research and Quality. (1995, March). *Using clinical practice guidelines to evaluate quality of care: Vol. 1.* (AHCPR Pub. No. 95-0045). Washington, DC.

Anassi E. O., Egbunike I. G., Akpaffiong M. J., Ike E. N., Cate T. R. (1994). Developing and implementing guidelines to promote appropriate use of fluconazole therapy in an AIDS clinic. *Hospital Pharmacist, 29*(6), 576–586.

Apter A. J., Reisine S. T., Affleck G., Barrows E., ZuWallack R. L. (1998). Adherence with twice-daily dosing of inhaled steroids: Socioeconomic and health-belief differences. *American Journal of Respiratory and Critical Care Medicine, 157*(6), 1810–1817.

Associated Press. (1999). *HMOs find a new way to restrict access to your doctor.* Retrieved May 1999, from *http://www.insure.com/health/zzhmodocs599.html*

Bassetti S., Battegay M., Furrer H., Rickenbach M., Flepp M., Kaiser L., Telenti A., Vernazza P. L., Bernasconi E., Sudre P. (1999). Why is highly active antiretroviral therapy (HAART) not prescribed or discontinued? Swiss HIV cohort study. *Journal of Acquired Immune Deficiency Syndrome, 21*(2), 114–119.

Buchner D. A., Butt L. T., De Stefano A., Edgren B., Suarez A., Evans R. M. (1998). Effects of an asthma management program on the asthmatic member: Patient-centered results of a 2-year study in a managed care organization. *American Journal of Managed Care, 4*(9), 1288–1297.

Burton R. A., Joffe G. M. (1998). Neonatal outcomes from a comprehensive prematurity prevention program. *Disease Management, 1*(2), 65–75.

Citrome L. (1998). Practice protocols, parameters, pathways, and guidelines: A review. *Administrative Policy in Mental Health, 25*(3), 257–269.

Collins T. (1998). In search of evidence: California system adopts clinical guidelines, finds quality approach is cost-effective. *Modern Healthcare, 28*(45), 108.

Field M. J. and Lohn K. N. (1990). *Clinical practice guidelines: Directions for a new program*. Washington, DC: National Academy Press.

Hershberger P. J., Robertson K. B., Markert R. J. (1999). Personality and appointment-keeping adherence in cardiac rehabilitation. *Journal of Cardiopulmonary Rehabilitation, 19*(2), 106–111.

Institute for Clinical Systems Integration. (1999). *About ICSI*. Retrieved September 2003, from *http://www.icsi.org*

Khoury A. T. (1998). Support of quality and business goals by an ambulatory automated medical record system in Kaiser Permanente of Ohio. *Effective Clinical Practice, 1*(2), 73–82.

McCulloch D. K., Price M. J., Hindmarsh M., Wagner E. H. (1998). A population-based approach to diabetes management in a primary care setting: Early results and lessons learned. *Effective Clinical Practice, 1*(1), 12–22.

McDowell K. M., Chatburn R. L., Myers T. R., O'Riordan M. A., Kercsmar C. M. (1998). A cost-saving algorithm for children hospitalized for status asthmaticus. *Archives of Pediatric and Adolescent Medicine, 152*(10), 977–984.

Natsch S., van Leeuwen S. J., de Jong R., Hekster Y. A. (1998). Use of albumin in intensive care unit patients—is continuous quality assessment necessary? *Journal of Clinical Pharmacy and Therapeutics, 23*(3), 179–183.

Shrake K. L., et al. (1994). Benefits associated with a respiratory care assessment-treatment program: Results of a pilot study. *Respiratory Care, 39*(7), 715–724.

Thomas L. H., McColl E., Cullum N., Rousseau N., Soutter J., Steen N. (1998). Effect of clinical guidelines in nursing, midwifery, and the therapies: A systematic review of evaluations. *Quality Health Care, 7*(4), 183–191.

Tilney C. K., et al. (1998). Improved clinical and financial outcomes associated with a comprehensive congestive heart failure program. *Disease Management, 1*(4), 175–183.

◆ # Additional Reading

Bowling A. (1997). *Measuring health: A review of quality of life measurement scales*. Philadelphia: Open University Press.

Bowling A. (2001). *Measuring disease: A review of disease-specific quality of life measurement scales*. Philadelphia: Open University Press.

Centre for Health Evidence. *Users' guides to evidence based practice*. Retrieved September 2003, from *http://www.cche.net/usersguides/main.asp*

Chapter 9

Strategies for Implementing Quality Improvement

DONALD E. LIGHTER

◆ Introduction

Taking a quality improvement project from the planning stages to implementation entails unique challenges. Most medical professionals are convinced that they are performing optimally, and the very thought of having someone provide oversight of their work often provokes an angry response. One reason for this natural reaction is the environment that has evolved over the past two or three decades in the health care delivery system. Physicians are no longer esteemed for their knowledge and insight into human disease; rather, they are viewed by some payers as villains with unparalleled control of the health care system and solely motivated by profit. In a grand oversimplification, some payers have lumped all elements of the health care delivery system into a category called "providers," in spite of the fact that each of the provider sectors has distinctive characteristics that must be addressed. Rather than integrating providers into a cohesive delivery system, some payers have only alienated physicians, making cooperation more difficult. This chapter addresses these issues and provides insight into promoting teamwork and cooperation in the health care delivery system.

◆ Deming's 14 Principles Applied to Health Care

W. Edwards Deming will be recognized as one of the great pioneers of quality improvement (QI) in American industry. Through his long career, spanning nearly 50 years, he promoted the tools of QI that are discussed in earlier chapters, and he also helped contribute an even more important concept to American management: respect for the worker's capability and motivation. Through his many books and publications (Deming, 1986), he promoted 14 principles of QI that have become the cornerstone of effective management. These principles, adapted to health care, form the basis for the approach to implementation of health care QI.

Principle 1: Stay in Business

"Create constancy of purpose toward improvement of product and service, with the aim to become competitive and to stay in business, and to provide jobs."

Many health care organizations, from providers through payers, are working very hard to regain the competitive edge that was lost in the days of cost-based reimbursement when hospitals, physicians, and other health care vendors were essentially paid whatever they charged. During that era, incentives tended to favor those with higher costs because that was the basis on which organizations were paid. Few incentives existed to improve efficiency and effectiveness, and many health care organizations, in adapting to the environment, lost their competitive edge.

American industry gradually came to realize that the health care sector was little more altruistic in managing resources than the industrial sector, and market forces were imposed on the health care industry that produced significant changes. A customer focus grew from these economic constraints, making the industry much more responsive to customer demands for improved services and greater convenience. At the same time, the industry became more adept at functioning within budgetary constraints that rewarded efficiency and cost reductions. Of course, these limits entailed dramatic changes in the industry, leading to such strategies as downsizing and the elimination of unprofitable services. The turmoil in the system was sometimes profound. Cost containment as an overarching strategy failed to achieve the long-term goal of producing value in the system.

QI promises to add back the important numerator in the value equation

(9.1) Value = Quality/Cost

Although reducing costs improves value, when cost reductions also reduce quality at the same rate, value is unaffected. Conversely, improvements in quality may increase costs somewhat, but improvement efforts must be directed at improving quality to a greater extent than increasing costs; i.e., the efforts must be cost effective. Thus, cost reduction efforts, in the absence of QI interventions, can lead to decreased value for payers.

Following Deming's first principle, organizations should focus on improving the quality of products and services while always considering the costs associated with improvements. Deming stressed the need for remaining competitive, and for American industry, competitiveness has become a global problem. American health care still tends to maintain local or regional markets, making the market dynamics different, even if the principle is the same. Importantly, Deming implies the need for providing jobs as one of the imperatives of the first principle. Efficient and effective organizations will grow, particularly in the health care industry, because the demand for health services continues to grow as the population ages (see Chapter 1, "Principles and Methods of Quality Improvement in Health Care"). Thus, new job creation must come from growth in the industry, not from inefficient work rules and staffing requirements. A dynamic workforce such as this must be flexible, i.e., able to adjust to varying hours of operation and skill set requirements for optimizing services. Health care organizations must be geared to listen to all customers, internal and external, and respond to their needs for improved services. The effective health services organization must be just as prepared to make services available outside regular business hours as it is to provide ongoing training opportunities for staff members who are trying to improve their skills.

Principle 2: Adapt to the New Economic Age

"Adopt the new philosophy. We are in a new economic age. Western management must awaken to the challenge, must learn their responsibilities, and take on leadership for change."

Deming worked in Japan extensively after World War II, helping that country become an economic giant after its devastating defeat in the war. He observed immense differences between Japanese and American manufacturing management, and this second principle was directed at sending a wake-up call to American managers. This same wake-up call can be modified for American health care managers, providers, and payers. The health care delivery system is profoundly different than it was just a few years ago. The new economic age in health care has removed many of the illogical economic incentives that led to inefficiencies in the system. The challenge is clear: the system must adapt to the new economic age in health care, just as American industry adjusted to the economic realities of the global marketplace. Health care managers must lead change and find innovative new ways to deliver care.

Change is rarely easy to achieve. Ingrained methods of conducting business take on inflated importance, with substantial investment by all stakeholders in the status quo. Physicians rely on fees to maintain their practices and incomes; hospitals base management decisions on the assurance that any increased costs for services will be automatically reimbursed by payers; insurers find refuge in paying claims and ignoring rising costs. All of these realities must be changed if the system is to make the conversion to the new economic order. Deming realized this for American industry and sounded the alarm. Now the health care delivery system faces the same mandate for change. Dynamic leaders are emerging to lead the industry, using many of the techniques for producing change that are described in this book. One of the first responsibilities that these leaders face, however, is a global understanding of the system, rather than a parochial view based on the needs of a single sector. Just as the demand for health services knows few limits, the unfettered growth in the supply of services leads to inappropriate practice patterns. Health care industry leaders, from both the provider and payer segments, must understand all segments of the marketplace to properly balance the allocation of resources with appropriate demand.

Principle 3: Eliminate the Need for Inspection

"Cease dependence on inspection to achieve quality. Eliminate the need for inspection on a mass basis by building quality into the product in the first place."

Regulation and inspection in the health care industry have evolved into a huge business. From large oversight organizations, such as the Joint Commission on Accreditation of Healthcare Organizations (JCAHO) and the National Committee for Quality Assurance (NCQA), to state and federal agencies, such as the Centers for Medicare and Medicaid Services (CMS; formerly the Health Care Financing Administration) and the Occupational Safety and Health Administration (OSHA), the health care industry is awash in regulation and inspection. All of these regulatory and accreditation requirements add to the cost of providing care, as well as overhead for insurers and managed care organizations that often seek certification as a requirement for contracting with large payers. Outcomes from these efforts have not been measured to determine the economic value added, and so there is no hard evidence indicating that the regulations have had a salient effect on the quality of care or improved value in the health care delivery system. On the other hand, reports like the one produced by the Institute of Medicine in 2001, which indicated that as many as 98,000 people a year may be dying in US hospitals as a result of medical errors, sustain regulatory efforts to reduce error and waste (Institute of Medicine, 2001).

The value of accreditation and the resulting standards remain unproven but accepted by the US health care system as a cost of doing business. Few employers use accreditation as a significant factor for deciding on the value of a managed care organization (Medscape, 1998). Although health plans that reported Health Plan Employer Data and Information Set (HEDIS) measures to the NCQA's Quality Compass tended to perform better on these measures (Albritton, 1998), that performance has not been equated with better-quality care or lower overall cost of care in objective studies. The NCQA has been increasingly criticized for the intensity of the review process, and many managed care organizations are reevaluating the decision to undergo review (Bocchino, 1999). As Deming's principles indicate, managed care organizations that seek NCQA accreditation might concentrate on improving HEDIS scores rather than improving the quality of care for members based on objective evaluations of the member population. Further study will be necessary to demonstrate value for accreditation by these organizations.

Principle 4: Reward Quality

"End the practice of awarding business on the basis of price tag. Instead, minimize total cost. Move toward a single supplier for any one item, on a long-term relationship of loyalty and trust."

Deming emphasized in this principle a well-known tenet in health care: suppliers of services must be trustworthy. Physicians and other providers in the system work diligently to garner patient trust and loyalty, but these same types of relationships must exist throughout the supply chain in the health care delivery system. Vendors of pharmaceuticals, durable medical equipment, financial software—indeed, all products and services in the system—must be reliable and worthy of the consumer's trust. Because health care consumers are rarely cognizant of many of the intermediary steps and products necessary to the delivery of health services, the task of health care managers entails assurance of quality throughout the system. Consumers must be assured that every vendor in the health care system is working toward improving the quality of care.

Managers, then, must find methods of enhancing the ability of suppliers to continually improve the quality of the raw materials and products that ultimately produce consumer products and services. One method, suggested by Deming in this principle, is sole-sourcing supplies and developing trust relationships with vendors. This approach can be ideal in some situations but may not be practical for all vendor relationships. The concept of establishing trust relationships with vendors can be advanced, however, by instituting quality expectations for products and services obtained from each supplier. Many industries are now exploring supply chain integration, in which relationships with suppliers are actively managed to improve a producer's operations through physical proximity or operational support (Alberty, 1999; Bhargava, 1999). Although this aspect of integration in the health care industry has not been exploited in the past, such relationship building will be critical to satisfying consumer demands in the future.

Principle 5: Improve Constantly

"Improve constantly and forever the system of production and service, to improve quality and productivity, and thus constantly decrease costs."

One of the most critical tasks for the health care industry is the conversion from a quality assurance framework to one of QI. Most health care managers with tenure in the industry are familiar with the quality assurance paradigm: set targets, meet targets through interventions with staff and providers, find new projects. Typical quality assurance projects would involve endeavors such as reducing the infection rate in an operating suite to a specific level or ensuring that at least 50% of the staff receive continuing education during a year's time. These projects attempt to ensure that organizational performance meets some minimum requirement, rather than encouraging employees to continually improve performance beyond the minimum requirement.

The new approach engendered by QI involves not being satisfied with meeting a specific goal but rather having the organization make continual progress toward 100% compliance. In other words, a mammography rate target for a health plan should be 100% of women at risk, rather than 85%. Staff members should inculcate the "zero defects" concept articulated by Phillip

Crosby (Crosby, 1979), working to provide the very best care possible with available resources. Crosby also encouraged production systems to move toward the goal of no rework, closely adhering to Deming's third principle.

The six sigma concept also applies to continuous improvement in health care (Chassin, 1998). Developed by Motorola in the 1980s, the six sigma concept sets specification limits to six standard deviations, rather than the usual three sigma limits. A six sigma specification allows only 3.4 defects per million units or opportunities, and almost no health care providers, payers, or institutions meet those levels of performance presently. Reaching the six sigma goal requires a firm commitment to quality. Chassin notes in his 1998 article that studies of quality indicators such as use of beta blockers after a myocardial infarction demonstrate that many health care processes have not even reached a one sigma level yet, and most providers have not implemented QI interventions to deal with the manifold problems in the delivery system. Payers are becoming increasingly vocal about these levels of defects, making the need for change more critical than ever.

Another important feature of this principle involves continually minimizing cost. Although the current approach to quality in health care tends to add cost, properly applied QI techniques should reduce costs in a number of ways, including

◆ less waste
◆ reduced rework
◆ improved customer satisfaction
◆ reduced inspection
◆ less supervision

Reducing (or even better, eliminating) waste decreases the cost of goods and services required for production, leading to lower cost per unit produced. Eradicating rework similarly triggers greater productivity by making each input unit create new outputs, rather than recycling processes to produce the same output unit over and over again. Higher quality products and services invariably lead to greater customer satisfaction, improving sales and increasing demands on production that allow optimization of the production process. By reducing inspection and supervision, significant management costs can be eliminated, again leading to greater profitability.

These tenets have demonstrated effectiveness in manufacturing, but are they also applicable to health care? Although the nuances of medical care sometimes can make the task of implementing QI efforts more difficult, these endeavors can be rewarded with lower costs and improved productivity. Virtually every segment of the industry can benefit from reductions in rework, elimination of supervisory oversight, and eradication of inspection. In health care, the mistakes leading to rework also can create medical malpractice risks that add to costs and can tarnish a provider's image and marketability.

Deming's principles are almost universally applicable to health care, and this principle is particularly germane for the health care industry.

Principle 6: Institute On-the-Job Training

"Institute training on the job."

Providers are accustomed to on-the-job training (OJT). Much of a graduate physician's residency training consists of working in an environment with supervision and educational opportunities at the work site. Upon completion of a training program, the number of educational opportunities expands exponentially, but they become increasingly difficult to access. Continuing education suddenly moves from the work site to expensive and inaccessible sites. Nurses and other health professionals have similar problems, because many institutions and employers are cutting back on continuing education budgets in response to shrinking revenues. The goal of the system must be to find creative ways of providing continuing education for practitioners that pique interest and challenge intellects. Newer technologies can help address these problems. Universal Internet access brings interesting and current multimedia education to the site of care inexpensively. Continuing education credit is available to virtually all medical professions. (Table 9.1 provides a sampling of continuing education sites on the Internet.) In addition to these sites for online continuing education credit, additional resources exist in cyberspace, from scientific papers to compendia of pharmaceuticals and much more. The wealth of information in cyberspace sometimes makes finding information difficult, but online search engines have simplified the process.

Most medical facilities have a computer network, facilitating access to the Internet and also providing the infrastructure for distribution of information across the network. Many resources available on media such as CD-ROM and DVD can place textbooks and other references at the disposal of health professionals, making decision support feasible even in small organizations. With better communications modalities through the Internet or telemedicine technology, online consultations with experts can provide clinical and educational support for even the most remote locations. Additionally, computerized decision-support tools are becoming more powerful as their knowledge bases grow, providing tremendous educational and clinical support. Providers will need to update skills in acquiring and evaluating information, but the tools for using these resources have become exceedingly straightforward.

OJT and continuing education have always been an important part of the health care industry. With the volume of medical research and publishing increasing exponentially (Wilkie, 1996), even more sophisticated methods of distributing and finding new information will become mandatory. Customers and payers are demanding current, scientifically valid care, and the providers who will succeed in the new health care economy will be able to

Table 9.1 Continuing Education on the Internet

Target Audience	Content	Address
Physicians	Emergency and critical care, pediatrics, internal medicine	http://www.cmeweb.com
	Critical care, pulmonology	http://www.vh.org/Providers/CME/CMEHome.html
	Radiology, ultrasound	http://www.acuson.com/cme/index.html
	General medical, infectious diseases	http://arcmesa.com
	Internal medicine, primary care	http://www.vlh.com
	General medicine	http://main.uab.edu/uasom/show.asp?durki=14847
Nurses	General nursing education	http://www.ce-web.com
	General nursing education, nursing journals	http://www.nursingcenter.com/prodev/ce_online.asp
	Clinical nursing subjects	http://www.rnceus.com
Pharmacists	General pharmacy topics	http://www.vh.org/Providers/CME/CMEHome.html
	General pharmacy topics	http://www.rxce.org

provide such care conveniently and economically. Additionally, providers who are bringing the best care to their patients tend to be more satisfied with their jobs and consequently more productive.

Principle 7: Help People and Machines Do a Better Job

"Institute leadership. The aim of supervision should be to help people and machines and gadgets to do a better job. Supervision of management is in need of overhaul, as well as supervision of production workers."

Deming and many others recognized in the 1960s and 1970s that the old paradigm of management was changing. Managers were being redefined as coaches and mentors, and the oversight function of their jobs was dramatically reduced. Rather than simply cajoling a workforce to improve productivity, managers were now trying to encourage workers and provide the support necessary for workers to improve their own levels of productivity. The 1982 bestseller, *In Search of Excellence* (Peters and Waterman, 1982), brought these concepts from the best American companies to the general management curricula of business schools, revolutionizing American industry and changing the role of managers.

The goal of health care managers, then, must be to optimize output from people and machines. Although it appears that this task should be relatively simple because most workers in health care are highly educated and motivated, the incentives in the system have become distorted over the years so that physicians often have incentives that conflict with those of hospitals and other institutions. In many cases, an adversarial relationship has built up between providers and payers because of techniques applied by managed care organizations to advance their needs for cost containment. These conflicting relationships complicate management's task, but they also provide the impetus for improving efficiency and effectiveness.

The complexity of the manager's job in health care produces a substantial motivation for implementing QI concepts. Cost containment has been a prominent feature in the industry for the past two decades, and the results have been untoward for patient and physician satisfaction, as well as efficiency in the system (Reinhardt, 1999; DeBakey & DeBakey, 1999). Because the paradigm of QI has proven to be efficacious in reducing costs and increasing satisfaction in American industry, many payers are putting pressure on the health care industry to implement QI methods for both administrative and clinical processes. Some health care organizations have adopted QI with great success (Cooperative Cardiovascular Project Best Practices Working Group, 1998; Zinn, et al., 1997; Brailer, et al., 1997). In virtually all of the organizations that have succeeded in these efforts, managers have changed the organizational focus from reducing costs to improving quality. Greater emphasis on quality should optimize the efforts of staff and use of resources to achieve organizational goals.

Principle 8: Drive Out Fear

"Drive out fear, so that everyone may work effectively for the company."

Perhaps one of the least motivating tools available to management is fear. Although fear may promote short-term gains, longer term accomplishments become unlikely. In fact, workers who are motivated by fear often opt out of the organization as soon as they can, robbing the organization of talent as well as crushing morale. Workers spend more time inventing ways of avoiding difficult situations than in finding methods of increasing output. Fear never improves productivity.

Managers must empower workers to perform optimally rather than threaten retribution. As noted in Chapter 7, "Advanced Statistical Applications in Continuous Quality Improvement," QI data can be used for retribution as well as for improvement. QI studies should be targeted at finding process problems that impede worker efforts, rather than identifying which workers cannot conform to the process. By emphasizing this philosophy and incorporating workers into QI studies, managers can reduce fear in the organization and improve productivity.

Fear pervades the health care industry at the beginning of the 21st century. Hospitals face shrinking utilization rates and increasing costs. Physicians have seen their professional authority and prestige undermined by managed care and consumer dissatisfaction. Health insurance companies must continually contain costs to maintain market share while avoiding litigation and sanctions from providers, consumers, and regulators. Falls in the returns on investment portfolios have put heavy pressure on financial management in all sectors of the health care industry. A QI approach can be an ideal solution to drive fear out of the system. A collaborative approach to making the system more efficient can overcome many of the barriers that have inhibited constructive progress toward improvement. If each of the stakeholders can recognize the strengths of the others while acknowledging their own shortcomings, a cooperative environment could be created that would reduce fear in the system and improve value for consumers.

Principle 9: Break Down Barriers

"Break down barriers between departments. People in research, design, sales, and production must work as a team, to foresee problems of production and in use that may be encountered with the product or service."

Barriers exist throughout the health care system, from barriers for patients accessing care, to barriers between institutions that could share expensive resources, to barriers between departments in health insurance organizations that lead to inefficiencies in payment. Deming's insight into barriers transcended the usual impediments in communications and included both physical and psychological barriers to improved productivity. Managers must recognize these issues and develop strategies to eliminate conditions that lead to problems with worker efficiency. Health care managers must understand the dynamics of the delivery system to be capable of optimizing the work environment.

As illustrated in Figure 9.1, barriers arise at several levels in the health care industry. The adversarial relationships that create fear in the system present a prime opportunity for improvement. By demonstrating the advantages of cooperation between the health care financing and delivery systems, health care managers can force through barriers that increase costs and decrease quality of care. Within organizations, health care managers can work to align incentives so that the entire organization and major suppliers can work toward the same goal: patient and customer satisfaction. Work units can also benefit from managerial influence to decrease interpersonal barriers to growth and development. As workers reach self-actualization through

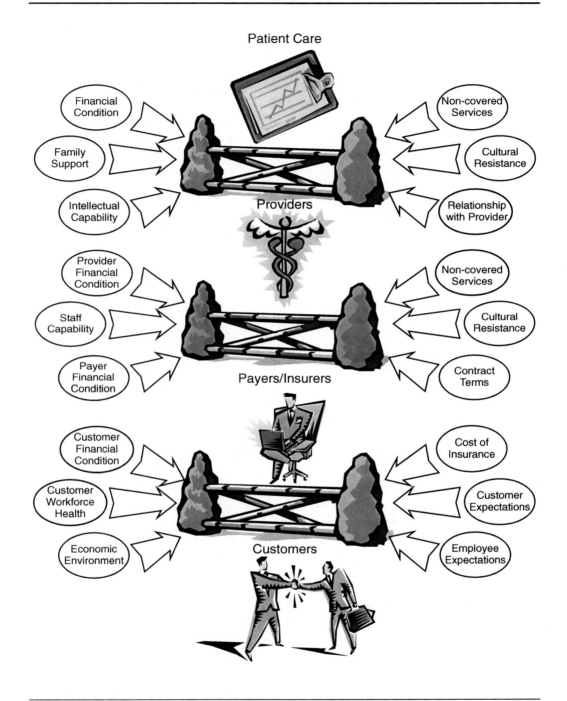

Figure 9.1 Barriers in the Health Care Industry

their work, they will become more productive and contribute to organizational goals.

Barriers to patient care occur, for example, when services recommended by the physician are not covered by the patient's insurance plan. Most people are not financially capable of paying for expensive services, so a denial by the payer usually means that services will not be rendered without a lengthy appeal or grievance process. Lack of insurance coverage presents only one barrier to patient care, however. A number of other issues have persisted throughout the history of medical care, e.g., the physician–patient relationship, cultural inhibitions and their effect on patient adherence to treatment regimens, the patient's intellectual ability, and family support of the therapeutic regimen. All of these factors affect the willingness of the patient to take a drug regularly, change dietary habits, or stop a harmful health practice. Skilled physicians have learned to manage many of these problems, but the system must also be designed to reduce inhibitions to care. For example, if patients cannot leave work to undergo a test, then the procedure must be available after normal work hours, necessitating longer hours of availability at hospitals and testing facilities.

Serious barriers have arisen between providers and payers in the era of managed care. Payers have exerted more control over the care provided patients through the mechanism of "covered services"—denial of payment for services that are considered not medically necessary by the insurer. Because most patients do not have the financial resources to pay for these denied services, they forgo the treatment or test, despite recommendations by the physician. Such denials have driven a wedge between insurers and providers because providers resent having insurance company staff supervise patient care. On the other hand, insurers often have no other alternative than to contain escalating costs of care. Thus, this adversarial relationship has created a barrier between these two important stakeholders. Physicians devise methods of circumventing insurance regulations while insurers become increasingly restrictive to counter physician efforts. These machinations have led to increasing costs as insurers add staff to implement increasing numbers of regulations and physicians add staff to deal with the upsurge in rules. Deming's philosophy would urge a removal of regulations and barriers that separate providers and payers.

Insurers have special problems, in addition to their travails with providers. Customer expectations have increased to include demands for quality care at prices that are affordable, and insurers have been placed in a position of decreasing the cost of care and increasing quality. Regulators have placed increasing demands on health insurers to achieve specific levels of performance on clinical, as well as administrative, measures. Customer demands and regulations can sometimes place barriers between insurers and the employers who purchase coverage. Employee expectations drive employers to require greater coverage for shrinking insurance premiums, leading to substantial pressure on insurer finances. Regulators often rate insurers using subjective criteria that then are interpreted by employers to reflect lower quality. These barriers can prove onerous for insurers, who must continually adjust to market pressures.

Managers in the health care industry face numerous challenges because of these barriers, and one of the first tasks of effective management involves gaining an understanding of the underlying sources of these obstacles. Although innovative approaches to barriers in the system can help improve the efficiency of the health care industry, compromise will be necessary for the system to succeed. Managers in each sector of the system, as well as employers and consumers, must be willing to cooperate with one another to ensure that value will be created in the industry.

Principle 10: Eliminate Slogans, Quotas, and Management by Objective

"Eliminate slogans, exhortations, and targets for the workforce asking for zero defects and new levels of productivity. Such exhortations only create adversarial relationships, as the bulk of the causes of low quality and low productivity belong to the system and thus lie beyond the power of the workforce. Eliminate work standards (quotas) on the factory floor. Substitute leadership. Eliminate management by objective. Eliminate management by numbers, numerical goals. Substitute leadership."

Deming disdained the use of slogans and similar invocations to improve productivity. Many organizations rely on these types of interventions as a means of improving productivity and simultaneously ignore process evaluations. Workers often find themselves in an environment that inhibits optimum productivity, and because slogans cannot change the environment, productivity will not improve. Management expectations will usually be unreasonable, leading to worker frustration and increasingly adversarial relationships between management and the workforce. Deming recognized this problem in American industry and designed a group exercise, the red bead experiment. In this exercise, he demonstrated that management interventions of setting goals for the workforce and cajoling workers to improve are ineffective when the environment does not support productivity gains. The following example illustrates a similar problem in health care.

Example 9-1

The administration at St. Anywhere Hospital was becoming progressively more concerned about dropping patient satisfaction scores in the emergency department. Surveys of patients treated in the department indicated that the most significant factor was the waiting time for services. A Pareto analysis then defined the problem (Figure 9.2). The figure demonstrates that long waiting times and staff discourtesy were among the most prevalent reasons for patient dissatisfaction. The administration placed a number of signs around

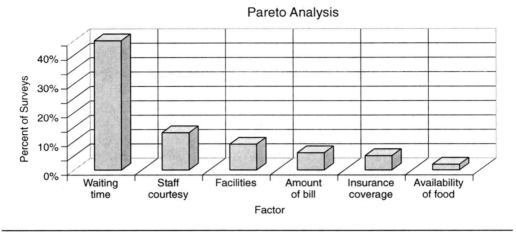

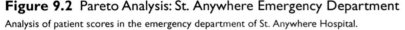

Figure 9.2 Pareto Analysis: St. Anywhere Emergency Department

Analysis of patient scores in the emergency department of St. Anywhere Hospital.

the emergency department staff rooms, with slogans such as "The Patient Is Our First Priority" and "Rapid Care Is Excellent Care," among others. Over the next few months, administrators noted that survey scores actually dropped slightly, rather than rising in response to the "customer first" campaign. At this point, they polled staff in the emergency department, who noted that scheduling patterns left the department understaffed during the early evening hours when the number of emergency visits increased. Administrators delegated scheduling to department managers, and over the next several months, patient survey scores improved by 30%, and waiting time and staff courtesy complaints disappeared from the Pareto analysis.

Once scheduling problems were identified and corrected by emergency department staff, waiting times decreased, and with improvement in patient satisfaction and better distribution of the workload, emergency department staff satisfaction improved, leading to better scores on staff courtesy. Deming stressed the primacy of workers' ability to solve logistical problems, and he repeatedly encouraged managers to create an environment in which workers can demonstrate proficiency.

Principle 11: Restore Pride of Workmanship for Hourly Workers

"Remove barriers that rob the hourly worker of his right to pride of workmanship. The responsibility of supervisors must be changed from sheer numbers to quality."

Although Deming initially referred to production line workers with this principle, he could easily have included health care workers in positions that pay hourly. Workers with basic skills perform much of the work in hospitals, health plans, and physicians' offices, and these people are often the most visible to the public. Receptionists, maintenance workers, nurses' aides, and transport staff all spend copious time with patients, and their attitudes and demeanor can have significant influence on patient perceptions of an institution or provider. A receptionist who treats customers rudely will have tremendous negative influence on a medical practice in much the same manner as a hospital environmental services staff member who does not thoroughly clean a room.

Deming started with the observation that hourly workers want to perform well and that job performance depends on the need to have pride of workmanship. Recognizing this need, managers should uncover any impediments to workers' achievement of excellent performance, regardless of organizational function. Whether the task involves better allocation of resources or minimization of interpersonal conflict, any barriers to optimum performance must be identified and overcome through cogent management.

Principle 12: Restore Pride of Workmanship for Managers

"Remove barriers that rob people in management and in engineering of their right to pride of workmanship. This means, inter alia, abolishment of the annual or merit rating and of management by objective."

What was stated in Principle 11 regarding hourly workers should apply to managers as well. Managers also must feel empowered to perform optimally. Management personnel are usually chosen because of their ability to lead, but if that ability is thwarted by other influences, e.g., executive management or environmental influences, managers will lose the pride of workmanship that drives performance. Deming posited that some management techniques popular in the 1970s and 1980s, such as management by objective and annual merit evaluations, deprived managers of the empowerment that they needed to achieve pride of workmanship. Organizations that have executive managers setting goals for each individual middle manager remove one of the important factors that drive managers: the desire to achieve self-actualization through achievement of self-determined goals.

This principle is particularly germane to physicians. During the first half of the 20th century, doctors became increasingly revered for bringing the scientific method to the care of their patients, and during the 1960s and 1970s, physicians were given nearly free rein to apply these scientific advances to medicine, regardless of cost. As society recoiled at the cost of the resulting largesse, increasing controls were placed on the ability of physicians to direct the vast resources of health care for individual patients, and the physician was gradually displaced from a position of preeminence in the health care delivery system to that of a provider or supplier of services. This change led to increasing dissatisfaction among physicians (Gallagher, 1998; Morain, 1998;

Gold, 1999) because of loss of autonomy, prestige, and income. This principle would indicate that physician performance should suffer, and managed care organizations have increasing difficulty with physician behavior within these restrictive systems.

Health care managers also can lose autonomy because of changes in both the internal and external environments. Restrictions instigated by upper management or by industry regulators can deprive managers of autonomy and replace job satisfaction with desperation. Health care managers now face decreasing job security as the industry changes dramatically nearly every year. Reorganization of work units, management turnover, and economic changes have created instability in the industry that has profoundly altered the health care environment. This lack of security has forced many managers to focus on short-term (1 year or less) financial performance, sometimes at the cost of diminishing quality of care and long-term viability of organizations. Senior management must buffer these stresses to provide managers with an environment that fosters quality.

Principle 13: Institute Education and Self-Improvement

"Institute a vigorous program of education and self-improvement."

Change requires education. From advances in health care to advances in management science, changes in the practice of medicine and management require continuing education to succeed. Physicians are required in many states to have at least 50 hours of continuing medical education for licensure renewal, and some management organizations require postgraduate education for membership. New ideas and techniques can revitalize organizations and workers, as well as improve the quality of the organization's efforts. The concept of continuing education is replete throughout medicine and the health care industry, but Deming touched on a more personal consequence of education and self-improvement.

Education not only facilitates change, it promotes personal growth. Workers who continue to learn more about their professions tend to be more satisfied and empowered because they can bring new concepts to improving the quality of their work. More knowledgeable workers usually are allowed more independence because they can assume greater responsibility for their performance. Managers can create the environment in which workers are encouraged to continually improve through education, as well as through personal experience.

Principle 14: Make Quality Everyone's Job

"Put everybody in the company to work to accomplish the transformation. The transformation is everybody's job."

Quality must become a cultural value within any organization. Deming realized this fact by articulating Principle 14, which calls on managers and senior executives to suffuse the organization with a QI focus. Quality assurance has traditionally been performed in designated departments, but the QI paradigm moves the responsibility to every department in the organization. A major change in the organization such as this requires strong and continuing support from upper management. Senior managers must stress that quality is expected from every worker and restructure the organization to reflect that philosophy. Performance incentives must be realigned to reflect the emphasis on quality, and everyone in the organization must be involved in enhancing processes for QI.

◆ Approaches to Implementation

Perhaps the most critical aspect of QI in any organization is obtaining an abiding commitment from senior management. If executive managers internalize the QI philosophy, success is much more likely. In practice, however, most senior managers are at least initially motivated by financial considerations or regulatory agency requirements. Nearly every facet of the health care industry is regulated in some way, either by government agencies or by independent regulatory bodies like the JCAHO or the NCQA. These agencies have promulgated standards and regulations that mandate QI activities, and these requirements often stimulate senior management to adopt QI solely to satisfy accreditation standards. A QI manager often must capitalize on the need for accreditation as a means for securing initial senior management support, but relying on that factor for long-term support usually fails. Once a QI program has begun, projects and interventions should be selected that have financial effects, as well as that improve a performance measure. It is important, however, that any QI project have a primary goal of improving the output of a process at a reasonable cost, thus adding value to the organization. QI must never be conceived as a series of projects, however. A true QI program involves everyone in the organization and pervades all organizational processes.

◆ Phases of Organizational Change

A QI transformation seems for most people to be almost trivially logical, but for others, any change in normal routine can prove vexing. Coupled with the requirement of most businesses for justification of substantial resource allocation, the transformation must be ordered and well documented. The sequence of events leading to permanent changes includes

1. awareness of need
2. identification of needed changes
3. planning
4. implementation
5. measuring impact
6. institutionalization of new approaches

These steps in the process of change are nearly always necessary to gain long-term improvement in a process. Some organizations may truncate or eliminate some of these steps at times, but success requires completion of all steps in the process of change.

Awareness of Need for Change

Even acknowledging the natural desire to perform a job better can be threatening for some people. Particularly in very busy institutions, the need for improving the quality of outcomes or processes usually does not find support because many in the organization would assert, "If we weren't doing a good job, then we wouldn't be so busy, right?" Health care organizations frequently find themselves in this situation. As the demand for health care services has expanded in the past three or four decades, most institutions and medical practices find themselves overwhelmed with large volumes of patients, all of whom have some sort of insured payment mechanism. With such a robust market and virtually assured payment for any services that are provided, many providers cannot justify the cost of trying to improve the system. Health care has traditionally been one of the few industries in which rework and defects are subsidized, affording few financial incentives to encourage elimination of defects. The advent of newer payment systems has changed the incentives, however, and the health care industry has vigorously incorporated cost containment, sometimes to the detriment of quality. Focusing the organization on quality, rather than just on cost containment, can eliminate many of the problems that the industry has produced through aggressive cost cutting. The growing awareness among health care managers of this basic tenet of business provides an opportunity for fueling a QI transformation.

As these changes are being studied, rumors and fears often permeate an organization. Workers learn that management is studying a "reorganization" or "reengineering" project and immediately fear for their jobs. This quandary presents a real opportunity for management to present the concepts of QI for employees, as well as to gain input from workers on many of the implementation issues that arise. Leaving workers with no other information but rumors inevitably leads to dissatisfaction and fear, clearly counter to Deming's Principle 8. During this period, management can initiate informational sessions that describe the QI process, the customer focus that the organization will foster throughout the workforce, and the need for everyone in the organization to be willing to change their traditional work habits to meet the new challenges. Worker input should be encouraged during these sessions, with open discussion of apprehensions and misgivings. Additionally, if the organization has departments, the leaders in each department must be continually included in the process of planning and updated on progress toward the goals of other work groups. In short, open communication is the key to allaying worker fears and providing a firm foundation for the changes to come.

Identification of Areas for Improvement

Most organizations have numerous opportunities for improvement, and because resources are always finite, QI interventions must be prioritized. Regardless of which opportunity rises to the top of the list, however, the QI philosophy must continually be reinforced throughout the organization, and some funds must be allocated to enhance awareness of the need for quality in every department. The methods of evaluating alternatives include the following:

◆ company data analysis
◆ customer feedback and surveys
◆ competitor data
◆ industry data
◆ employee surveys

These methods all require varying amounts of resources, and some organizations, e.g., small medical groups, may want to have consultants perform the tasks, rather than develop these capabilities internally. Consultants sometimes are valuable for larger organizations as well, to augment areas in which the company may be deficient, such as data collection or analysis.

The differences between administrative and clinical data are discussed in Chapter 3. The type of data required will depend on the QI focus, but every health care organization can benefit from analysis of both types of data. Table 9.2 lists criteria for prioritizing QI opportunities. In both clinical and administrative improvement systems, cost often assumes primary importance because every organization must survive financially. Thus, if a program can evaluate quality issues that are also the most costly, QI interventions can address two problems simultaneously. The most expensive clinical conditions, for example, often are replete with QI opportunities (Denton, et al., 1998; Tucker, et al., 1998; Balas, et al., 1998). Analyzing a data set for the most costly clinical conditions requires administrative data.

Another important criterion that differentiates clinical improvement efforts is the morbidity, i.e., the degree of illness and disability caused by a disease, and the mortality (death) associated with a clinical condition. Although these two concepts are distinct, they are often considered together as a means of identifying clinical conditions of importance for QI. Clinical conditions with high morbidity or mortality rates are often chosen for intervention, and performance measures that reflect these two attributes are used to gauge the success of the interventions. National programs for clinical QI have been implemented for these reasons, such as the Cooperative Cardiovascular Project initiated by the federal government (Marciniak, et al., 1998). The rationale for these programs emanates from evidence indicating that reducing morbidity improves quality of life and also from the unending quest of the medical profession to reduce mortality from disease.

Table 9.2 Selection Criteria for QI Opportunities

CLASS	CRITERIA
Clinical	• Cost of condition
	• Morbidity and mortality
	• Customer demand
	• Importance to providers
	• Ability to change
	• Regulatory or accrediting requirements
	• Cost of change
Administrative	• Cost of process
	• Degree of dysfunction
	• Cost of errors and rework
	• Importance of quality lapse to customers
	• Regulatory or accrediting requirements
	• Ability to change
	• Importance to management

Although these issues are of importance in determining priorities for QI interventions, other factors may supersede cost and health issues. Nearly all health organizations are regulated in some way or participate in accreditation by independent agencies. For example, the NCQA certifies health plans, physician organizations, and credentials verification organizations. Their HEDIS measures drive the QI activities in organizations that they review, so presently, health plans interested in NCQA certification have projects for heart disease, behavioral health, immunizations, and other conditions included in the HEDIS measures. The federal government is exerting similar influence through its QI System for Managed Care (QISMC) for Medicaid enrollees who have chosen or have been placed in managed care plans. Each year, CMS selects a disease, such as diabetes mellitus, as its target disease for quality management, so all health plans with a Medicaid or Medicare health maintenance organization option must implement programs to improve the care of the chosen condition. Another approach, taken by JCAHO, which evaluates hospitals and health plans, does not only mandate a small number of core measures at the present time but allows health plans and hospitals to choose many of their own metrics based on issues for intervention specific to the organization. Regulatory and accrediting agencies thus exert substantial influence on an organization's choice of QI targets.

Consumer and provider preferences may also be important determinants of QI focus. A hospital may select a specific QI project because of community interest in the problem. Medical groups may be required by a health plan to participate in a chart review for a clinical condition included in the HEDIS measurement set. Health plans may find that a large employer is interested in a specific disease because many of its employees lose work due to the illness. Physicians may demand improvements in a health plan's payment system to produce shorter turnaround time for reimbursement. As QI projects are being evaluated, internal and external customer input is invaluable in narrowing down important issues, even to the point of determining performance measures. Customer rankings can be weighted in a scoring system to define project priorities, as in Example 9-2.

Example 9-2

The ABC Clinic designed a system for selecting a QI project that included information about cost, physician preference, patient preference, health plan requirements, and state regulations. The practice manager created a scoring system that measured each of the disease entities of interest on standardized scales so that all variables would be measured in the same manner. The board of directors placed weights on each of the measures based on their assessment of the importance of the measure to the clinic. Table 9.3 contains the weights, scores, and weighted scores, and Figure 9.3 illustrates the aggregate information graphically. Based on the weighted scores, *disease 1* would be targeted as the most likely to satisfy most of the clinic's requirements. Interestingly, *disease 3* has the highest raw score, primarily because the performance measure is well documented and valid. However, because that item was weighted lower than others, the final weighted score placed it second.

This example emphasizes the usefulness of applying a weighted scale to analysis of this type of data. If raw scores are employed, *disease 3* would be the target of the clinic staff, but the first disease was chosen to reflect the hierarchy of importance of the measures.

Customer information can be obtained in a number of ways, such as analyzing complaints received, performing surveys, or polling employees about customer encounters. Surveys tend to be the most reliable, because a properly performed survey should randomly sample the population of customers to provide an unbiased estimate of customer opinions. Surveys can be simple—four or five questions on satisfaction with the products and services of the organizations—or they can be much more detailed, entailing collection of many pages of information for a more thorough understanding of problems and successes.

Extensive customer surveys are sometimes mandated by regulatory agencies such as the Consumer Assessment of Health Plans Survey (CAHPS), which is part of the HEDIS measures promulgated by the NCQA. Originally sanctioned through a grant by the Agency for Healthcare Research and Quality (AHRQ), the survey was developed by Harvard Medical School, the RAND Institute, and the Research Triangle Institute. It has been

Table 9.3 ABC Clinic: Weighted Scores for Selection of QI Project

FACTOR	WEIGHT	DISEASE 1		DISEASE 2	
		RAW	WEIGHTED	RAW	WEIGHTED
Physician choice	0.1	6	0.6	12	1.2
Patient choice	0.25	4	1	6	1.5
Health plan choice	0.25	10	2.5	7	1.75
Morbidity and mortality	0.05	3	0.15	10	0.5
Cost	0.2	14	2.8	6	1.2
Validity of measurement	0.05	4	0.2	5	0.25
Ease of data collection	0.1	10	1	4	0.4
Patient volume	0.1	3	0.3	5	0.5
Ability to change	0.2	3	0.6	4	0.8
Total	1.3	57	9.15	59	8.1

FACTOR	WEIGHT	DISEASE 3		DISEASE 4	
		RAW	WEIGHTED	RAW	WEIGHTED
Physician choice	0.1	3	0.3	4	0.4
Patient choice	0.25	8	2	6	1.5
Health plan choice	0.25	3	0.75	5	1.25
Morbidity and mortality	0.05	8	0.4	4	0.2
Cost	0.2	1	0.2	4	0.8
Validity of measurement	0.05	10	0.5	6	0.3
Ease of data collection	0.1	3	0.3	8	0.8
Patient volume	0.1	9	0.9	8	0.8
Ability to change	0.2	15	3	3	0.6
Total	1.3	60	8.35	48	6.65

adopted by the NCQA and in a modified form by the CMS as a means of measuring consumer satisfaction with elements of health plans, such as interactions with providers, assistance from the health plan in obtaining needed care, etc. (Agency for Healthcare Research and Quality, 1999).

Complaints can serve as another useful source of information. Although the information is biased, it can often provide insight into some of the problems that the organization is having with customers. Most health plans keep complaint logs, analyzing them every few months for trends in types of complaints. As clusters of complaints indicate a particular problem, e.g., delayed handling of claims for a certain customer, managers can focus on a solution to the problem. Large government agencies, such as state Medicaid bureaus, can use this same information to determine if particular segments of the

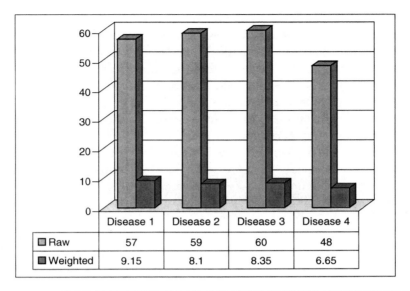

	Disease 1	Disease 2	Disease 3	Disease 4
▣ Raw	57	59	60	48
▦ Weighted	9.15	8.1	8.35	6.65

Figure 9.3 ABC Clinic Scores for Clinical Intervention Selection

population are having difficulty with access to care or finding an appropriate provider. Although the information is more problem oriented, complaint information can serve almost the same purpose as focus groups for identifying quality obstacles and allow managers the opportunity for directing efforts for improvement. One of the functions of good management, however, is to view these issues as symptoms of process errors, rather than just brush fires to be extinguished.

Employees can provide information about customer attitudes as well. Because frontline employees frequently receive the brunt of patient complaints and problems, these workers should be included in an analysis of the system. Usually, this information suffers from some filtering by the employee—e.g., to avoid retribution from management or to avoid appearing inept or unable to cope—but if an open environment for sharing information without recrimination can be established, employees can offer significant aid in improving quality. Several methods may be used to achieve this goal, such as allowing employees to submit information anonymously through a suggestion box or by establishing regular meetings with managers to discuss issues that arise with customers. Good managers will keep lines of communication open so that customer problems are handled expeditiously.

Although competitor data are rarely easy to obtain, in some markets that data can be found through business coalitions; surveys performed by local governments, news media, health care institutions, or individual customers. Some community business coalitions have established local report cards for providers or health plans that list aggregate information such as health plan enrollment figures, major customers, performance on HEDIS measures, and other helpful data. Physicians can frequently find data about competitors at hospitals or from health plans through reports and comparisons of medical practices and characterizations of practice patterns. Hospitals frequently obtain information about competitors from state and national hospital associations, as well as from public health departments and state regulatory bodies. Although much of this information tends to be aggregate data used to compare competing organizations, it can be used to benchmark the organization against local and national performance standards. As the QI paradigm spreads through the health care industry, competitors should become more willing to share performance data to improve the quality of care for the population.

Industry wide data have become easier to obtain with the advent of the Internet. A number of sources have been made available on Web sites that contain industry data useful for benchmarking individual organizations against national standards. Some of the available sites are listed in Table 9.4. Web sites usually contain either local or national data, and the federal government maintains the most useful national sites at the present time. The most comprehensive guide to government Internet information sources is FedWorld at *http://www.fedworld.gov*. The site is maintained by the US Department of Commerce and provides search facilities for all federal government Internet resources. Consumer action groups, business coalitions, and state and municipal governments publish sites with local data, and frequently this information is available at each state's Web site.

Finally, because employees are internal customers, they should be surveyed regularly to define potential QI issues. Employees live with organizational processes every day, and they often have constructive suggestions for ways to improve the system. Regular meetings or surveys are useful in obtaining information on workers' views, and health care industry workers should include providers such as doctors, nurses, and specialty service providers, as well as administrative staff. Workers will vary in their willingness to share, so avenues for providing input and opinions should be flexible, open, and nonpunitive. Using some of the group techniques discussed in Chapter 2, senior management can obtain a wealth of data from frontline workers.

Planning for Change

Once quality targets are identified, the processes underlying the problems must be analyzed using tools that were described in detail in Chapter 3. Each process should be analyzed and described using a flowchart developed by the managers and workers involved with the process, with a QI professional serving as an expert consultant. Most workers will not initially have in-depth understanding of the science of studying processes, so assistance from a QI professional can be of value. The following steps provide a sound approach for the planning procedure.

Table 9.4 Sources of Industry Information on the Internet

INDUSTRY	SITE NAME	CONTENT	URL
Health insurance	NCQA Quality Compass	HEDIS measures for participating health plans	*http://www.ncqa.org*
	IPRO quality data	Medicare+Choice HMO HEDIS data	*http://www.ipro.org*
	NY State Health Accountability Foundation	HMO report cards for New York state	*http://www.nyshaf.org*
Skilled Nursing Facilities	Medicare nursing home survey results	Results of surveys of nursing homes by state	*http://www.medicare.gov/Nhcompare/Home.asp*
Hospitals	Hospital Wage Index Survey File	Information on wages in hospitals used to calculate reimbursement rates	*http://www.cms.hhs.gov/providers/pufdownload/default.asp*
	Nationwide Inpatient Survey	Hospital inpatient utilization data	*http://www.ahcpr.gov/data/hcup/hcupnis.htm*
	Michigan Hospital Report	Statistics from hospitals in Michigan—one state's approach to data sharing	*http://www.michiganhospitalprofiles.org*
Physicians	HealthScope	Medical group comparisons in California	*http://www.healthscope.org/Interface/med_groups/default.asp*
	HealthPages	Medical group, physician, health plan, hospital comparison data—consumer-oriented	*http://www.thehealthpages.com*

NCQA, National Committee for Quality Assurance; HEDIS, health plan employer data and information set; HMO, health maintenance organization.

1. Teams of management and workers should convene.
2. Each team should receive information about the quality issues identified for intervention.
3. Teams create flowcharts of processes related to the target issue.
4. Using the flowcharts, teams identify potential sources for quality issues.
5. Teams identify performance measures for the problems identified in step 4.
6. QI staff and teams collect baseline data to verify that proposed problem sources are correct.
7. Teams design interventions and present ideas to senior management.
8. QI staff and senior management work with teams to develop implementation plans.

These steps conform to the Shewhart plan-do-study-act approach described in Chapter 1 and emphasize inclusion of everyone in the organization to accomplish the transformation.

The first step involves selection of the appropriate team for the task. Team membership depends on which areas in the organization are affected by the project. Workers and managers from all departments that work with the process should participate in the flowcharting exercise, although subgroups may assume responsibility for specific aspects of the analysis. The help of a QI professional at this stage can expedite the creation of the flowchart, because team members would not need to learn the details of flowcharting in addition to learning to work within the group and produce the important results of the planning process. Depending on the familiarity of the group members, some time for team building may be helpful in improving the quality of the final product.

The first substantive task after the team has coalesced is creation of a flowchart for use throughout the planning and implementation phases. As the key component in the planning phase, the flowchart should reflect the process in its current state as accurately as possible. All of the information gathered during the evaluation phase of the project should be available to the planning team so that the group can readily identify the processes that must be examined in more detail. Teamwork principles become crucial to ensuring input from all participants on the team, and a QI professional can often help achieve this objective. At times, this part of the planning process can become an exercise in defensive strategy as each department or work group strives to make its portion of the process appear problem free; however, the facilitator of the planning group must create an environment in which all participants can provide honest input without retribution from another department or management. Process problems that are ignored at this stage can sabotage the final implementation if the improvement intervention is misdirected.

If the process is very complex, then the flowchart task can be divided into smaller, more manageable subtasks, and subgroups can be formed based on the departments or work groups affected by each subtask. These subgroups must also operate in a blame free environment and encourage input from all team members. Responsibility for coordinating these subgroups usually falls to the QI professional, and a subcommittee of the larger group can sometimes put all of the pieces of the flowchart back together into a cohesive whole. Prior to finalizing the flowchart, the group should reconvene to ensure that the final draft of the flowchart reflects the reality of the system in the organization and come to a consensus regarding the flowchart before the final analysis of potential problems. The team facilitator should make certain that everyone in the group feels comfortable with the flowchart before it is used to identify process issues.

Although this step may seem somewhat academic, it is important for adequate planning. Often, improvement efforts are based on reports generated for senior management that may focus on only one facet of the overall process and lead to an erroneous conclusion that a particular part of the process is flawed. Without an understanding of the entire process, however, the conclusions made by management can ignore important events that actually cause the aberrant results, leading to inappropriate interventions and unexpected outcomes. Although senior managers may feel comfortable about their understanding of the process without performing the flowcharting step, in most cases, operational details of these processes are better understood by workers actually involved in day-to-day operations. Thus, establishing the true nature of the process using flowcharts is an essential step in the QI procedure.

Once the flowchart is completed, the same group may be called upon to identify problems in the process or another group may be convened. For example, if the team determines that a specific portion of the process is the source of all of the problems with outcomes, then the department that is involved in that segment of the overall work flow may be assigned to create solutions. Rarely do company wide process problems localize to specific departments, but if they do, then the departmental approach may suffice. For most problems, however, some coordination between departments or work groups will be necessary, and the planning team that evaluates the flowchart for problems should include workers from all potentially affected areas.

These deliberations often produce conflict. As interventions are discussed and recommendations made for solving the problems, resource allocation and budgets will usually be affected. Workers and managers in each department may not want to devote some of the budget to this activity, feeling that the problem is more appropriately handled in another department's budget. Compromise is key in these situations, and the group process techniques discussed in Chapter 2 can be used to help the group agree on a final plan. When conflicts are certain to arise, it often helps to have an outside consultant involved at this stage to improve the willingness of the group to cooperate.

Once potential process problems have been defined, the team should analyze the way in which these problems interact, perhaps even collecting data to verify these hypotheses. At this stage, a problem in one section of the process may be determined to emanate from another part of the workflow, leading the team to focus on the underlying problem, rather than the obvious symptom. Health care workers are very familiar with the concept of examining symptoms to identify an underlying disease state. Using the same tools of deductive reasoning, effective QI teams discern causes of problems and create solutions that address root causes, rather than simply treating symptoms. This stage of the planning procedure should also include evaluation of costs involved with each alternative intervention, as well as the performance measures that will be used to evaluate outcomes of the interventions. Useful performance measures will encompass revenue, cost, and operational outcomes, satisfying the needs of senior management as well as frontline workers. Senior management will be interested in bottom-line issues such as revenue and cost, while workers will want additional information about the efficiency of the process. With this groundwork in place, interventions can be designed to optimize performance measures and ameliorate the problems in the process.

Once the proposed interventions have gained consensus, budgets can be codified and the entire package presented to senior management. As mentioned previously, senior management support is crucial for QI programs to succeed, and gaining commitment at this stage generally ensures that the project may be taken to completion. Having senior managers involved at this stage can also serve to provide them with a feeling of involvement, even ownership, of the QI effort, leading to a stronger commitment to company wide QI efforts as the scope of QI broadens.

Implementation

Implementation plans should focus on the effects of interventions on workers involved in the process. Because resources may need to be reallocated, senior managers are often involved in the implementation planning phase of the project. Bringing plans to fruition involves the following issues:

◆ addition or removal of capital equipment
◆ staff training
◆ altered work patterns, e.g., hours of operation, worker skills
◆ customer interactions
◆ management/staff relationships

Most QI interventions are most economically successful when little additional funding is necessary for success. However, in some cases, capital expenditures are simply unavoidable, such as replacing aging computer equipment or outdated machinery in operating rooms. In the event that capital equipment purchases are necessary, these costs must be amortized, rather than expensed to the project because, in most cases, the equipment will be used even after the project is completed. This accounting approach will appropriately lower the cost of the project and make the outcome more cost effective.

Almost any revision in the established workflow will require some staff education. In some cases, the education will be extensive, e.g., training workers to use a new software package, but in others, the time commitment to retraining will be minimal. The costs of training will usually be allocated directly to the project, unless the education has some value in other areas of the organization. Altering other parameters of the workers' jobs may prove more complicated, however. Changing hours of operation or requiring a different skill set may indeed prove difficult for some workers to accept, leading to staff attrition and dissatisfaction. Having workers involved during the planning process should help minimize these issues, however, because the representatives on the planning team should address these problems before the implementation plan is finalized.

Customer interactions with the organization can also be altered as the implementation plan is executed. Many organizations will have customers represented on the implementation design team to anticipate any problems with customers as the process improves. Having customers involved with the team can help prevent making any major mistakes during implementation, and keeping a focus on customer needs at the heart of the entire planning process can ensure that implementation will not damage customer relations.

Finally, with change comes stress on relationships. Previously harmonious interactions between workers and managers may suffer during a transitional period. The approach to the entire planning process can influence the effects of change; workers and managers who have been involved in designing the change are much more likely to cooperate with the new methods of operation than those who have been ignored throughout the process. Team building during the planning and transitional phases can prove to be the most important factor for facilitating the success of a QI intervention.

Measuring Impact

Two important aspects of measuring the results of an intervention must be considered: time for the intervention to take effect and the extent of the effect on selected performance measures. As a project is being designed, these two factors must be considered, because failure to deliver expected results within a reasonable time can damage the credibility of the organization's entire QI effort. Senior managers often assume some political and financial risk in the organization to foster the growth of a QI effort, so the results of a project must be timely and substantive.

Once a program has been implemented, nearly everyone eagerly awaits the first reports to demonstrate the efficacy of the new approach on the system. Effects of interventions often take more than one cycle to demonstrate efficacy, so as the project is being rolled out, the team must include a conservative time schedule for reporting results to workers and management. The flowchart and a program evaluation and review technique (PERT) chart (see Chapter 3) can prove useful for this task because these tools contain the ideal work flow and the critical path times for achieving the desired output. Using this information, and capitalizing on tools such as storyboards (see Chapter 2), the expectations for the project can be reasonably set and effectively communicated to the organization. Ambitious QI teams and managers often overestimate the effects of an intervention, so the rate of any changes should be attenuated to conservative levels that help make management expectations achievable.

Performance measures are of utmost importance in measuring the impact of an intervention. These measures should have a number of characteristics to be useful: they should be valid, unbiased, reliable, low in variability, and low in cost. Performance measures with these attributes will inspire confidence in senior management and workers that changes will be judged appropriately.

Valid measures are those that actually measure what they purport to measure. In some cases, these may be direct measurements, such as a serum sodium level, but in many others, particularly in health services research, measures often are used as surrogates for a parameter. An example of such a measure is the use of immunization rates in 2-year-olds as a means of determining if the population at risk is adequately immunized. This measure may be valid for the cohort of 2-year-olds in the study, but it is often used as a surrogate to gauge the effectiveness of a health plan or medical group in immunizing a population of patients. As a proxy for overall efficacy of an immunization program, the rate of completed schedules for 2-year-olds would need to be validated with other data, e.g., rates of completion of recommended immunizations at each age up to 2 years of age, reaction rates to vaccines, and breakthrough instances of the diseases for which the immunizations are given. Frequently, new measures must undergo extensive validation to become acceptable metrics for a QI application.

Bias can damage the validity of a measure. In statistical terms, bias occurs when a metric consistently and systematically estimates a parameter inaccurately. For example, an office scale must be frequently recalibrated to avoid a biased or incorrect weight. If the scale is not recalibrated, then the weights from the scale may be consistently inaccurate. Similarly, a number of factors can cause bias in quality measures. Data recording techniques may be incorrect, leading to inaccuracies in the information used for analysis. For example, as health plans use administrative or insurance claim data (see Chapter 3) for evaluating clinical parameters, numerous errors typically occur. As providers record information for medical bills, they tend to code services to maximize the amount charged to the insurer. This phenomenon, known as code creep or upcoding, distorts administrative data and biases results of analyses. Similarly, as data are being collected from clinical charts, the reviewers often must interpret the information in the charts to make it fit the data collection criteria. Misinterpretation of the information in the charts leads to another form of bias. Similar problems occur with financial data, because line items in accounting systems may have different meanings in different companies. For example, some companies may record a line item of "marketing" and include costs of advertising as well as other marketing costs, whereas others may break down specific marketing items into several components. Thus, comparisons may be difficult because of the data recording bias inherent in these different accounting approaches.

Measures must also be reliable, meaning that the measure must produce the same results for a given value, regardless of the time that the metric is recorded or who records the data. One way of improving the reliability of performance measures involves creating operational definitions, detailed descriptions of performance measures that specifically depict the methods by which data are collected, what data are collected, and how the data are analyzed. The HEDIS measures used by the NCQA for evaluating health plans provide an excellent example of operational definitions. The definitions for these measures are very specific regarding data to be collected and the methods for analyzing and reporting the measures. The specificity of these operational definitions removes much of the ambiguity associated with reporting HEDIS measures, allowing better comparisons between health plans. Reliable measures provide the basis for appropriate QI interventions and are invaluable to the success of a project.

Nearly all measures have some degree of variability inherent in measurement or reporting. The basis of much statistical process control theory relates to evaluating data sets for "normal" levels of variation and determining when variation becomes abnormal. Measures with large degrees of variability are unpredictable, making the results of interventions difficult to assess. Changes in these types of measures often occur randomly, so if a change is noted after a QI intervention, the change could be a result of random error rather than an effect of the intervention. Figure 9.4 demonstrates this point. The graphs labeled High Variability Measure and Low Variability Measure show the data points and means for *parameter 1* and *parameter 2*. The means of each of these data sets change an equal amount at the same time. However, the large degree of variation in the high variability measure "hides" the change in the mean, while the change in the mean for the less variable measure appears much more clearly. The likelihood that the change in the mean is due purely to chance is much greater for the high variability measure. With all of the background noise in the high variability parameter, the change in the mean is much harder to detect. Thus, one important criterion for selection of performance measures for QI should be relatively low variability in the metric.

Finally, the cost of collecting and analyzing data for the measure must be affordable. Virtually all functions in QI have a financial cost. This cost may stem from a number of sources, including staff time required to collect, store, and analyze data; capital assets used in the process; and overhead charges

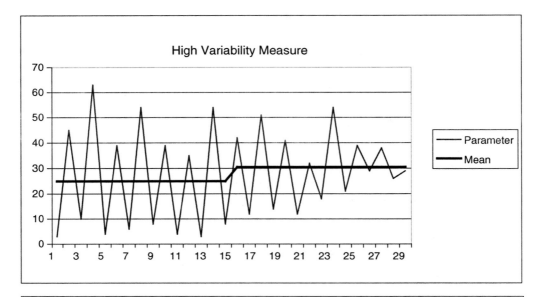

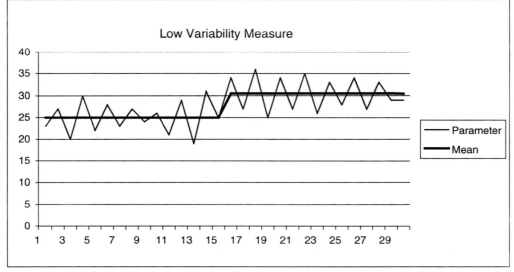

Figure 9.4 Effects of Variability on Interpretation of Changes in Performance Measures

(utilities, rent, supplies, etc.). As a budget for the project is being created, all of these costs must be included to perform an appropriate cost–benefit analysis. If data collection can be simplified, or preferably automated, the project will cost less and be more likely to produce useful outcomes.

QI succeeds only when outcomes can be measured. A traditional aphorism in quality management is usually stated "You can't manage what you can't measure," and demonstrating the impact of interventions provides the only means of confirming the efficacy of the QI approach.

◈ Institutionalization of Change

The ultimate goal of QI projects is to demonstrate the value of the approach to the fiscal and operational health of the organization so that the quality focus can permeate the company's culture. As stated in Deming's 14 principles, effective quality management will reduce costs, improve performance, and ensure the future of the company. Although these concepts may be intuitive to most QI professionals, they must be demonstrated to the remainder of the organization. Thus, the results of a QI project must be disseminated throughout the company to establish the effectiveness of the approach in achieving improved financial and operational performance. The ultimate goal of change, however, must be internalization of the new approach so that the quality approach underlies all of a company's operations.

To achieve this goal, the successful changes must become integral to the operations of the organization. Everyone in the company, from senior management to the newest employee, must be convinced that the QI approach will provide the best opportunity for reducing costs and enhancing productivity and then internalize that philosophy so that it can be applied throughout the organization. This essential alteration in attitudes and philosophy should lead to other salient changes in the company's operations, including (1) different approaches to work, (2) alignment of incentives, and (3) improved information dissemination. These changes reflect the transformation of the organization from an internally focused, cost-directed company to one that is externally focused and customer-directed.

Once a QI philosophy has assumed greater importance in the organization, all workers will fearlessly adopt a customer focus, subordinating short-term personal gain for customer satisfaction. Workers will not blithely disregard their own needs and desires indefinitely, but management must ensure that workers who embrace the "customer first" philosophy are rewarded. This concentration on customer needs will lead to the company's success, and workers must be recognized as the results of their efforts are realized. Innovation by the workforce should be encouraged through appropriate acknowledgment by managers and effective strategies to facilitate communications between workers and management.

In the quality-focused organization, incentives for workers, vendors, and customers will be aligned to reflect the needs of each group. Many health care companies suffer from conflicting incentives among stakeholders, leading to increased costs and inefficiency. For example, the reimbursement system for most providers adds to the overhead and financial cost of health insurers, and most health insurance companies are paid by customers in a manner that conflicts with the long-term goal of providing good patient care. These misaligned incentives have created serious discrepancies in the health care finance and delivery systems. Through appropriate renegotiation of payment mechanisms, the incentives can be brought into a more harmonious relationship and relieve the current conflicts in the industry. Incentives within a company can be similarly dysfunctional. Hospitals are frequently paid a fixed amount by a diagnosis-related group, whereas physicians are paid for each service they render. The hospital has a fixed payment for a patient's hospitalization, with an incentive to treat the patient quickly and efficiently to reduce costs of care, but the physician is paid more when the patient stays longer in the hospital. Because physicians must concur with decisions to discharge patients from the hospital, these conflicting financial incentives lead to inappropriate use of inpatient services. Health plans that manage contracts with both parties must recognize these problems and work to correct them through contract restructuring. Many such problems with incentives exist in the health care delivery system and must be corrected. A quality-focused organization will recognize these problems and work to ameliorate them as a way of improving the quality of customer service.

One key feature of all of these issues is the need for information to be disseminated to all relevant stakeholders in a timely manner. Most organizations have a wealth of information hiding in databases, and converting data into information presents a major technological challenge. Systems are available to manage this effort, and management must find ways of funding the transition of the company's data repositories into information resources. Once the information has been appropriately formatted, dissemination through intranets and extranets can provide the communications backbone to link customers, employees, and managers in a cohesive network that capitalizes on the strengths of each stakeholder. Information sharing becomes an important component of a quality-focused organization, and most expenditures on information technology are rapidly paid for through improved decision making.

The ultimate result of these transformations is the internalization of a customer orientation in the organization that reflects the drive for quality. Excellent companies meet the needs of their customers through innovation, but they ensure customer satisfaction by aligning incentives and effective communications. When the tenets of QI are part of the institutional culture, these elements become integral to the operations of the company.

◆ Balanced Scorecard Approach to QI

Around the beginning of the 1990s, David Norton and Robert Kaplan published a series of articles in the *Harvard Business Review* regarding a concept of strategic management that they termed the balanced scorecard (BSC). The ideas that they advanced were based on their research with a number of different companies and industries but very limited analysis of the health care industry (Kaplan & Norton, 1995). Although not many examples exist, some institutions are beginning to use the BSC to develop strategic plans based on QI principles.

BSC Structure and Implementation

The BSC provides an amalgamation of all the parameters necessary to formulate a QI plan and implement the infrastructure to achieve the strategic goals of the organization. Norton and Kaplan recognized very early that the planning process is imperfect, but the process must also be dynamic; i.e., if a performance measure or strategic goal becomes obsolete or inappropriate, substitutes should be identified and implemented. The process of ongoing monitoring of the BSC must become a primary goal of management to ensure continued competitiveness of the organization.

The structure of the BSC integrates four primary functions of business: (1) financial, (2) customer, (3) business processes, and (4) innovation and learning. The rationale for these four parameters is well established.

> Financial—The primary function of the business is to produce consistent excellent financial results that maximize the value of the firm and continually improve shareholder value.
>
> Customer—Businesses recognized very early that success in customer acquisition and retention translated frequently into financial gains.
>
> Processes—In order to achieve the goals of customer orientation and subsequent financial ramifications, business processes must be designed to optimize the responsiveness, efficiency, and effectiveness of the organization.
>
> Innovation and learning—Even though a business performs well, without innovation and learning by all segments of the organization, the success will be short-lived. This parameter places emphasis on the future of the company through gains in organizational knowledge and experience, rather than relying simply on immediate returns.

Use of the BSC by management involves integration of these four areas into an organizational paradigm that emphasizes identification and response to customer needs and QI. Management then must relate all of the organization's performance measures to these goals and create incentives for managers and workers to ensure progress toward the goals. The activities surrounding the creation of an enterprise-wide BSC involve nearly every segment of the organization, and coordination of these efforts falls heavily on management. Each of the four perspectives relies substantially on QI concepts of measuring performance, implementing a customer-oriented philosophy, and continuously improving the organization. The BSC uses appropriate performance measures that are selected specifically for their relationship to the strategic objectives of the organization, rather than just to satisfy short-term financial exigencies.

BSC Interrelationships

The formulation of the BSC by Kaplan and Norton has brought a new level of definition to relationships between functional areas of the organization. Managers are familiar with the trade-offs necessary in any economic decision made by the firm, such as the capital expenditure for a new piece of equipment with a fixed economic life. On the other hand, managers often do not recognize the symbiosis between financial- and customer-related parameters and the business processes and learning culture of the organization. Certainly, the relationship to cost profiles is obvious, but the benefits to long-term viability of the business are often overlooked. The BSC clarifies these relationships, with the result of improving the overall effect on organizational performance. Figure 9.5 demonstrates the interaction among BSC perspectives. The focus of the model is the strategic vision of the organization for improving quality. Without a clear understanding of the strategic vision, development of measures for the BSC will lead the organization to make errors in decisions because of inadequate information. All perspectives must relate to the strategic vision, and each perspective relates to the others through the central vision driving the company. As tactics are implemented, the data collected in the BSC reflect the progress of the company toward achieving the goals delineated by the strategic vision. Even though all four perspectives have equal importance, the financial perspective usually assumes prime importance for most managers and so will be considered first.

Financial Perspective

Financial results frequently assume utmost importance in the current business environment, often to the exclusion of other outcomes of business activi-

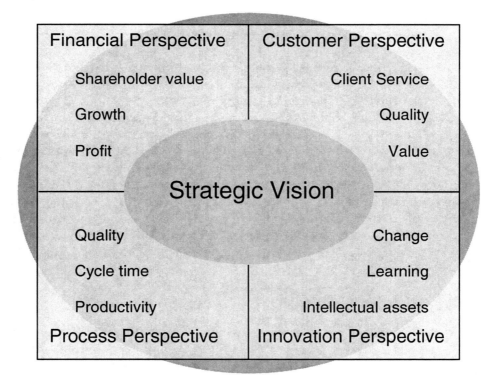

Figure 9.5 Balanced Scorecard: Relationships of Key Components

ties; thus, financial measures end up as an important consideration in any QI formulation. Organizations usually find themselves in one of three stages in the business cycle: (1) growth, (2) maintenance, or (3) harvest.

Enterprises that are in the growth stage have financial profiles that are characteristically problematic when viewed out of context. These business units usually have products or services that possess significant growth potential, so they require significant capital and management resources in order to achieve their potential.

Example 9-3

A new computerized scanner designed to evaluate patients for coronary artery disease will require substantial education of the medical staff and the community before the use of the service will increase. The hospital needs to invest capital to purchase and implement the technology to perform the test. Additionally, the hospital will need to make capital expenditures to disseminate information regarding the test to the medical staff and perhaps to the community. Once the technology is in place, the hospital would continue to subsidize the new service by employing technical staff to perform the test, as well as providing the administrative and facility overhead required to create the environment for the evaluation. All of these expenditures are unreimbursed until the test is ordered by physicians and paid for by insurers, leading to negative cash flow in the initial stages of the program.

In the example of a growth-stage enterprise within a hospital, negative cash flow is expected in the early phase of development, but the quality of the service must be conclusive. The most important financial aspect of the new test is the production of sales revenue to cover the initial costs, and quality considerations include efficacy and morbidity related to the procedure. Thus, the relevant quality measures of early success are the diagnostic accuracy of this new technology compared with more traditional methods and possible complications from the procedure. Physician, employee, and patient satisfaction with the new modality are also key measures of quality. Although the return on investment is important to hospital management, the BSC helps managers consider all of the potential returns generated by the new technology, e.g., customer and provider satisfaction, earlier detection and lower cost of care for patients with heart disease, and the benefit to employee growth in caring for patients with cardiac disease as a result of the new technology.

During the maintenance stage, companies find themselves with a line of business that generates substantial revenue but still requires some capital investment. The maintenance stage is perhaps the most common position for most organizations such as mature medical practices because products and services are well developed and well accepted, and sales are usually brisk.

Example 9-4

Physicians at the Oakmont Clinic started performing "executive health evaluations" in 1987, and since then, the service has grown at a rate that exceeded their expectations. They are now facing a new opportunity because one of the major employers in their area is interested in implementing the service for their 1200 executive and middle management staff. To maintain the current level of quality, the contract would require an expansion of the facilities to handle the increased volume, as well as hiring three additional employees. Analysis of the clinic's current and projected cash flow and renewed negotiation with vendors indicates that the contract could be serviced with no increase in debt and only about half of the next 6 months' net cash flow. Performance measures were adopted to evaluate patient and provider satisfaction, as well as financial measures to track costs and revenues. The contract is signed.

Any changes in the services of a maintenance-stage organization must ensure that the quality services or products that led to success are not compromised by the change.

Finally, harvest-stage enterprises have mature products or services that have few or no prospects for increasing market share. These products and services have a significant margin, as well as sufficient cash flow, and the primary uses of capital are to maintain the quality of the staff and facilities that provide the current return.

Example 9-5

A long-term-care facility with a broad array of services for residents is considering modernization and expansion of its physical plant. The population in the referral area has decreased over the past 10 years, and the facility has not experienced an increase in its population for at least 8 years. The marketing staff did not see any chance that the facility would increase its population in the foreseeable future, and with constraints imposed by third-party payers, revenue growth was not expected to exceed inflation in costs. Thus, the executive management of the facility decided to allocate funds to improve the quality of services but not expand the physical plant.

Harvest-stage organizations often have little potential for growth, but substantial risk of loss of market share, making investments in QI important for preserving the current business level.

The financial perspective cannot be ignored in a QI framework, and the BSC ensures that these issues are addressed. As QI interventions are being designed, the business phase of the organization must be considered, and assets allocated to quality interventions should reflect a strategy appropriate to the business stage of the organization.

Customer Perspective

The market share of an organization relates to two important factors: customer acquisition and customer retention. Acquiring new customers is often an expensive, time-consuming process. Many clients of health care providers or institutions are fiercely loyal, making a change to another provider very difficult to achieve. The personal nature of the provider–patient relationship creates a level of loyalty that is unmatched in most of the business world, and most providers are reticent to gain market share by aggressively attracting patients from competitors.

Marketing efforts are often directed toward primary care physicians and their staffs to promote referrals to certain specialists, but these relationships are gradually being replaced by contractual arrangements with insurers. Most insurers now have established panels of physicians from whom members of the health plan may access care. If the member wishes to see a physician outside the plan, the plan may not pay some of the cost, and in some cases will not pay any of the cost of care. Thus, market share depends on contractual arrangements with third-party payers even more than on individual patient selection. On the other hand, providers on a health plan's panel still must compete for patients. Additionally, in some markets providers must also compete for health plan contracts by demonstrating value—i.e., high quality and low cost. Thus, customer acquisition has become increasingly dependent on the ability of a provider to demonstrate quality to health plans, employers, and patients.

Customer retention helps maintain the market share base so that an organization can grow. Patients usually leave a provider's organization as a result of perceived lapses in quality of care or adverse outcomes of care. Inability to retain patients leads not only to shrinking market share but also to difficulty attracting new customers to the organization. Thus, customer retention is a key element in maintaining and expanding market share. More health plans and patient advocacy groups are demanding quality information from providers, including cost and performance data. As QI systems are implemented in health care organizations, the effect of the interventions on customer satisfaction has become a vital consideration.

Measures for these important customer parameters can take many forms, depending on the nature of the institution. Any intervention should include a measure for customer satisfaction with the new product or service. Additionally, every health care practitioner may want to measure satisfaction parameters specific to the institution. A hospital might want to measure customer loyalty by performing a survey or by tracking customers for return visits to the institution. Medical practices should measure record transfers to determine trends and ask departing patients why they are transferring their care. Durable medical equipment organizations may want to track referrals from providers and determine patterns of orders by specialty or product line. Each measure should be sufficiently capable of determining changes quickly so that problems may be detected and solved before large shifts occur.

Unfortunately, customer satisfaction rarely lends itself to easy measurement. Surveys often become the only method of measuring satisfaction, and in health care, the concept of well-being is an additional factor that is usually included in patient surveys. Some surveys, such as the SF-36 or SF-12, have been designed to quantitate patient well-being, but they do not measure satisfaction with health care. The CAHPSs used by the NCQA as part of the managed care organization measurement system provide some objectivity, and newer versions, e.g., the CAHPS-H, are being used by hospitals to access patient satisfaction. Many institutions and practices now administer customized satisfaction surveys targeted to determine specific information about potential problem areas such as waiting times, but sometimes they are more complex to administer and less statistically reliable.

Customer satisfaction is such an important issue in modern health care that it must be considered in any QI system. Because customers should benefit from improved processes, the value of including these measures in the evaluation of systems should be obvious. Institutions that are focused on cost containment often forget this important point, and changes that contain costs decimate customer satisfaction and devastate market share.

Business Process Perspective

Although most health care executives are aware that their businesses must be efficient to be profitable, creating the processes to achieve that goal present major challenges. Many managers exert the majority of their professional effort trying to optimize use of resources in the organization, but, often, without a systematic approach, they only emulate firefighters trying to stamp out the latest conflagration. Most health care organizations have well-defined departments with nominally clear processes, and the traditional method of planning in business has been to optimize the functions of these departments. However, by evaluating the financial and customer components of the organization's efforts before the business processes, the health care manager may effect a more efficient reengineering of the organization by identifying completely new processes or even departments needed to appropriately service these new market requirements.

Processes in the organization must be directed at serving customers and promoting efficient use of resources, and measures of effectiveness should relate to these two issues. As noted before, customer reactions to any proposed improvements can be measured by customer satisfaction surveys, but process efficiency measures will depend on the individual process being evaluated. A generic measure used in manufacturing can be adapted for use in gauging process efficiency in service organizations.

(9.2) PCE = processing time/throughput time

where PCE is process cycle effectiveness,
        processing time is time for the actual process elements, and
        throughput time = processing time + inspection time + movement
        time + waiting time + storage time

The PCE measure can be used for virtually any process in the organization, as shown in the following example.

Example 9-6

A patient was sent to the laboratory for a blood test ordered by her physician. To obtain the blood test, she had to register at the outpatient department, proceed to the laboratory phlebotomy room, wait for the phlebotomist, have the blood drawn, and then wait in the hospital outpatient department for the results. Times were measured for the process as follows:

◆ travel to outpatient department: 5 minutes
◆ register in outpatient department: 15 minutes
◆ travel to laboratory: 4 minutes
◆ await phlebotomist: 20 minutes
◆ blood draw: 5 minutes
◆ blood transfer to chemistry lab: 30 minutes
◆ inspection of sample for labeling: 3 minutes
◆ perform blood test: 2 minutes
◆ generate report to physician: 15 minutes

The end result was

◆ process time: 5 minutes (blood draw) + 2 minutes (perform blood test)
= 7 minutes
◆ throughput time = 99 minutes
◆ PCE = 0.07

Breaking a process into components in this manner helps identify inefficiencies, and the PCE can then be tracked as a measure for the process perspective.

    Although the PCE is a rather generic measure, more specific metrics can be identified for any process. Using these measures in conjunction with those designed for the other elements of the BSC provides a more complete picture of the effects of a QI program. Organizations often use several measures in this domain to determine process effectiveness, and changes in financial and customer metrics can be related to process effectiveness measures with the BSC approach.

Innovation and Learning Perspective

Any health care organization hoping to survive in the emerging marketplace must develop innovative business approaches. Innovation frequently emanates from workers, so continuing education is critical for organizational survival. This concept is well accepted for health care professionals, but it must be extended throughout the workforce to hourly workers as well. Deming's principles stress this point several times, and the nature of the marketplace in demanding new and improved services emphasizes the issue.

Nearly any QI effort will entail staff education and growth, and these issues should be included in deliberations regarding a potential approach to improvement. Where possible, OJT should be made part of every department in the organization, and the success of these efforts should be gauged using performance measures such as continuing education hours per worker or by measuring some skill set that workers are expected to gain as part of the quality intervention. Hospitals are at the forefront of these activities, with such offerings as educational programs on infection control for all workers to help prevent the spread of potentially devastating illnesses. Medical groups can provide similar education. Opportunities to educate health professionals in new and innovative disease management techniques can expand the market of a medical practice and improve the quality of care. Home health providers must continually update all workers on new methods of caring for complex illnesses outside the hospital.

Not only should the actual training be measured, but the results of the training should be tracked. For example, if employees in a medical practice attend a seminar on new methods of training asthmatic patients to use metered dose inhalers, the effect of the training should be measured by evaluating patient use of inhalers, e.g., through the use of data regarding repeat prescriptions or the incidence and severity of acute exacerbations. Effective methods of training can be better identified and repeated with such measures, and results of quality interventions can be attributed to these educational efforts.

◆ QI Implementation in Complex Organizations

As demonstrated in the section on the BSC, QI interventions must be evaluated from several different perspectives to ensure that changes in one area are not detrimental to other areas. Nowhere is this issue more important than in large and complex organizations. An implementation plan must attempt to consider all possible implications of an intervention, not only for a particular department, but for all departments in the organization. With the strategies outlined in this chapter, including the BSC approach, interventions in organizational processes can be properly evaluated and improvements measured. Only through an organized, systematic approach can long-term gains in quality be achieved.

◆ Discussion Points

1. Deming articulated 14 principles of quality improvement. Briefly describe each one and give examples from your own experience.
2. What did Deming mean when he stated in Principle 8, "Drive out fear?" How can managers achieve this goal?
3. Principle 9 in Deming's list indicates that managers should break down barriers. What barriers exist in organizations, and what can managers do to eliminate them?
4. List the phases of organizational change. At what stage is your organization?
5. Name the four perspectives of the balanced scorecard. How are they related?
6. Choose a business process in your organization that requires improvement. Using the phases of organizational change, evaluate the process and design an implementation plan. Using the balanced scorecard, define performance measures to track the success of your implementation plan.
7. What issues are most important to senior management in a quality improvement program? How can a quality improvement team address the issues adequately?

◆ Notes

Agency for Healthcare Research and Quality. (1999). *Consumer Assessment of Health Plans (CAHPS): Overview*. Retrieved September 2003, from *http://www.ahcpr.gov/qual/cahps/dept1.htm*

Alberty J. (1999). *Achieving supply chain integration through outsourcing*. Retrieved June 1999, from *http://ryder.ascet.com*

Albritton J. (1998). NCQA sets the standard for health plan evaluation. *Northern Colorado Business Report*. Retrieved June 1999, from *http://www.ncbr.com/oct98/health.ncqa.htm*

Balas E., Kretschmer R., Gnann W., West D. A., Boren S. A., Centor R. M., et al. (1998). Interpreting cost analyses of clinical interventions. *Journal of the American Medical Association, 279*(1), 54–57.

Bhargava P. (1999). *Supply chain integration*. Retrieved July 1999, from *http://www-personal.umich.edu/~pbhargav/overview.html*

Bocchino C. (1999, April). *Letter to NCQA regarding Accreditation 2000 Public Comments*. Retrieved June 1999, from *http://www.aahp.org/services/health_care_delivery/a2000ltr.htm*

Brailer D., et al. (1997). Physician-led clinical performance improvement: A new model for quality management. *Journal of Clinical Outcomes Management, 4*(5), 33–43.

Chassin M. (1998). Is health care ready for six sigma quality? *Milbank Quarterly, 76*(4). Retrieved September 2003, from *http://www.milbank.org/quarterly/764featchas.html*

Cooperative Cardiovascular Project Best Practices Working Group. (1998). Improving care for acute myocardial infarction: Experience from the cooperative cardiovascular project. *Joint Commission Journal on Quality Improvement, 24*(9), 480–490.

Crosby P. B. (1979). *Quality is free: The art of making quality certain.* New York: Mentor.

DeBakey M., and DeBakey L. (1999, July 7). Should physicians unionize? Yes, it would curb HMO abuse. *Wall Street Journal.*

Deming W. E. (1986). *Out of the crisis.* Cambridge, MA: MIT Press.

Denton T. A., Luevanos J., Matloff J. M. (1998). Clinical and nonclinical predictors of the cost of coronary bypass surgery: Potential effects on health care delivery and reimbursement. *Archives of Internal Medicine, 158,* 886–891.

Gallagher M. (1998, March 7). Presbyterian's prescription for change. Retrieved July 1999, from *http://www.abqjournal.com/news/pres/1pres3-8.htm*

Gold M. (1999). The changing U.S. health care system: Challenges for responsible public policy. *The Milbank Quarterly, 77*(1). Retrieved September 2003, from *http://www.milbank.org/quarterly/7701feat.html*

Institute of Medicine (Ed.) (2001). *Crossing the quality chasm: A new health system for the 21st century.* Washington, DC: National Academy Press.

Kaplan R., and Norton P. (1995). The balanced scorecard. Boston: Harvard Press.

Marciniak T., et al. (1998). Improving the quality of care for Medicare patients with acute myocardial infarction: Results from the cooperative cardiovascular project. *Journal of the American Medical Association, 279*(17), 1351–1357.

Medscape. (1998). Why organizations select their HMOs. *Drug Benefit Trends, 10*(1), 8. Retrieved June 1999, from *http://www.medscape.com/SCP/DBT/1998/v10.n01/d4310.trend/d4310.trend.html*

Morain C. (1998, October/November). *Collective action. Between rounds.* Retrieved July 1999, from *http://www.betweenrounds.com/volume2/issue4/collective/index.htm*

Peters T. J., and Waterman R. H. (1982). *In search of excellence: Lessons from America's best-run companies.* New York: Warner Books.

Reinhardt U. (1999, July 7). Should physicians unionize? No, patients would pay the price. *Wall Street Journal.*

Tucker A. W., Haddix A. C., Bresee J. S., Holman R. C., Parashar U. D., Glass R. I. (1998). Cost-effectiveness analysis of a rotavirus immunization program for the United States. *Journal of the American Medical Association, 279*(17), 1371–1376.

Wilkie T. (1996). Sources in science: Who can we trust? *Lancet, 347*(9011), 1308–1311.

Zinn J. S., Brannon D., Weech R. (1997). Quality improvement in nursing care facilities: Extent, impetus, and impact. *American Journal of Medical Quality, 12*(1), 51–61.

◆ Additional Reading

Barry R., Murcko A., Brubaker C. (2002). *The six sigma book for healthcare.* Chicago: Health Administration Press.

Collins J. (2001). *Good to great: Why some companies make the leap...and others don't.* Toronto: Harper Collins.

Chapter 10

Making Continuous Quality Improvement Work: Care Management

DONALD E. LIGHTER

◈ Introduction

Quality health care can be difficult to discern in the health care delivery system. The Institute of Medicine of the National Academy of Sciences in Washington, DC, has worked steadily since the 1980s to bring the tenets of quality improvement science to the American health care system. In a report of the National Roundtable on Health Care Quality (Chassin & Galvin, 1998), the Institute of Medicine concluded that quality of care, not managed care, lay at the root of the problems in American health care. They emphasized that quality could be measured with the same level of precision as other measures of patient care in medicine, and in spite of significant gains by some institutions, many still lagged in both quality efforts and measurement. The RAND Corporation came to similar conclusions, but they also examined the methods by which quality information was collected and disseminated throughout the system (Schuster, et al., 1998). After an exhaustive review of the medical literature, they concluded that a large gulf existed between the care that people should receive and the care that was actually delivered, regardless of whether the services were for preventive, acute, or chronic care.

Although the US health care system is the envy of many nations around the world, there is always room for improvement. Many of the preceding chapters detail the science of quality improvement, but implementation can present unique challenges because of the diversity of practice settings, consumers, and providers. Perhaps one of the greatest challenges for quality improvement teams is actually bringing quality interventions to the site of care. Although originally proposed by the pharmaceutical industry as disease management (Boston Consulting Group, 1993), the concept of an organized approach to care has now evolved into care management so that preventive care and services can fall within the same framework as diagnosis and treatment of diseases. Dr. John Lucas, president and chief executive officer of St. Francis Health System in Tulsa, OK, recently defined disease management as "a comprehensive system of coordinated patient care that includes prevention strategies, addresses process issues, and includes the analytical as well as the educational disciplines" (Byrnes, 1998a). This definition of disease management is broad enough to include the tenets of care management, which expand the scope of interventions to include preventive population care. Care management is expected to bring the elements of quality and efficacy to the health care delivery system (Bernard & Frist, 1998). In short, care management represents quality improvement taken to the limit in health care.

◆ Care Management: A Contemporary Approach

The health care delivery system has been plagued with fragmentation over the past few decades. Consumers with complex diseases often have several physicians providing necessary services, and at times those services could be duplicative, or interactions between drugs or services could often be potentially harmful. Coordinating care has traditionally been the purview of primary care physicians, who have become exceptionally busy because of changes in reimbursement, with resulting lapses in the ability of these providers to effectively manage such complex patients. Over the past few years, care management programs have begun focusing on diseases that are high cost or have a high potential for morbidity if not closely managed. Conditions such as diabetes mellitus, asthma, hypertension, and congestive heart failure have received a great deal of attention because of their wide distribution and high cost. Although designed to provide coordination of care and improve quality, managed care organizations and insurers have also embraced care management as a means of reducing the cost of care. Numerous studies have demonstrated the economic benefit of disease management programs in these and other clinical conditions (Doxtator & Rodriguez, 1998; Drea, 1998; Gonzalez, 1998; McDowell, et al., 1998; Liptak, et al., 1998).

The traditional health care delivery system has evolved into what payers and the public recognize as an increasingly dysfunctional hodgepodge of services and products that can benefit from the application of quality improvement (QI) science. The current system is designed to provide treatment, rather than encourage prevention; most physicians have been trained to provide services to cure disease rather than prevent clinical problems. Health insurance reimbursement subsidizes expensive treatments such as cardiac bypass surgery but will not pay for nutritional counseling, weight loss programs, or smoking cessation programs that can limit the need for such expensive interventions. Consumers suffer when their care is not coordinated; missed appointments, failure to take medications as directed, lack of success in making needed lifestyle changes—these and many other consequences of uncoordinated care lead to disease progression and the need for more costly, invasive care. The resulting conflicts between providers, who are focused on individual patient care, and managers, who have responsibility for maintaining cost-effective services, have been very damaging to the morale and prestige of the health care system. The Institute of Medicine, in its 2001 landmark book, *Crossing the Quality Chasm* (Institute of Medicine, 2001), cites ". . . coordination of care across patient conditions, services, and settings over time" as one of its key recommendations for improving the quality of care and reducing medical errors.

The goal of care management is to integrate the health care industry into a cohesive, efficient system of care that improves the quality of health care services and enhances the health of the population. Physicians accustomed to the relatively narrow focus of individual patient care now influence larger cohorts of consumers with a particular disease or risk factor, extending the doctors' influence over larger groups of individuals. Managers can allocate resources based on the greatest return on investment, measured in health outcomes, rather than simply reacting to unconstrained demand. Consumers assume greater importance and responsibility in the new system of care management. No longer passive recipients of care, consumers now can be proactive in finding the best preventive care to maintain function and extend useful life while, at the same time, improving the quality of life. Consumers will have access to outcome information that can help them make informed decisions regarding the type and site of care that they receive. A new system for ensuring that care is rendered appropriately and effectively can restore consumer and payer confidence in the health care delivery system. The most appealing feature of a care management model for American health care is the ability to apply the approach to diverse environments and populations.

♦ Care Management: Theoretical Framework

Another definition of care management that has gained wide acceptance is that of Peter Juhn of Kaiser-Permanente, who states that care management is "a comprehensive systems approach to medical care that combines the latest medical knowledge on the best clinical methods, population-based outcomes measurement and evaluation, and advanced practice tools" (Juhn, et al., 1998). Several attributes of care management can be inferred from this definition and from knowledge of the needs of a care management program.

♦ The care management approach is **comprehensive**. The disease or preventive care options are well understood and characterized as scientifically as possible. Thorough literature searches and consensus panels have identified best practices, idealized patterns of care, optimum outcomes, objective measurements, and appropriate diagnostic and therapeutic modalities.

♦ **Data are available to identify consumers at risk**. The target populations with the disease or risk factor can be identified with data available to the care management organization. Populations are generally identified by several data sources, including demographic information, diagnosis categories, resource utilization, costs, and epidemiological markers.

◆ The **focus of care management is on prevention and/or cure** of a disorder. Cohorts of consumers in the population that are at risk for a disease entity should receive educational interventions to help prevent the disease, and diagnostic and treatment regimens should be customizable for individuals based on good medical practice and the scientific literature.

◆ **Educational interventions** should be funded and promoted. Consumers who are armed with knowledge of their disease and are made responsible for their own care tend to have better outcomes (Morgan, 1998; Byrnes, 1998b). As patients assume greater responsibility for their own care, they have lower costs of care, as well as greater satisfaction.

◆ **Continuity of care** must be promoted. Consumers with complex medical illnesses require ongoing, oftentimes intense, management to ensure that they adhere to treatment recommendations. That need necessitates a care manager who can establish a rapport with the patient so that the patient will feel comfortable providing feedback on sensitive issues as well as cooperate more fully with sometimes difficult treatment recommendations. A care manager able to establish these important relationships can pick up on subtle cues given by the patient of impending problems, thus forestalling any complications that would increase morbidity or lead to untimely death.

◆ **Data management systems must include clinical information**. Typical insurance data management systems are inadequate for care management, and traditional paper charts maintained by providers fall far short of supplying enough information to perform care management. Population-based interventions, such as educational programs on prevention, can be initiated using administrative databases, but for true care management and risk reduction, much more information will be necessary. Automated systems for clinical recordkeeping, telemedicine facilities, and advanced Internet communications strategies will prove to be the central nervous system for care management programs.

All of these attributes will be found in a truly effective care management program. Many organizations implement *case* management programs to deal with chronically ill people with specific illnesses, but these programs lack the comprehensiveness required for *care* management. Clinical practice guidelines (CPGs) have been implemented in some managed care organizations, but without the accompanying resources to effect successful implementation, practice guidelines are of little value.

Unfortunately, the type of organization implementing a care management program has an influence on the goals of interventions. Pharmaceutical companies initiated many disease management programs in the early 1990s, but in many cases, these programs were designed to increase utilization of the company's pharmaceutical products. Managed care organizations then jumped into the care management arena, but the primary goal for most of those companies was to reduce costs. Provider organizations that implemented disease management programs frequently sought to increase utilization of specific equipment or facilities that they owned. Each of these organizations used measures that served their goals, e.g., drug sales, service revenues, or net profit, which nearly always involved short-term targets that failed to capitalize on the long-term benefits of care management. Although care management programs have the potential to achieve lower costs and to optimize use of services, these endpoints generally cannot be achieved over two or three fiscal quarters; changing consumer health care utilization habits will be achieved only gradually through education and improvement in overall health status.

Key Elements of a Care Management Program

As part of the planning process, several key components of a care management program must be secured to improve the chances for success. Table 10.1 lists and categorizes these elements. Ensuring the availability of essential resources for a comprehensive care management program requires forethought and planning, as well as management support. Each of the components listed

Table 10.1 Key Components of a Care Management Program

TYPE OF ELEMENT	ELEMENT
CQI Infrastructure	◆ Data collection instruments
	◆ Data base resources
	◆ Data analysis tools
	◆ Data management software
	◆ Computing systems for analysis and information dissemination
Clinical	◆ CPGs
	◆ Risk-assessment instruments
	◆ Diagnostic aids
Educational	◆ Patient education materials
	◆ Physician education materials
Personnel	◆ Registered nurses
	◆ Physicians
	◆ Physician extenders
	◆ Other health professionals
	◆ Health care administrators
	◆ Insurance administrators
	◆ Suppliers and vendors

CQI, continuous quality improvement; CPG, clinical practice guideline.

in Table 10.1 has particular importance for the success of a care management program, and together they can be considered the basic infrastructure for QI. Lacking these resources, a care management program will most probably not even be able to measure the effect of interventions, much less demonstrate their efficacy.

A sophisticated information system serves as the primary component of any QI infrastructure. Three elements of data management are important to a care management project: collection, storage and validation, and analysis. Data collection processes have tended to be mostly manual systems, consisting of forms completed by staff responsible for gathering information, with data entered into computer systems in batches. Newer portable computer systems with user-friendly software are replacing paper systems and eliminating an expensive and time-consuming step in data management. Rather than filling out paper forms, care management team members can now enter data directly into a computer database, making the data immediately available for validation and analysis. Database management systems have become much easier to configure and use, allowing users with even rudimentary computer skills to structure data sets for QI projects.

For smaller projects, e.g., those involving only a few hundred records, spreadsheet programs provide an alternative data management system. Powerful features of spreadsheet programs now allow statistical analysis of data sets that previously required expensive and arcane statistical analysis programs. The most important disadvantage of using a spreadsheet function for database management is the inability to easily normalize the database. Database normalization is a process that reduces redundancy by configuring the database so that repeated data are entered only once. For example, an electronic medical record/billing system would need to have patient demographic information entered only once but that same information can then be related to numerous transaction records. Spreadsheets can be configured to reduce this redundancy but not as easily as database management programs. On the other hand, spreadsheet data can be transferred to most database management programs, so if a care management project starts using a spreadsheet for data collection and analysis, the data set can later be transferred to a more sophisticated database.

Another useful feature of contemporary database management programs is the ability to filter data as they are being entered. For example, a data field for zip codes could allow only five- or nine-digit numbers within a specific range of values. Such capabilities allow validation of the data as they are being entered, rather than using computer programs to screen the data after they are already in the database. Prescreening data can improve the quality of the database because anyone entering information into the database can be prompted at the time the erroneous entry is being made to correct the item. Data validation filters performed on existing databases can only identify records to be eliminated from the database because they are corrupt. Thus, if an error was made consistently during data entry, the entire database could be lost.

With more sophisticated data management systems, huge amounts of data can now be stored and accessed for more effective analyses. Distributed database systems now provide local storage of data elements at each data collection site and provide automated transfer of local data to a central repository that combines multiple data sources, merging records for advanced analyses that can correlate treatment programs and disease states. Many of these data repositories have become very large (terabytes of data), leading to strategies for improving access to data, including data marts, which are extracts of the repository germane to a particular functional area (e.g., internal medicine, pediatrics, or general surgery) that reside on dedicated servers to improve access speeds and avoid direct access to the immense data repository. An organization with a large data repository may have multiple data marts to serve the needs of various departments throughout the enterprise.

If an automated entry system is not available, then paper forms must be used for data collection. In spite of the disadvantages of paper forms, they frequently require less time and training for staff because most people are accustomed to this method of data collection. The design of paper forms can be somewhat complex, however. Because most data collected on paper forms will ultimately make their way into a computer system, the form should be designed to expedite data entry. Form entries should be organized in the same order as the data entry fields on a computer screen so that skilled entry clerks can input the data more efficiently. Additionally, any data entry form, whether paper or computer, must be designed to reduce the possibility of bias in the data collection. Complicated forms sometimes induce data collectors to enter information mechanically in a certain pattern, leading to bias in the data set. Forms should be as straightforward as possible, without any complex elements to confound data collection personnel. Pilot testing of the forms with data collection personnel can help in this regard. Additionally, all forms should be accompanied by a list of operational definitions to allay any confusion about the data that are to be collected.

Computers continue to evolve into increasingly sophisticated systems that can perform advanced analyses at little cost. Although huge population studies may still require mainframe computers, most care management systems can be run on personal computer systems with relatively inexpensive software. These new systems can import data from a variety of sources and integrate them for creating insightful reports to use for decision making. Statistical analysis programs have also become much easier to use. A basic knowledge of statistics is still helpful, but many programs now suggest the analytical approach based on the data set. A listing of commonly used statistical programs and associated Web sites is included in Table 10.2.

Health statistics and demographic data can be obtained in electronic format from a number of sources, some of which are listed in Appendix 10A,

Table 10.2 Statistical Analysis Programs for Computer Workgroups

PROGRAM	URL
SAS	*http://www.sas.com*
SPSS	*http://www.spss.com*
Minitab	*http://www.minitab.com*
Statistica	*http://www.statsoftinc.com*

along with their URLs. Most data sources are either free or can be purchased inexpensively. Additionally, the National Center for Health Statistics provides summary data online at *http://www.cdc.gov/nchs/fastats/Default.htm*. This site has information in a number of different formats, from state comparisons to individual statistics reported nationally and by state. In addition to these federal government sites, most states publish their vital statistics data (birth and death) on their state Web sites. Examples of a few of these sites can be found in Table 10.3.

Data analysis focuses the care management process on key issues for intervention, and the information that emerges from these investigations should direct the team's efforts and resource allocation. Precision in data collection and accuracy in the evaluation of the data sets must be an important objective of the care management process.

As noted in Table 10.1, the next important element of a care management program can be termed the clinical aspect. CPGs are discussed in Chapter 8, but the importance of these instruments cannot be overstated. After clinical guidelines are created, they must be converted into usable instruments, e.g., by designing forms and databases for collecting information about patients in the program. The CPG will contain an operational definition of the patient groups for which the guideline was developed, and in some cases, a risk assessment questionnaire can be of help in clarifying whether a patient should be included in the program. Risk assessment tools generally consist of a questionnaire and a scoring method. Patients who achieve a specific score are considered at risk, whereas those who have scores below the threshold are considered not to be at risk. Health risk appraisal (HRA) tools can be general in nature or focused on specific diseases (Goetzel, et al., 1998; Hornsby, et al., 1997; Powell, et al., 1996; Weaver, et al., 1998). Many organizations now perform HRAs for a number of reasons, such as to stratify populations for health education programs or to identify patients in a medical practice for specific interventions. Most important, though, HRAs serve as useful tools for finding groups at risk within a population. A sample of HRA instruments is included as Table 10.4.

Finally, once groups at risk have been found, clinical strategies must be available for clinicians to deal with the problem. In fact, this issue may be of primary importance in selecting a care management program to implement.

Table 10.3 Selected State Vital Statistics Web Sites

STATE	URL
Master State List	*http://www.cdc.gov/nchs/howto/w2w/w2welcom.htm*
Michigan	*http://www.mdch.state.mi.us/PHA/OSR/index.asp*
Colorado	*http://www.cdphe.state.co.us/hs/hsshom.asp*
Minnesota	*http://www.health.state.mn.us/stats.html*
California	*http://www.dhs.cahwnet.gov/org/hisp/chs/chsindex.htm*
Virginia	*http://www.vdh.state.va.us/epi/newhome.asp*
Oregon	*http://www.dhs.state.or.us/data*
New Jersey	*http://www.state.nj.us/health/hcsa/hlthstat.htm*
Montana	*http://healthinfo.montana.edu/msu/statistics.html*
Texas	*http://www.tdh.state.tx.us/bvs/health.htm*
Pennsylvania	*http://www.dsf.health.state.pa.us/health*
Oklahoma	*http://www.health.state.ok.us/program/phs/ohs/index.html*
Kansas	*http://www.kdhe.state.ks.us/hci*
Tennessee	*http://www2.state.tn.us/health/statistics/index.html*

If the care management process can successfully detect individuals or groups at risk but no intervention is available to deal with that risk, then the program will not be able to achieve its goal of influencing care and outcomes. Thus, care management program selection should include an analysis of the ability to influence outcomes. Not only should the interventions be available, they should also be feasible. For example, a recommendation that individuals with head injuries be evaluated with computed tomography (CT) should be made only when a CT scanner is available at the site of care. If the intervention is not technically feasible, then the care management program will not be successful. Interventions that are well accepted by clinicians and easy to implement are preferable to those that are more difficult for clinicians to accept or perform—the concept of the low-hanging fruit. As with any innovation in medicine, practitioners want to be certain that a new approach is successful before it becomes widely accepted. As clinicians gain increasing understanding of the care management process and form collegial relationships with care managers, more difficult interventions can be promulgated.

If the intervention is acceptable to physicians and available at the site of care, the care management team often needs to make the intervention easy to use. The mechanism for enhancing access depends on the organization implementing the program. A managed care organization might remove economic or medical management constraints from the procedure, whereas a medical group might assign a staff member to expedite a procedure. For example, to encourage eye exams in diabetic patients, a managed care organization could

Table 10.4 Sample of Health Risk Appraisal Instruments

HRA	REFERENCE	DESCRIPTION
PRA and PRA Plus	Boult, Dowd, McCaffrey, Boult, Hernandez, and Krulewitch, 1993	Risk appraisal tool for determining the risk of hospitalization
SF-36	http://www.sf-36.com	General risk appraisal for health problems and general well-being
SF-12	http://www.qualitymetric.com/demos/SF-12.html	Short version of the SF-36
Child Health Questionnaire	http://www.healthact.com/chq_content.asp	Multifactorial survey of children's health status
Duke Health Profile	http://www.heritage-info.com/mocaidrx/files/dm/Duke_health_profile.doc	Multifactorial screening tool for adult physical and behavioral health
London Handicap Scale	http://www.medal.org/adocs/docs_ch37/doc_ch37.05.html#A37.05.09	Screening survey for individuals with physical challenges

HRA, health risk appraisal; PRA, probability of repeat admissions.

remove the need for approval of the referral to an eye specialist, and a medical group might assign the task of making the referrals to a staff nurse rather than require a physician visit or intervention prior to the referral.

The key to making a care management program succeed can be summarized briefly as the need to streamline and enhance the process of care. A systematic approach to the disease or risk factor and its treatment can provide the basis for a productive program, and by encouraging excellent care, payers, consumers, and providers should find the program rewarding.

◆ Development of a Care Management Program

As with any QI intervention, the success of a care management system relies on the amount of planning and preparation that an organization performs before implementing the program. Effective programs require a systems approach, which considers the approach to a disease or risk management program comprehensively, rather than as just a consortium of individual components. The systems approach provides insight into the interactions of all of the elements of a care management program, guaranteeing that as changes are made in one component, ensuing changes in the others are anticipated. A systems model of a care management program is included in Figure 10.1. The model emanates from strategic management approaches to planning and implementation, and each step in the process enhances the success of the program.

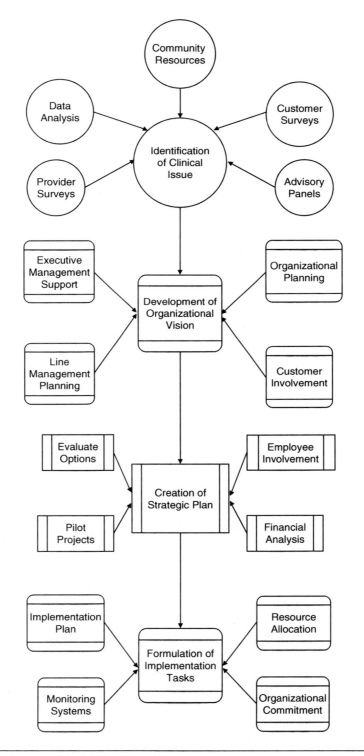

Figure 10.1 Systems Model for Care Management

The first task in the process is to determine a clinical problem of concern to the organization. A number of factors are germane to this step, including the focus and mission of the organization. A pediatric endocrinology practice, for example, would choose a program for diabetes, rather than one for rheumatoid arthritis. A number of input sources should be consulted for discerning the most important clinical issues for an organization to consider. Customers should be a seminal resource for organizations as they home in on potential programs because customers are the ultimate beneficiaries of these innovations. In addition to ideas regarding potential projects, customers can also serve as a source of implementation barriers. If barriers are significant, a program may be doomed from the start and should be either revised or eliminated. Key selection criteria for most organizations include clinical conditions with

◆ high cost
◆ high volume
◆ high risk of quality problems
◆ high profile with providers and customers
◆ high potential for changing the process of care
◆ high potential for satisfying the requirements of customers, regulators, and accrediting bodies

These criteria help direct the selection of the disease or risk factor that will be the focus of the care management program, and final selection should be predicated on thorough data analysis.

Most organizations recognize the need to collect and analyze data as the means of determining what care management projects to initiate. Depending on the type of organization, data sources can range from medical charts to computerized business records. For clinical applications, medical data are of greatest value, but managed care organizations rarely have unfettered access to medical records. Hospitals have inpatient clinical data, as well as information from outpatient services such as home health, ambulatory surgery, etc., but the bulk of medical care is provided in medical offices. Thus, a comprehensive care management program is best designed with data from all sites of care. Programs that focus on just one segment of care of a disease or risk factor will invariably ignore important ramifications of interventions in another area. For example, an asthma program that focuses on inpatient care will fail because lack of appropriate outpatient management simply returns patients to the hospital for more of the same expensive care. Similarly, a diabetes program that focuses only on acute exacerbations will fail to recognize the long-term care issues of retinopathy, renal failure, and foot ulcers that lead to costly and debilitating complications. Properly implemented, a care management program should evaluate all aspects of a clinical condition to determine the best methods of intervention.

Other sources of data such as provider and consumer surveys and advisory panels can prove useful. Surveys can be expensive to design and deploy, so they should be used judiciously to obtain specific feedback. Many organizations maintain advisory panels of consumers, suppliers, and payers to obtain ongoing opinions about issues of importance to management. Panels can be composed in any way that is useful to obtain needed information, generally at greatly reduced costs compared with surveys and chart reviews.

The next step in the care management process entails gaining organizational support for the care management effort. These programs almost always require change, and they often produce financial and personnel costs that require senior management support. After a QI team has defined a care management plan, the next task involves gaining buy-in from management and sometimes from other departments. Small organizations such as two- or three-physician medical groups may want to include all members of the staff, but large organizations such as hospitals or health maintenance organizations (HMOs), will often require several meetings to reach all affected staff members. The team will usually create a professional business presentation, including

◆ a rationale for the project, including data leading to the selection of the clinical condition
◆ an outline of the major milestones for the project with a timeline
◆ a clinical approach to the problem, including a CPG
◆ financial projections, including cost of the project and projected savings in the cost of care
◆ performance and outcome measures, with operational definitions

A business presentation for a project of this magnitude usually includes a written report, as well as a slide presentation that summarizes important features for senior management.

Gaining organizational support is a key factor in the success of a care management program. Senior managers will be concerned about costs, but they are usually also interested in other aspects of the program, such as customer satisfaction and improved market share. The concerns of middle management encompass operational issues, particularly assurance that necessary resources will be available to accomplish the goals of the program. Frontline personnel will be particularly interested in ensuring that adequate resources are available so that their workloads will not become excessive. Finally, customers may be enthralled with the program, but they often require reassurance that other services will not be interrupted.

Once committed, the organization will begin making strategic plans to implement the project. Using the tools and techniques described in Chapter 2, the care management team involves various stakeholders in the organization to design the processes required for implementing the program.

Team work and group processes are of utmost importance for a number of reasons. First, including the same staff members who will be responsible for implementing the program will ensure that the procedures and timetables are realistic and achievable. Only the people who actually do the work are cognizant of workloads and slack resources. Second, as staff members become involved in the project, their level of commitment should increase, improving the likelihood of success. People who design programs are most often also committed to making them work. Finally, during the planning stages, staff members who have not worked with each other can begin to form relationships that will prove useful during implementation of the project. The benefits of the group process are detailed in Chapter 2, and creation of a viable care management program requires group commitment and participation.

The final step in the care management program creation process, formulation of implementation plans, makes the strategic plan come alive. Managers and workers convert the strategic outline into executable functions, creating budgets and allocating resources. As before, group processes are of utmost importance to ensure success. Staff members who are responsible for putting the plan into action must be involved at this step to design or modify the systems needed to put the plan into operation.

Figure 10.2 illustrates a flowchart for a care management project. Initial tasks include selection of a disease entity or risk factor to manage, followed by population selection, and then selection of a CPG to use. The guideline often provides some direction on how to stratify the population, and in the figure, four typical categories are displayed. Stratification criteria can have many dimensions, including

◆ cost
◆ risk level for complications
◆ incidence of complications
◆ risk of mortality
◆ types of therapy and interventions
◆ index of severity criteria
◆ specific lab or x-ray findings
◆ disease stage

Cost is an important factor for most organizations. The driving force in managed care organizations is reducing cost, ideally by decreasing the incidence of expensive complications and progression of disease. Provider groups that initiate care management programs often are at financial risk for patient care through capitation, diagnosis-related groups, or per diem reimbursement arrangements in which providers are paid a fixed amount for a patient's illness, regardless of resource use. Thus, screening the administrative database for high-cost diseases is often the first step in identifying candidates for different levels of intervention.

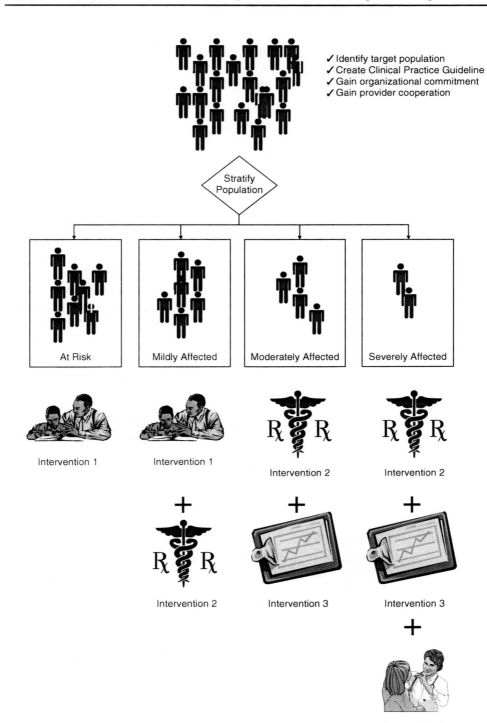

Figure 10.2 Care Management Program Development

Other methods of stratifying the population consider the complication rates or incidence of complications for a subpopulation. Complications of an illness often increase cost and diminish the ability of an individual to continue functioning in a job or activities of daily living, so segregating the population of affected individuals into groups according to the presence or risk of complications can be a useful strategy. Interventions then would be designed to prevent or ameliorate the complications. Similarly, separating groups in the disease population by risk of mortality could provide another method of designing effective interventions.

Some systems of stratification consider measures such as an index of severity, which is a scoring system that has been adopted by the medical profession to determine the extent of patient illness. These indexes can take many forms and are routinely used by providers and payers alike to gauge the clinical condition of each individual (Brunelli, et al., 1999; Moler and Ohmit, 1999; Doody, et al., 1999; Lassere, et al., 1999). In some situations when the index of severity has too many categories, more advanced groups can be formulated using advanced statistical techniques (Luke, et al., 1996). Numerous indexes have been created and are commonly used in medical practice, and the CPG should include any of these scoring systems that are useful to practitioners. Use of these systems to aggregate patients into groups can make the care management program more logical for providers because they can match interventions with stages of disease with which they are familiar.

Another common method of differentiating individuals with a disease involves using laboratory or imaging findings or therapeutic interventions. Patients with a certain level of a diagnostic marker or a particular finding on x-ray can be placed into categories because they often require a specific type of intervention. For example, a finding of lobar consolidation in an elderly person with community-acquired pneumonia would dictate a particular therapeutic approach. Similarly, individuals with diabetes can be grouped by insulin requirements, e.g., insulin dependent and not insulin dependent. Whichever classification system finally prevails should be easily identified with the use of data analysis tools available to the care management team and should also be logical for the provider community that will be implementing the program.

Gaining management support requires that the care management team demonstrate a return on investment for the project. The return can be financial, or it can be measured in marketing terms such as increased market share or improved patient satisfaction levels. In some environments, reduced needs for staffing can be established, although those situations are relatively rare. Generally, however, a business analysis must be performed and presented to senior management in order to procure funds for the project.

Interventions will almost always be suggested by the CPGs. Figure 10.2 presents a scenario with four potential interventions. As the severity of the disease increases, so too does the intensity of the interventions. *Interven-*

tion 1 could be an educational program that addresses risk factors for the disease, with direct mailings for those at risk and perhaps a direct educational program for those with mild manifestations of the illness. The educational program promotes prevention and early diagnosis so that if the disease appears, medical attention can start as early as possible. Additionally, the educational program can include

◆ a layman's description of the pathophysiology of the disease
◆ techniques for managing the illness
◆ medications or surgical interventions
◆ lifestyle modifications to attenuate the disease
◆ complications
◆ procedures for getting medical help
◆ information for families of individuals with the illness

Educational materials must be culturally and educationally appropriate for the population that will receive the information. Frequently, these materials have been developed by any of a number of organizations, such as drug companies, special interest organizations, universities, and governments. For common diseases such as asthma, diabetes, and heart disease, in particular, there are multitudinous educational materials, including computer programs and videotapes, available from special interest organizations and the federal government.

In addition to educating patients, care management teams must also inform providers of the program. One of the most effective ways of teaching physicians and nurses is to become involved in their regular continuing education programs such as grand rounds and workshops. Continuing education credits make these educational programs attractive, and in some cases, the care management team will budget funds to train physician leaders in the program. These physicians act as mentors to their peers and can be effective educators. As the CPG is being developed, the care management team can identify physician leaders who understand the program and can communicate the goals, objectives, and operational characteristics of the program to their peers. Additionally, physician leaders in the community can be enlisted to serve as resources for their colleagues, making information about the program readily accessible to all providers who will be caring for patients in the program.

Team members should also be thoroughly familiar with the program. Because care management teams may include nonmedical people, these team members must be educated about the program and its ramifications. Although they are involved throughout planning and implementation, the nonmedical members of the team may not have an in-depth understanding of the nuances of the system of care, and because they may represent the team in the community, it is important that they are prepared for the inevitable questions. Sometimes a 1- or 2-hour seminar might allow enough time for the team members to learn about the disease, but if the problems are particularly complex, then a day-long retreat can help.

After educational interventions, many care management programs will implement drug management systems, as in *intervention 2,* to improve adherence to medication regimens and reduce adverse reactions and drug–drug interactions. Nurses or other care managers generally monitor patient drug compliance by examination of drug claims data, direct interaction with patients, or reports from pharmacists and physicians. Managed care organizations collect immense amounts of data, and a significant component of this information is from pharmacy transactions. Computer programs can track individual prescription refill patterns, and when a medication refill is overdue, care managers are alerted to take action.

Often, specialized care managers, called case managers, are involved in these interventions. Case managers are usually nurses or other allied health professionals with special expertise in a disease entity. They are able to evaluate data regarding patient care and determine if the care is appropriate, and they often are able to interact with patients to obtain important clinical data. Case managers use algorithms for care based on the CPG and are prompted to call the patient's provider when care seems to be deviating from an expected pattern. Thus, if a patient fails to refill a prescription, the case manager may call the patient or the provider to remind him or her of the needed refill, sometimes even having the drug delivered to ensure that the patient receives the drug. Some protocols call for the case manager to call the patient on a regular basis to determine that the patient is following instructions from the provider. Case managers are usually involved with interventions only for the most seriously ill individuals, but they may be involved with less severely ill patients as well. In some systems, pharmacists may act as case managers, and in a primary care gatekeeper model of managed care, the primary care physician assumes this responsibility (Boland, 1993; Self & Demirkan, 1999).

The next level, labeled *intervention 3* in Figure 10.2, usually entails more aggressive case management, and the case manager becomes more intensively involved with the care of the patient. Complex, chronically ill patients often have several providers and take multiple medications, even when they are not severely afflicted with a disease process. Case managers monitor patient care, sometimes with electronic medical records, and intervene periodically with educational programs and interactions with the provider to ensure that drug regimens are appropriate and specialty care is obtained when necessary. Case managers maintain an ongoing relationship with the patient, often calling several times a month to check on the status of the illness and the condition of the patient. Any problems are immediately relayed to the patient's physician for rapid follow-up and intervention.

The final level of intervention, *intervention 4,* saved for the small number of individuals who are most severely afflicted with the disease, involves the case manager to an even greater degree. These patients or their providers may be contacted as often as daily to ascertain any changes in clinical condition. The case manager is usually a close ally for the provider, who often cannot sustain this level of interaction. As automated systems become more widespread, technologies using the Internet will become standard methods of obtaining patient data rapidly and conveniently (Redford & Parkins, 1997; De Vreugd, 1997; Rooney, et al., 1997). Not only will these new technologies improve access and the quality of care, but after the initial cost of the technology has been amortized, the cost of care should also fall.

The flowchart in Figure 10.2 works for many disease processes. Although some care management programs are much more extensive, the basic configuration of a program should follow these steps. There are many challenges within the outline, as stated earlier, but a care management team with management support and members drawn from various areas of the organization, customers, and providers should be able to foresee most of the barriers to a successful program. The next section discusses some of the more common problems that the team may encounter.

Barriers to Implementation

Even a perfect plan faces problems in the real world. Providers, insurers, consumers, staff members—all have an integral role in making the care management system work; but these groups do not usually share the same incentives. Many barriers lie in the path of implementation, and these issues should be addressed before the program starts. Table 10.5 lists several of these potential problems. As the care management team moves to deploy the program, a barriers analysis can be performed to determine which of these potential problems are significant and what can be done to eliminate the problems.

Providers have some specific issues with care management programs, but they often verbalize just a few. One of the most common complaints is that of a "cookbook medicine" approach to patient care. Physicians learn the workup for many diseases in medical school and graduate training, but most doctors develop practice patterns that vary from those codified approaches

Table 10.5 Barriers to Implementation of a Care Management Program

STAKEHOLDER	BARRIER
Provider	◆ Lack of scientific validation of proposed interventions
	◆ Lack of appropriate feedback system to determine success
	◆ Inability to visualize the disease process beyond a specific area of expertise
	◆ Little or no experience with working in teams

continues

Table 10.5 *continued*

Stakeholder	Barrier
Provider (cont.)	◆ Professional prestige
	◆ "Cookbook medicine" perception
	◆ Inadequate communication with disease managers
	◆ Time commitment to program
	◆ Misaligned incentives
	◆ Financial effects
	◆ Malpractice liability
	◆ Regulatory agencies and requirements
	◆ Skills and competencies
Payer	◆ Regulatory agencies and requirements
	◆ Cost of program
	◆ Shareholder concerns
	◆ Financial concerns
	◆ Liability for medical care
	◆ Resource utilization
	◆ Internal skills and competencies
	◆ Contractual relationships threatened
Consumer	◆ Lack of individualized care
	◆ Inadequate resources
	◆ Restrictions on services
	◆ Changing providers
	◆ Denied access to care
Suppliers	◆ Declining revenues due to changing practice patterns
	◆ Damaged relationships with providers
	◆ Decreasing market share
Employees	◆ Job security
	◆ Work overload
	◆ Inadequate skills
System	◆ Lack of consistency in incentives among all stakeholders
	◆ Lack of scientific evidence regarding diagnosis and treatment of disease or risk factor
	◆ Measurement systems inadequate
	◆ Data systems inadequate
	◆ Communication systems inadequate
	◆ Difficulty obtaining appropriate data
	◆ Gaps in service availability for population

through changes in medical science, practice experience, and peer pressure. Presenting a physician with a CPG almost immediately dredges up the feeling that the physician will have little latitude in treating the patient, and most physicians will rebel. Although the practice patterns of most doctors are internally consistent, many deviate from current credible standards, leading to the wide variations in medical practice noted by Wennberg and others (Austin, 1997). Thus, physicians do not change readily, even in the light of new scientific evidence. In general, physicians must be convinced that four criteria are met before change will occur.

1. Patient care and outcomes will improve.
2. Malpractice risk will not increase and preferably will decrease.
3. Practice income will not suffer.
4. Uncompensated workload will not increase.

If these issues can be dealt with to the doctor's satisfaction, then the most important hurdles are surmounted. Even the issue of cookbook medicine will not be an impediment if the physician can be assured that these four issues are addressed.

Some other concerns shared by providers include the need for scientific validation of the recommendations made in CPGs. In most cases, the fact that recognized local and/or national experts created the guidelines provides reassurance that recommendations are current and valid. However, some physicians want input into the process of guideline creation, and in those situations, having the physician participate on the committees that produce CPGs can have a very positive influence on the physician's cooperation and buy-in by others in the medical community. This problem also relates to the difficulty physicians have with the loss of prestige in care management programs. Many physicians perceive that using a guideline makes them less intellectual in their approach to medicine, so the rigorous scientific basis for the program must be emphasized to overcome this barrier. Additionally, if the practice recommendations differ substantially from a physician's traditional practice patterns, patients in the practice may perceive that the physician has not been providing proper care, leading to malpractice risk and transfers to other providers. Thus, the educational component of the care management program may need to address any significant disparities between the current practice patterns of the physician and the new recommendations.

The practice of medicine has become more hectic in the recent past due to the economic constraints placed on the system, primarily by managed care. Busy physicians are besieged on all sides by managed care organizations that need to perform QI studies that enhance managed care organization profit margins and satisfy accreditation standards. The time commitment from each of these programs may be small, but in the aggregate, the time commitment can become untenable. Coordination of care management programs within a region could promote good medical care and data collection without placing an undue burden on physicians. Managed care organizations, hospitals, disease management companies, and state agencies must work to standardize approaches to disease entities and data collection so that physicians are not hampered in using the programs because of different guidelines or disparate forms. Without this kind of cooperation between organizations with care management programs, physician compliance will be erratic at best.

Physicians are traditionally team leaders, but in care management programs, they are placed in a position of being a team member instead. Most physicians have little experience working in groups, leading to significant conflicts as they attempt to assume their usual position of leadership within a care management workgroup. At times, care management program directors may feel alienated from the physicians involved in the process, but these situations demand good team-building skills and interventions. Physicians must not be placed in adversarial positions in care management programs or the programs will fail. Team-building exercises, such as those discussed in Chapter 2, can be helpful in gaining physician cooperation with the changes required by care management.

Perhaps one of the greatest barriers to physician participation in care management systems is the perceived or actual risk of medical malpractice. As noted above, physician compliance is often driven by four factors: patient care, malpractice risk, income loss, and increased workload. Most physicians are inherently afraid of the malpractice risk, not just because of the potential for economic loss, but also because their professional competence is threatened, along with their standing in the community. Thus, every precaution should be taken to mitigate malpractice risk, and any questions that arise should be taken seriously and dispelled.

Any areas of the care management program that have potential for liability should be identified to the practitioner, along with the way that the care management program has dealt with the risk. In general, however, malpractice risks in care management programs should be lower than in traditional medical practice because the program should be based on evidence in the medical literature or expert panel consensus.

Physician incentives should be examined in relationship to the care management program. The health care delivery system consists of disorganized, market-driven contracts between providers and payers, with market imperfections in the relationships based on a number of factors, including geography and specialty. Thus, a care management program may recommend that a certain type of care traditionally delivered in an office should now be shifted to a hospital outpatient center instead. The effect on the physician's practice income could be striking, a clear disincentive for the physician to participate in the program. In a fee-for-service system, any recommendations that decrease the amount of care delivered will reduce physician income, whereas in a capitated system, any recommendations that increase the amount of care that the patient requires will usually decrease practice income. Thus, the care management planning team must fine-tune the program to ensure that physician incentives—indeed, incentives for all stakeholders—match the goals of the program.

As with any segment of the health care industry, physicians are regulated by a number of different agencies and bureaus, which vary from state to state. The obvious candidates are state licensing bureaus, but many other organizations now are involved in physician oversight. For example, many managed care organizations now have contract provisions that stipulate requirements for the physician's office environment, and most physicians must comply with the arcane rules and regulations of agencies like the federal and state Occupational Safety and Health Administration. The list of regulatory bodies seems endless to many practitioners, so the care management program must be reviewed for any potential conflicts with all of these regulatory bodies.

The design of the program also needs to include provisions for excellent communication between the care management team and providers. A physician faced with a patient in the program needs to make decisions rapidly, and if information is not immediately available, then the physician will make a best-judgment determination, which may not comply with program guidelines. Updated information must be readily accessible, and contemporary modalities such as the Internet ensure that providers can quickly obtain the most current information. Use of the Internet for information dissemination has become increasingly appealing because most providers have ready access to it. In some cases, the care management team may want to provide "unconnected" physicians with the tools for accessing a Web site as an inexpensive means of improving information distribution.

Physicians can sometimes be dissuaded from participating in a care management program because they lack the skills or resources for providing the services required by the program. As the CPG is being adapted for the program, physicians involved in the process should be polled continuously about the ability of the medical community to actually deliver the services recommended by the guideline. If gaps appear between the capability of the system and the guideline recommendations, then the guideline may need to be revised, or one of the interventions included in the care management program may have to be an educational program to help providers comply with the current recommendations. For example, if a guideline recommends a specific imaging test for diagnosis or follow-up of a clinical condition but only an older technology is available because practitioners have not been trained in the new procedure, then the care management program may need to focus initially on training providers for the new method.

Payers must also deal with constraints and barriers to implementation. Most payers have ambivalent relationships with their providers, based on contracts that have compromises that providers have accepted only grudgingly. Contract provisions that allow chart reviews, office inspections, and medical management have made providers restive participants in managed care programs, so a care management program that adds to the burden of the provider can sour a payer's relationship with its physicians and hospitals. In some cases, providers may use participation in a care management program to gain other concessions from the payer, adding to the cost of implementing the program. The care management team must be sensitive to these relationships and attempt to minimize any disruption in the existing system.

No stakeholder in the health care delivery system can escape regulatory and accreditation bodies, and health insurance companies are no exception. From state insurance commissions to federal agencies such as the Centers for Medicare and Medicaid Services (formerly the Health Care Financing Administration) to accreditation organizations such as the National Committee for Quality Assurance, health insurers are beset with regulators on many fronts. The cost of complying with these entities is enormous, so most payers are very sensitive to any changes that could jeopardize compliance. Care management programs that enhance the ability of the company to satisfy the regulations and standards provide an added incentive for plans, and any program that threatens compliance will meet stiff resistance. Thus, the care management development process must include analyses of the regulatory environment of target payers with an eye toward easing the burden of regulation.

Cost issues take a variety of forms for payers. The direct cost of the program must be borne by some budgetary line, and distribution of the cost throughout the organization can be troublesome. Payers generally have a process for budgeting, and once the budget is set for a fiscal year, significant costs such as care management programs can rarely be accommodated until the next budget cycle. Thus, the budget process may stall implementation of the program by as much as 1 to 2 years. Additionally, for payers that are owned by stockholders, the cost of the program must be justified by a commensurate return on the investment, usually measured in dollars and not patient satisfaction. Not-for-profit organizations may be at a slight advantage in this regard, but even though there are no shareholders in the not-for-profit company, the company still must generate a profit to continue to grow.

In addition to the direct costs of the program, many indirect costs can accrue to the company. Almost any new program will require dissemination of information throughout the organization, including manuals and educational materials for the staff. In some instances, new skills will be needed, necessitating educational programs and the hiring of new employees with the requisite skills. Computer equipment and software may need to be upgraded, or telephone systems may require replacement. A number of improvements that are required by the program but can be amortized over several projects could create substantial indirect costs. As mentioned previously, one of the steps in the care management development process is the creation of a business presentation that itemizes all of the direct and indirect costs so that senior management can make a fully informed decision. Lack of sufficient funding can deal a death blow to a promising care management project.

A growing concern in the health insurance industry is the increasing liability for patient care that is being foisted on the industry by litigation and legislation. A number of recent cases have placed greater responsibility for adverse outcomes of care on insurers because these companies often make decisions that determine a patient's access to care (Court, 1998; Sedgwick, et al., 1999; Smith, 1998; Physician Insurers Association of America, 1998). Any interventions that increase that liability will most likely be rejected by managed care organizations, presenting a substantial barrier to implementation. Recommendations made by provider groups in CPGs should be thoroughly documented with citations from the medical literature or, absent any credible scientific evidence, by consensus among recognized experts in the field. Even with these assurances, the risk of litigation remains problematic.

Consumers usually have different but related concerns. The lawsuits brought against physicians and managed care organizations generally allege that care was denied because of a decision made by a medical director or the attending physician in collusion with the medical director of the managed care organization. These legal actions are often a symptom of consumer dissatisfaction with the procedures and outcomes of managed care. The concerns of consumers revolve around access to care and cost of services. Demand for most health services is fairly insensitive to price because health insurers assume much of the cost of care. The increasing use of rationing through prior authorization has diminished access to services, leading to consumer dissatisfaction (Kilbourne, 1998; Miller, 1998). Thus, any care management programs that restrict access to care should be accompanied by substantial consumer education. Additionally, many care management teams find that consumer input during the design process helps anticipate some of the problems that may arise later with consumers.

Another common consumer concern is the fear that physicians could start treating patients in a manner that does not consider an individual's specific circumstances. A cookie-cutter approach to medical practice is as discomfiting for consumers as it is for physicians, so as care management programs are brought to the marketplace, physicians and consumers alike will need reassurance that the programs will be used only when applicable to a particular clinical circumstance. Finally, consumers are especially sensitive to the need to change providers as a result of new terms of coverage or specific circumstances related to the program. A program that forces people to change physicians or hospitals in order to participate could face a consumer backlash that adds to the difficulty of making the program work.

Suppliers, such as medical equipment vendors and pharmaceutical companies, may present particular barriers to care management programs. If the supplier's economic interest is threatened, e.g., through restrictions on a type of equipment or a drug, the supplier may react by attempting to forestall or completely eliminate the program. Suppliers may have strong relationships with providers or even legislators, allowing them to exert influence on the implementation process. Gaining key supplier support during the design process can help prevent these reactions from occurring. Suppliers can sometimes bring otherwise inaccessible data to the planning process and improve the quality of the project. In those instances where many suppliers may be affected, a representative from an industry association may be able to effectively represent their interests.

Employees of organizations implementing care management programs can also provide resistance to the project. Although change is inevitable, it is rarely welcomed. Employees facing substantial changes in their jobs can create barriers to implementation by slowing work flow, creating false information, delaying response times, and creating other types of problems. Many of the techniques discussed in Chapter 2 are designed to incorporate employees into the planning and implementation processes, thus gaining employee concurrence with the program. Having employee input throughout the planning phase allows more accurate determination of resource needs and costs, as well as allaying employee concerns about job security and workload.

Finally, system problems can create barriers to advancing the care management program. As detailed previously, one of the most important facets of a project is the quality of the information used to make decisions. Data must be accessible and valid; otherwise a project cannot proceed. One of the early tasks of a planning team is to ensure the quality of the data that will be used to determine targets for intervention. Deming's concept of tampering, i.e., treating a common cause variation as a special cause, would be especially applicable if data provided erroneous results (Balestracci & Barlow, 1996). Additionally, the data must be analyzed appropriately. Statistical analysis of data can take many forms, and the assistance of a biostatistician can prove invaluable to the success of the project.

Another data-related barrier for the care management team to consider is the lack of salient process and outcome measures for the condition. Clinicians, consumers, and administrators will frequently have strong opinions about the ability of certain measures to reflect important outcomes or process capability. If the selected measures do not adequately gauge the effects of interventions, support for the project will rapidly fade. Because a number of outcome measures exist for measuring the results of interventions, as well as general health status, the selection of an outcome measure for a particular project may require substantial forethought. Two excellent references by Anne Bowling on disease-specific outcome measures and health-related quality of life measures are included in the Additional Reading section. Each measure must also have a precise operational definition to prevent confusion regarding the results of the care management program. All stakeholders in the program must have confidence in the measures for the project to succeed. Additionally, the communications systems to relay results to all stakeholders must be effective in conveying information in a manner that is meaningful to each group.

Some care management programs are implemented over a wide geographic area, usually with wide variations in the availability of certain key resources needed for the program. For example, if a diagnostic positron emission tomography (PET) scan is recommended as one step in the evaluation of a condition, the PET scanner must be within a reasonable travel distance for the consumer. Programs that are implemented over wide geographic areas with disparate resources often must tolerate greater discrepancies in patterns of care because of the lack of appropriate facilities or specialists at each site of care. Failure to consider this issue when analyzing data from a project can lead to spurious conclusions.

The many barriers to implementation described here can delay or even stop a care management program. If performance measures are inadequate, leading to incorrect analysis or interpretation of the outcome of the program, inappropriate care may result, a result that can doom future efforts at care management. Attention to details and thorough analysis can preclude many of the errors that arise and keep a project running smoothly, and in this respect, the responsibilities of the care management team are very substantial.

Process and Outcome Measures

QI efforts hinge on data, and the important informational components of a care management program are measures of the process of care and the outcome of care. Performance measures assume utmost importance in any QI system, and invariably these measures are difficult to define acceptably in health care. The American Academy of Family Physicians defined the desirable attributes of performance measures for health care as follows (American Academy of Family Physicians, 1998):

◆ scientifically valid
◆ capable of improvement
◆ prevalent in the population
◆ significant enough to need intervention
◆ significant enough to influence population health
◆ important to physicians and patients
◆ capable of improving value for patients, payers, and providers

The Institute of Medicine recently emphasized that measures of health care quality have been available and used quantitatively for the past 25 years and that these measures have a "degree of scientific accuracy comparable with that of most measures used in clinical medicine" (Chassin & Galvin, 1998). The frequent lament that health care lacks adequate performance measures is truly spurious.

Process measures target the means by which care is rendered; outcome measures gauge the ultimate effects of the processes. An ongoing debate in health care relates to which of the two types of measures is of greater importance. To a certain extent, determining which type of measure is most important depends on which position in the health care delivery system one takes.

For example, if a process causes great pain or discomfort for a patient to gain a small increase in probability of survival, then the process measure would be of greater importance to the patient. On the other hand, a provider in that scenario frequently would weight the outcome measure, survival, with greater importance. A payer would take a completely different view, perhaps assigning a greater weight to a cost–benefit measure. In short, any valid measure has significance to some stakeholder in the health care delivery system; the challenge is to balance the measures so that the process and outcome measures all contribute to a final group of measures in ways that are meaningful to the stakeholder using the measures.

Process measures are perhaps the most widely used because they can usually be collected concurrently with the delivery of care, and they have a much shorter time horizon. These measures are designed to quantify the efficiency and effectiveness of processes of care, and they are often reported as rates, such as cost per patient or time per procedure. Process measures can be clinically oriented or economically driven, depending on the focus of the care management process. Table 10.6 lists some process measures for care management programs. Defining process measures is one of the steps in creating the care management program, and these measures derive directly from the CPG. A flowchart of the clinical care process is a key component of the guideline, and process measures are inferred from the points on the flowchart that require measurement. An example flowchart for asthma is presented in Figure 10.3. The figure shows a home asthma management flowchart, with three performance measures indicated by the numbers on the flowchart. The measures are designed to evaluate the competence of the caregiver in managing a child's asthma. The first measure determines the ability of the educational process to train caregivers to evaluate a child's respiratory status by assessing the percentage of parents in the population of asthmatic children who can pass a test on evaluation of a child's respirations. The second is more of a systemic measure, i.e., the number of beta-2 agonist prescriptions per child per 6-month period, but it demonstrates the level of control of asthma in the population, with the added feature of stratifying the population by usage to design specific interventions. Finally, the third measure assesses the ability of the caretaker to properly evaluate the child's status after treatments have been completed. All three of these measures are process measures, and they illustrate the utility of the CPG for directing the data to be analyzed.

Outcome measures, on the other hand, attempt to gauge the effects of treatment interventions on short- and long-term parameters such as cost and health status. These measures usually fall into one of several categories:

◆ cost or expenditures
◆ health status
◆ complication rates
◆ mortality
◆ satisfaction with care or outcome

Table 10.6 Sample Process Measures in Care Management

Type of Measure	Measure	Definition
Risk	Cigarette smoke exposure in asthmatic children	Rate of parental smoking among asthmatic children >12 years of age
	Concentration of asbestos in workplace environment	Concentration of asbestos fibers in ppm in workplace air
	Alcohol misuse survey	Percent of population who have completed and returned an alcohol misuse survey
Process	Peak flow usage in asthmatics	Percentage of patients with asthma who measure peak flow according to schedule
	Diabetes education	Percent of patients with Type II diabetes who have undergone at least one educational session for diabetes care
	Diabetic foot exams	Percent of diabetic patients who report having a foot examination within a one-year period
	Beta blocker after heart attack	Percentage of patients with myocardial infarction who receive a beta blocker within 30 days of the event
Functional Status	Functional Status Measurement	Percent of patients in population with at least one provider encounter who were screened for functional status during the year

ppm, parts per million.

Society has placed increased emphasis on outcome measures over the past few years, primarily because health care processes still demonstrate tremendous process variance. By concentrating on outcomes, the variations between providers or health plans may be deemed irrelevant, if different processes can produce the same outcomes. However, divorcing the performance measurement system from process measures may prove short-sighted. The way that a process is designed has substantial influence on the ability to change the process. If health care processes have substantial variation, then, according to QI theory, they will not be stable over time and will not produce consistent results. Thus, process measures are important for determining if a system can sustain outcomes over a longer period of time. Additionally, this point also emphasizes the need to study processes over time, as noted in Chapter 5.

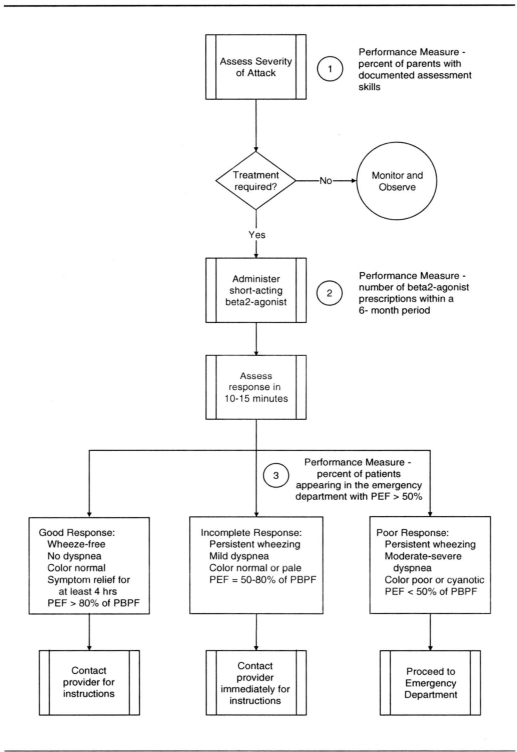

Figure 10.3 Flowchart for Asthma with Indicated Performance Measures

PEF, peak expiratory flow; PBPF, personal best peak flow.

A number of metrics that are used to measure managed care organizations can be deemed outcome measures. The clinical Health Plan Employer Data and Information Set (HEDIS) measures promulgated by the NCQA are nearly all outcome measures (National Committee for Quality Assurance, 1999). Measures like immunization rates for 2-year-olds provide an assessment of the process of primary care of children for a given health plan. Other organizations are implementing similar systems. In 1999, the Joint Commission on Accreditation of Healthcare Organizations (Joint Commission or JCAHO) has started a process of performance measurement for its accredited health care organizations called ORYX. The stated goal of ORYX is to "establish a data-driven, continuous survey and accreditation process to complement the Joint Commission's standards based assessment" (Joint Commission on Accreditation of Healthcare Organizations, 1999). Rather than establish a single measurement system such as HEDIS, the Joint Commission will certify contractors with measurement systems that can be used by health care institutions. The other major national organization that is currently establishing performance measures is the Foundation for Accountability. The Foundation for Accountability measures are similar to those of HEDIS but not exactly the same (Foundation for Accountability, 1999).

The selection of outcome measures for a care management program follows a procedure similar to that used for process measures. As the CPG is being developed, some measures will probably be suggested by the endpoints of the flowcharts. An example of a diabetes flowchart with outcome measures is found in Figure 10.4. The outcome measures chosen for this portion of the flowchart are glucose levels and rates of diabetic retinopathy. Each of these metrics will allow evaluation of the process of care outlined in the flowchart, but an important feature of these two measures should be noted. Blood glucose levels are monitored regularly, and a number of values will be available very quickly. On the other hand, the rate of retinopathy in the diabetic population will take much longer to measure adequately because that complication may take several years to develop. Thus, outcomes can be measured over a relatively short time period and over longer time periods. As most physicians will recognize, short-term fluctuations of blood glucose have substantially less importance than the long-term reduction in the rate of diabetic retinopathy. Unfortunately, the time horizon of most care management programs currently will not allow for 7-year follow up of patients with these problems, but for these programs to be successful, they must address outcomes that are important.

The types of measures adopted for care management projects depend on the organization implementing the program. Provider organizations will tend to concentrate on measures that gauge their ability to provide access to care, lower complication and mortality rates, and maximize net income. Managed care organizations will justifiably concentrate on financial and utilization measures but also will include measures needed to satisfy accreditation and regulatory agencies. Managed care organizations are becoming increasingly

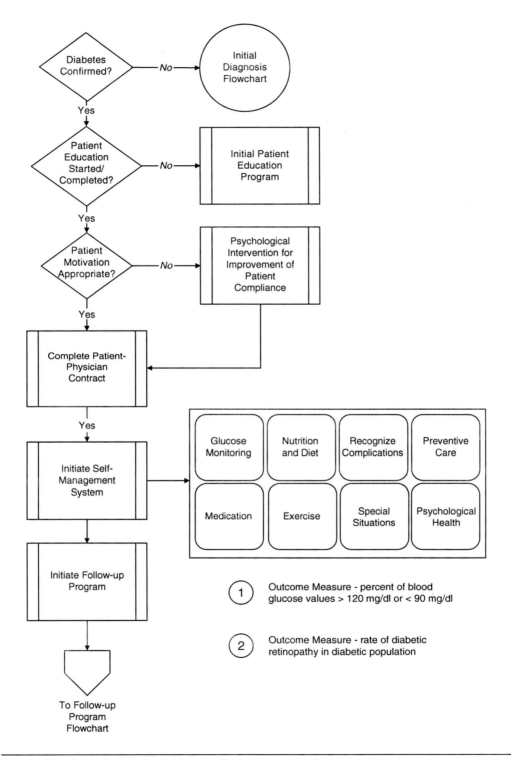

Figure 10.4 Portion of a Diabetes Flowchart with Outcome Measures

responsive to customer desires, including both employers and members, so any measures that are of interest to those groups will also likely be included in the measurement set. Hospitals and similar institutions will usually evaluate measures of efficiency and capacity utilization, with patient satisfaction included as a proxy for efficacy. Hospitals, however, serve many diverse publics. Because physicians are primary drivers in the hospital's market, the hospital will usually include measures that are important to providers such as complication rates and mortality rates. Hospitals must also answer to a number of accrediting agencies and regulatory bodies, so any measures that are required for ongoing certification will also be included in the measurement set. Finally, organizations such as hospitals must be particularly responsive to their marketplace, so community groups may also influence the choice of measures. In summary, internal and external customers drive the choice of measures. Any health care organization that is interested in surviving in the evolving marketplace should be prepared to find measures that optimize satisfaction of these many stakeholders.

Performance measures can be targeted at an overall process of care, e.g., rates of retinopathy or amputations among diabetics, or they may be more focused on episodes of care. Complex clinical conditions can often be subdivided into more manageable segments, termed episodes of care. These episodes usually connote an acute exacerbation of a chronic disease or some time-limited complication of the clinical condition. For example, diabetic care could include episodes for any of the following problems:

◆ ketoacidosis
◆ hypoglycemia
◆ treatment of a foot ulcer
◆ evaluation of microalbuminuria

The diagnostic and treatment procedures related to each episode could be considered together as the episode of care. Performance measures can be fashioned that reflect the quality of care for each episode, e.g., inpatient days for ketoacidosis or amputation rates for foot ulcers. In order to best allocate resources, many organizations will focus on a particular episode of care for intervention, rather than try to deal with the entire disease process. With appropriate analytical capabilities, the organization can define performance measures of interest and then analyze its database to target those episodes of care that have the worst outcomes. To achieve this level of care management, however, the organization must have a clear operational definition of each episode of care within the disease process, as well as the analytic capability to uncover aberrant patterns of care or outcomes.

Defining episodes of care for a complex disease entity can sometimes be a difficult task, but the rewards are substantial (Friedman, et al., 1998; Westerhof, 1998). Some definitions relate the episode to a hospital admission; others will include all prehospital and posthospital care (Lamberts &

Hofmans-Okkes, 1996; Nyman, et al., 1998). Because no standardized method of defining episodes of care has yet been established, each organization using the concept can effectively determine what constitutes an episode for each disorder. The definition of an episode is important, however, because it may tread on traditional patterns of care. For example, if a patient with diabetic ketoacidosis is to be referred to an endocrinologist in the care management schema, then the onset and conclusion of the episode must be accurately defined so that appropriate resources are available for the patient.

Because outcome measures are often used to assess the success of a care management program, the definition of these measures is important to the team and to management. Everyone with an interest in the outcomes of the program should be involved in determining what measures will be used for the assessment, and physician input will be necessary because of the clinical implications of the definitions of the outcome measure and the episode of care.

◆ Financial Analysis of Care Management Programs

All care management programs start with a budget. Unfortunately, most budgets are incomplete because they fail to include a number of costs or to adequately consider the potential benefits. Financial analysis has long been the purview of accountants and bookkeepers, but with contemporary computer tools, budgeting can be performed by care management teams as well.

Financially, care management programs can be broken down into costs and revenues, just as any other process in the organization. Appropriate assessment and allocation of costs become key in determining the true value of the care management program in the organization. The organizing financial relationship for the care management process can be characterized by the following equality

(10.1) cost of program = cost of program development + cost of interventions + administrative costs − savings on services − savings from decreased complications

The assumptions implicit in this relationship should be evident. The cost of the program will be calculated in dollars because all of the terms in the equality are dollar amounts. Factors such as customer and provider satisfaction, opportunity costs for choosing one clinical condition instead of another, and the increased costs for caring for individuals who live longer and develop other clinical problems are not included in the equation but can be significant. The care management team should particularly address the customer and provider satisfaction issues before committing resources to a project because a large-scale revolt among providers may not be worth the financial gains from even the most effective care management program.

Determining Direct and Indirect Costs

Table 10.7 lists costs associated with development of the program separated by stage of development. Development costs consist of the direct and indirect expenses of creating the care management program. As noted in the table, these costs include staff time for creating the framework for the program as well as time devoted to research and development of the CPG that serves as the foundation of the project. In addition to staff time, some organizations will compensate outside providers for assisting with guideline development, which frequently can mean meetings that include meals or overnight stays. Many organizations have separate staff members who perform the more sophisticated data collection and analysis functions, so the costs incurred by these staff members in creating data collection forms, database systems, and data analysis programs must be included in the development costs. Other personnel who may be involved in the project planning stage include financial,

Table 10.7 Costs Associated with Care Management Program

COST COMPONENT	DESCRIPTION
Development	✓ Staff time for meetings, research, and program creation
	✓ Data analysis, database development, and results reporting
	✓ Staff time for creation of CPG
	✓ Expert panel costs for creation of CPG
	✓ Staff costs for development and validation of performance measures
	✓ Financial analysis of program and interventions
Intervention	✓ Incentives for patients and providers to use program
	✓ Design, printing, and distribution of educational materials
	✓ Staff costs for case management
	✓ Telephone and communications (e.g., Internet site)
	✓ Equipment and instrumentation for improved clinical interventions
	✓ Costs for more sophisticated services
	✓ Data collection and analysis
	✓ Results reporting
	✓ Direct medical costs: hospital, physician, ancillary services
	✓ Drug costs
Administrative	✓ Clerical support
	✓ Information services support
	✓ Management time commitment
	✓ Overhead costs (utilities, rent, etc.)

marketing, and upper management staff. The costs for their time should be added to those for the staff directly involved in creating the program.

During the intervention stage, many of the same staff members will most likely still be working on the project. Additional staff will include people in the organization who produce the educational materials for distribution to providers and patients. Materials and printing costs, as well as the cost for any special media such as videotape or an Internet presentation, must be added to this cost category. As the program is put into place, professional personnel such as case managers and data collection staff will become important in making the project operational. Any special facilities or materials that they require, such as computer systems, telephone management devices, or printed protocols, will produce costs at this stage. If the CPG recommends a specific intervention that has not been used in the past, then the cost of that intervention will be incurred as the project proceeds. In some cases, the care management team can negotiate favorable rates for these new interventions, and after a few cycles of program operations, the actual costs can be incorporated into the calculations. With the use of development and intervention team estimates of the impact of each important element of the program (as in Table 10A in the Appendix), a cost–benefit matrix can sometimes help quantify the effects of the program on important cost parameters. The team evaluates each of the key interventions in terms of the expected effect on the most important outcome parameters, placing estimates of the percentage of change in each of the outcomes. These estimated percentages can then be used to approximate incremental costs resulting from the intervention. This work is useful for developing pro forma cost estimates and targets.

Returning to Table 10.7, the administrative costs for the program should also be considered in making the final cost determination. Many organizations will assess an overhead cost allocation per employee, but if this is not done, then actual cost estimates should be made to ensure that all costs are included. If a cost allocation system is used, then the team should carefully determine the precise number of people necessary for the project so that the cost allocation is correct.

The economic benefits from the program can attenuate the costs and, as shown in Table 10.8, the care management team can estimate these benefits. For example, an intervention may help patients care for themselves at home rather than make a visit to the provider's office (*intervention 3*, Table 10.8). Although the cost of care may be increased by the intervention, the benefit in reduced provider visits can be of value in situations where the provider is capitated—paid a fixed amount for caring for the patient regardless of the utilization of services by the patient. Savings will also be realized from a decreased complication rate, and the estimates of cost savings for complications can be especially effective if the team has data on the episodes of care costs for the adverse outcomes.

Traditional data analyses for these cost determinations involve evaluating diagnosis and procedure codes in a claims database, leading to aggre-

Table 10.8 Cost Benefit Matrix for Care Management Program

INTERVENTION	COST OF CARE	PATIENT VISITS	COMPLICATIONS	MORTALITY
1	+2%	+3%	−1%	0%
2	−3%	+2%	−3%	−1%
3	+8%	−4%	−1%	−3%
4	−1%	+1%	0%	0%
5	−4%	0%	+1%	0%
Total	+2%	+2%	−4%	−4%

gated costs by procedure. Unfortunately, these evaluations miss important information about the population with the disease or risk factor. Aggregating data by patient provides much more information about the characteristics of a disease entity and its management. For example, determining the cost of performing quantitative urinalyses for microalbuminuria in a health plan's membership will include diabetics and nondiabetics, and the information will not provide any information about the severity of kidney disease in the population. However, analyzing the same database by first sorting the data by disease codes and then aggregating procedural information by patients with the disease will provide a per-member cost of care, as well as a host of other information about the population of patients with the disorder. The team will nearly always gain substantial insight by grouping individuals within the population by any number of variables, e.g., cost of care, provider, numbers of procedures, types of procedures, diagnostic subcategories, and stage of disease.

Each of these categories provides a different view of the population that can contribute to the development and implementation of the care management program. As the team is evaluating interventions, characteristics of these categories will be instrumental in determining which interventions are most likely to succeed. As mentioned previously, populations of individuals with a clinical condition are often stratified for purposes of determining optimum interventions, and these categories exemplify a few useful ways of analyzing the data.

Although cost of care is frequently used as a surrogate for severity of a disease, it may only indicate inefficient practice patterns and thus requires further analysis. Providers who perform inappropriate tests or procedures can drive up the cost of care, making relatively unaffected patients seem more ill than their diagnosis would indicate. On the other hand, diagnosis coding is often inaccurate, so the severity of a group of patients within the population must often be evaluated using several different approaches. For diseases affecting relatively few individuals or with scoring systems for stage of disease, such as certain types of cancer, patients may be identified through individual chart reviews or physician reports. However, for large populations of patients, e.g., those with diabetes in a managed care plan, statistical analysis may be the only approach available to segment such a large group.

Other means of analyzing groups besides just cost can be gleaned from administrative data, such as provider analysis and diagnosis code subcategorization. Stratifying the population by provider will often reveal the presence of untoward practice patterns that can be the target of the team's interventions. Additionally the data from these analyses can enable the team to assess different practice patterns for efficacy. Using data from these analyses, the team can work with provider panels to review and possibly revise CPGs to reflect the most effective practice patterns. Diagnosis codes in claims systems conform to the International Classification of Diseases (ICD) coding system established by the US Department of Health and Human Services. These codes attempt to capture the breadth of diagnoses in modern medicine but often fall short because of lack of specificity. Revisions of the coding system are being developed, with the aim of improving the descriptive power of the system; however, the data that reach most insurance claims databases fail to attain a level of specificity that permits meaningful analysis of most disease states. Using ICD codes, however, can provide a rough cut of the administrative data and allow the care management team to begin the planning process. Additionally, ICD codes can detect patients with comorbid (coexisting) conditions that may place them in different risk categories or make them ineligible for the care management approach.

Risk Assessment

The concept of risk has a significant influence on the analysis of a care management program. Financial risk, to be discussed later in the chapter, is only one of several types of risk that care management programs incur. Other risks include

◆ medicolegal
◆ provider satisfaction
◆ customer satisfaction
◆ medical
◆ measurement

All of these risks threaten the viability of the organization, and quantifying the degree of risk within each category can be an important exercise to ensure the success of the program.

Medicolegal risk will be discussed in more depth in Chapter 11, "Legal and Regulatory Issues in Quality Improvement." The primary source of malpractice risk in care management programs stems from the increasing incursion into the physician–patient relationship by a number of organizations, primarily managed care organizations at the present time. Case law and legislative efforts alike are increasing the risk of medical malpractice for organizations that interpret medical findings and recommend medical therapies or even suggest what services may not be covered by an insurance plan. For many years, HMOs have promoted their ability to improve the quality of patient care, and when the decisions that are made by health plan medical directors do not serve the goal of QI, consumers will react by initiating lawsuits or prodding legislators to pass new laws. Recent lawsuits and legislative efforts point to greater liability for organizations performing any services that appear to have implications for medical care (Smith, 1999; Swanson, 1999; Thomas & Budetti, 1998). Because care management programs intervene in patient care, the potential for medical malpractice liability cannot be ignored.

Maintaining provider and consumer satisfaction can be particularly difficult for care management teams. As these projects are implemented, providers can feel an imposition on their time, and one of the goals of the care management team must be to optimize practitioners' time commitment to the program. Providers are being beset on all sides by organizations that want to implement these types of programs, so any efforts to coordinate these projects between care management organizations would likely be very well accepted by providers and patients alike.

Consumers also have conflicting messages at times. If the care management program appears to contradict the advice of the provider, then both consumer and provider will be confused and displeased. The care management team must have some feeling for the providers' conundrum, and involving the provider community through the development of the program should allow practitioners to keep the workload for their colleagues at a reasonable level. Similarly, keeping the consumers of these programs informed about the expectations of the program and emphasizing the cooperative relationship with providers should assuage their concerns.

The rate of the target disease in a population also adds risk to the care management venture. The budget for nearly any care management program will include a factor that adjusts for underestimates in the rate or severity of the disease, but even this estimate may be too low. Additionally, if a managed care organization conducts the program, then the addition of a new customer to the plan can change the configuration of the care management program if the new cohort of members has a disproportionate level of the disease. Care management programs that are structured to assume some financial risk for the care of patients in the disease category must be certain that payments are sufficiently structured to account for this risk. Thorough study of the current and historic rates of the disease, in addition to the costs incurred for affected patients in the intended population, as suggested previously, are of utmost importance in tempering this type of risk.

Another type of medical risk is related to the treatment regimen that a care management program may recommend. Nearly any medical regimen is accompanied by adverse reactions as well as health benefits, and those complications can add to the cost of the program. The medical literature often will provide information about expected rates of complications, but these rates may not be very precise because the studies have been conducted in specific cohorts of patients under controlled conditions. When treatment modalities are released for use in the general population, the rates may vary from the controlled studies, and a certain amount of variation should be expected. To account for this variation, the team should reevaluate complication rates during the project; this information will provide updates on costs as well as indicators for measuring quality of care.

Finally, the risk of measurement error is inherent in the care management process. Measurement error can occur in a number of ways:

◆ selection of the wrong performance measures
◆ inadequate data collection
◆ improper data collection
◆ incorrect data collection
◆ incorrect data analysis
◆ incorrect data reporting

All of these potential data collection and analysis errors can contribute to erroneous decisions, thus increasing costs, morbidity, or even mortality. The most important method of reducing these errors is to have well-trained and motivated staff involved in the entire process of care management program development and implementation using the principles of data collection and analysis that are discussed elsewhere in this text.

Approach to Data Analysis

The process of data analysis to determine the financial impact of a program requires access to cost and pricing data for care and normally must include data from one or more third-party payers. National data sets are available, as presented in Appendix 10A, but designing a local program using cost data from national sources can be fraught with difficulty and error. National data sets can be expected to have more coding variation due to the size and scope of the databases, and national databases will often not reflect local practice patterns. Thus, if population-specific data can be obtained for the analysis, the precision of the evaluation will be greatly improved.

The basic steps in data analysis using an administrative database include

1. Definition of patient selection criteria. These parameters are typically defined in the CPG to include patients in the care management program.
2. Determination of patient stratification criteria. These conditions create the subgroups for use in analyzing the data: The first sort of the data would be by patient identifier, grouping all of an individual's di-

agnoses, procedures, and costs for a given time period into a patient-specific record. These records are then sorted by other criteria selected by the team, including episodes of care, procedure types, diagnosis code or subcode, disease stage or severity, total cost of care for the period, or demographic characteristics like age and gender.

3. Validation of the selection criteria by other sources, such as provider advisory panels, consultants, actuaries, etc. Episodes of care should be organized logically into discrete summaries of specific instances of diagnosis or treatment for a disease entity, and the episode should make sense clinically, as well as administratively. Thus, providers with expertise in the disease entity should be involved in defining an episode of care. Actuaries are of particular help in evaluating demographic stratification issues.

4. Evaluation of the proportion of the population and cost by each stratum. Data processing systems should be able to provide this information very easily.

5. Determination of the growth of each stratum over time to allow projection of costs into the future. This analysis must use data from several time periods to establish a trend for each stratum.

6. Identification of coexisting clinical conditions that add to the total cost of care or confound the analysis of episodes of care by adding procedures and costs. As much as possible, these comorbidities should be screened from the data, unless they represent conditions closely associated with the disease. For example, coexistence of congestive heart failure and arthritis is less clinically significant than congestive heart failure and hypertension. Again, provider input is invaluable for determining which comorbidities are significant and which should be excluded.

Episodes of care include periods during which a particular drug is administered or certain types of therapy are provided, such as a course of chemotherapy or radiation therapy. Cost data for each episode will include expenditures for all of the resources and transactions that occur within that segment of the patient's care. Transactions include any encounters with the health care delivery system, e.g., inpatient care, outpatient care, emergency department care, or home health care.

Using this information, the costs for caring for a population of patients with a clinical condition can be estimated in a number of ways, but one of the most useful methods adopted by the health insurance industry involves calculating costs per member per month (PMPM). The equation used to determine PMPM cost is as follows:

(10.2) PMPM cost = C ÷ M
        where C is the total cost of services for the population, and
        M is member months.

Member months is the product of the number of individuals in the population and the number of months that the study was performed. For example, if there are 1000 individuals in a study for 12 months, then the number of member months is 12,000. Note that another statistic, per member per year (PMPY), could also be used, and for this example the PMPY value would be 1000. Using this approach, the cost of care can be put into categories based on PMPM or PMPY amounts.

Table 10.9 illustrates an example of the use of a distribution of costs by PMPY for diabetes. The data in the table provide some direction to the team regarding target groups for intervention. Although more information is necessary, *group VI* presents a tremendous opportunity for intervention because 6.5% of the population generates 36% of total costs of care. High-cost groups such as *group VI* often undergo case management as a means of trying to contain costs and improve the quality of care. On the other hand, *groups IV* and *V* usually have other types of interventions such as educational programs for patients or providers to improve patterns of care and utilization of services. Data like those in Table 10.9 provide a way for the team to determine which patient groups to target.

Activity-Based Costing

Modeling the costs in a care management project can take a number of forms, based on the costing model used by the institution. A model that is gaining increasing applicability in QI, activity based-costing (ABC), helps evaluate costs to determine if they add value for the consumer (Cokins, 1999). ABC is best applied in organizations with multiple diverse product or service lines because allocating aggregate costs to specific service lines often proves difficult. The ABC approach differs from traditional cost analysis by identifying the specific activities that are required to produce each product or service.

Table 10.9 PMPY Cost Distribution for Diabetes

GROUP	PMPY COST (IN $)	PERCENTAGE OF POPULATION	NUMBER OF INDIVIDUALS	EXPECTED COST (IN $)	PERCENTAGE OF TOTAL COST
I	0	0.3	3	0	0.00
II	0–150	0.8	8	600	0.04
III	151–350	3.5	35	8750	0.64
IV	351–1000	78.0	780	526,500	38.99
V	1001–5000	10.9	109	327,000	24.21
VI	5000–10,000	6.5	65	487,500	36.10
	Totals	100	1000	$1,350,350	

PMPY, per member per year.

These activities come from a variety of sources: administrative support, overhead, professional staff, maintenance staff, information services, and many more. The contribution from each source is analyzed for each product or service and then actual costs are assigned by the relative contribution of each resource. Through this assignment of resources, the care management team can better determine the true costs of the interventions in the program. A simple ABC costing exercise can be found in Table 10.10. Three resources are used to produce the service: *resources M, N,* and *P.* The resources are defined in units, which could be units of time, numbers of components, or any other resource measure. The number of units of each resource used in the service is then tracked and a proportion of the total number of units available for use is calculated and used as a weighting factor for calculating the actual cost of the resource used in production. From these activity-based costs, a total cost of the service can be discerned.

Substantially more information can be obtained from the table, however. Efforts to control costs are often directed at the component that is used in highest volume in the production design rather than cost drivers. ABC provides the information to determine which of the resources actually drives the cost of the service. In Table 10.10, the amount of *resource N* used in the service is relatively small, but the cost impact is relatively large because of the unit cost of the resource. On the other hand, *resource P* appears to be an essential component of the service, but because of its unit cost, the overall contribution to the cost of the service is somewhat lower. Although both of these resources would be considered cost drivers, *resource N* would be a better target for intervention because changes in the use of each unit of *resource N* would cause relatively greater changes in cost. However, if *resource N* cannot be changed easily or if changes will take a long time to implement, then the next most likely candidate for intervention would probably be *resource P* because of its contribution to total costs.

The trend of each cost driver is important as well. As with any QI parameter, costs must be tracked over time to discern the trend of the measure. Returning to Table 10.10, if *resource N,* the highest cost resource, were actually

Table 10.10 Activity-Based Costing Example

RESOURCE	UNITS FOR PRODUCING SERVICE	TOTAL UNITS AVAILABLE	PROPORTION OF UNITS USED	TOTAL COST OF RESOURCE (IN $)	TOTAL UNIT COST OF RESOURCE (IN $)
M	38	1390	0.027	1,039,423	28,415.88
N	67	3493	0.019	10,145,932	194,611.25
P	653	2456	0.266	543,324	144,458.70
Total					$367,485.83

showing a decline of 15% per year but *resource P* was growing at 20% per year, the latter would present a better target for intervention. A simple example will help clarify this principle. Suppose that caring for a particular clinical condition required three imaging modalities: planar x-rays, CT scan, and PET scan, represented by *M, N,* and *P* in Table 10.10. The growth in costs for the three entities is presented graphically in Figure 10.5. The total unit cost of CT scans is clearly greater than that of the other two, but the cost of PET scanning is growing rapidly as it is applied, sometimes inappropriately, to the care of the clinical condition. In spite of the fact that the total cost for CT scans is greater than that for PET scans, the care management team would most likely target PET scanning for intervention.

ABC systems can be somewhat complex, but they provide substantially more information than do traditional models. The ability to identify cost drivers becomes increasingly important as care management systems become more widely used. Targeting costs intelligently can help the team achieve large savings and increase the returns from the program, enhancing the value of the care management system to the organization.

Financing Care Management Programs by Risk Sharing

A number of approaches to care management have arisen in the health care industry. Managed care organizations often have care management programs

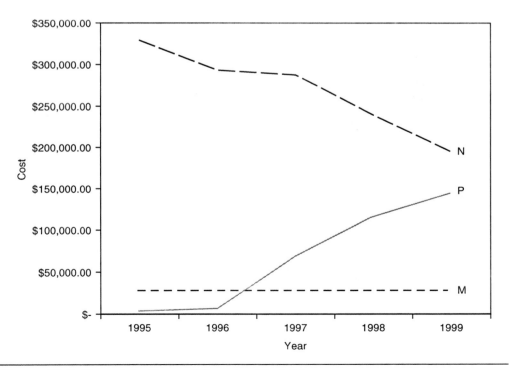

Figure 10.5 Growth in Costs of Scanning Modalities

that they manage internally, but provider organizations such as hospitals, physician organizations, and integrated delivery systems have also begun to integrate care management programs into their operations. Finally, commercial vendors have also established care management programs, often specializing in one disease or in the clinical conditions associated with a single organ system. These organizations often assume some of the financial risk associated with their care management programs, accepting capitation payments for carve-out services, i.e., services for a specific segment of the population at risk. For example, a diabetes disease management vendor would enter into a contract to provide services for all of the diabetics in the membership of a managed care organization, thus "carving out" those patients from the population of a managed care organization.

The types of payment systems vary greatly. Capitation contracts are by far the most popular because they cap the costs to the managed care organization and transfer virtually all of the financial risk for patients in the care management program to the vendor. These contracts usually entail a fixed contract price paid to the care management vendor to provide services for all of a payer's patients with a given clinical condition for a specific period of time. These payments do not vary with the number of patients, so the vendor assumes the entire financial risk for patients with a disease. Payers, of course, prefer these arrangements, because they have capped their costs for a particular disease, but the risk taken by the vendor can be immense. Pricing is critical in these contracts, because the risk to the vendor is very high and cannot be spread across a large population as is done in an insurance company.

A number of variations have also appeared to share the risk between the payer and the vendor. Contact capitation, in which a fixed payment is made when the patient is actually referred to the care management vendor, creates a system of reimbursement that removes the risk for the vendor of large numbers of patients being referred within a fixed reimbursement contract. The risk that the vendor bears in contract capitation relates to patient management, not numbers of patients. The payer assumes the financial risk if larger than projected numbers of patients present with the disease.

Other risk-sharing arrangements have been adapted from the managed care industry, e.g., withholds, risk pools, risk corridors, and stop loss agreements. Risk sharing by withhold arrangements involves placing a certain percentage of a capitation payment into a special account called a risk pool. The risk pool is maintained until a specified time when the total costs of the program are determined and the risk pool funds are used to pay any shortfalls in costs. Any excess in the risk pool is then distributed in some proportion to the payer and the vendor, according to the care management contract. An example of this type of arrangement is found in Example 10-1.

Example 10-1

The XYZ Care Management Company has entered into an arrangement with the MONEYHMO managed care organization to assume financial responsibility for all of MONEYHMO's asthmatic members, using XYZ's proven asthma care management program. The two organizations have entered into an agreement in which XYZ will be paid a total of $1,000,000 for this care, with a risk pool of $200,000 maintained by MONEYHMO for settlement of the account at the end of the year. If the cost of care exceeds one million dollars during the year, then the excess costs will be paid from the risk pool. If the cost of care exceeds both the contract payment and the amount in the risk pool, then XYZ assumes responsibility for any excess over the $1,200,000. On the other hand, if there is an excess in the risk pool after all expenses are paid, then 60% of the remainder is distributed to XYZ and 40% to MONEYHMO.

Withhold arrangements can be made for any type of payment system: capitation, contact capitation, or even fee for service. In the latter two types of payment systems, however, the amount in the risk pool varies by the payments made to the vendor.

A variation of the withhold arrangement that sometimes can provide more precision in the distribution of risk entails dividing the risk pool into several sections, depending on the type of service rendered. These agreements are particularly helpful when the vendor has different levels of control over various services, as in Example 10-2.

Example 10-2

CMI Care Management provides services for outpatient management of asthma and inpatient professional (physician) services. The company does not pay hospitals and has no arrangements for hospital services, so health care organizations that enter into contracts with CMI must arrange separately for hospital inpatient services. CMI has entered into an agreement with MONEYHMO for asthma care management, with shared risk for outpatient services according to a contact capitation arrangement with a 20% withhold. The risk pool for outpatient services will be split 70:30, CMI:MONEYHMO, at the end of each year. Because CMI is also liable for inpatient professional services, the contract contains a provision for another risk pool that has a 10% withhold and a 60:40 distribution of risk pool surplus annually. Finally, because CMI should have a distinct effect on hospital inpatient service costs, they negotiated an agreement for a third risk pool, consisting of 20% of MONEYHMO's average annual cost of inpatient services for asthma patients over the past 4 years. If MONEYHMO's costs for inpatient asthma care are reduced by 20% during the contract year, then CMI will receive half of the 20% risk pool; for each percentage point over the 20% reduction, CMI receives another 0.75% of the risk pool funds up to the limit of the risk pool.

Capitation contracts and withholds have become increasingly complex over the past several years, primarily because the risk–return relationships in health care are evolving to meet increasing demand for services with decreasing reimbursement.

An interesting concept that has gained increasing acceptance over the past few years is that of risk corridors (eHealth, 1999). Simply another method of sharing risk, the risk corridor establishes a target value for PMPM or PMPY costs and then sets the level of risk at plus or minus a percentage. The risk corridor is especially useful in fee-for-service systems but can be applied to capitated systems as well. Example 10-3 describes a typical risk corridor scenario.

Example 10-3

CHF, Inc. is a care management company that contracts with managed care organizations to manage patients with congestive heart failure. CHF pays all costs for the care of these patients and, in turn, receives a capitation payment of $6.00 PMPM with a 10% risk corridor. According to the contracts that CHF negotiates with managed care organizations, CHF assumes responsibility for costs as high as $6.60 PMPM but keeps any savings up to $0.60 PMPM below the $6.00 capitation payment. If medical expenses are below $5.40 PMPM, then CHF shares half of any additional savings with the managed care organization.

Risk corridor arrangements can be more complicated, with the addition of a withhold to cap upside and downside risk.

The final method of sharing risk is through stop loss insurance, which limits the care manager's liability, depending on the level of expenditures for either an individual patient (individual stop loss) or the population of patients in the care manager's contract (aggregate stop loss). The stop loss agreement can entail a charge PMPM with the payer assuming all liability if a patient's care exceeds a specified amount or if the aggregate loss for a cohort of patients exceeds a target. These arrangements can be made between a payer and a care manager, or the care manager can purchase stop loss insurance from any of a number of reinsurance vendors. Common stop loss agreements set limits of $50,000 per individual patient or a percentage of the expected claims amount per month. Example 10-4 illustrates approaches to stop loss insurance.

Example 10-4

DM, Inc., a care management company specializing in diabetes mellitus, was evaluating approaches to the problem of capping its financial risk. There were several options available, and they were performing an analysis of each. First, they could purchase stop loss insurance from BIGINSURER, Inc., a multinational reinsurance seller, that would start paying for an individual patient's care after costs exceeded $100,000 during any given year. Additionally, BIG-INSURER had another product, called an aggregate stop loss policy, that would pay any overages in expenses incurred during a quarter that exceeded 120% of the expected quarterly capitation payments. DM had spoken with its larger customers, who were amenable to the concept of reducing the capitation payment by 2% to assume self-insurance risk for any patient who exceeded $100,000 per year, i.e., an individual stop loss agreement. The customers, however, were unwilling to enter into an aggregate stop loss arrangement with DM.

A thorough financial analysis can be performed to determine which of these options would provide the greatest protection at the least cost, but the analysis will hinge on accurate assessments of probabilities of catastrophic cases within a patient population.

Attenuating Financial Risk

The financial risks of care management can lead to substantial rewards if the program is effective. Unfortunately, many care management projects take time to mature and proceed down the learning curve, and during that time, financial losses can be sizable. Risk sharing can ameliorate those potential losses, but other approaches may also be of value, such as

◆ exclusion of outliers
◆ adjustments for severity
◆ utilization caps
◆ membership caps
◆ gradual program implementation

Each of these approaches has specific advantages and can be applied to either an internal program or a contract with an external vendor.

Any care management program should carefully define the patient population to which it applies. The CPG serves that purpose, and most CPGs will include a section that defines patient characteristics in clinical terms or by ICD codes to ensure that only patients who could benefit from the program are included. Even with stringent selection criteria, some individuals who qualify for the program become extremely ill and exceed the resources of the program. For example, a hemophiliac who develops high levels of Factor VIII inhibitors and requires huge daily Factor transfusions and immunosuppressant therapy could rapidly deplete the resources of a hemophilia care management program. The program could purchase individual stop loss insurance to protect against this contingency, or it could specify in the contract that any patient in the program exceeding more than a certain level of costs per year would be excluded from the program. The contract may specify an amount or perhaps a certain percentage above the PMPM or PMPY costs as the level at which the patient would be excluded. Although these types of contracts may provide some security for a care management vendor, they are not particularly popular with payers because the payer will be left trying to find insurance for an essentially uninsurable individual. Thus, a care management company may find that a reinsurance policy is more economical and competitive in the current marketplace. If the care management program is conducted internally, however, high-risk patients will most likely remain in the care management program and simply move to a more intensive management level, unless the individual somehow develops conditions that are not within the purview of the program.

Any care management will apply patient interventions based on severity of the clinical condition. Just as a plan for outliers can be implemented, so too can a differential payment system determined by the severity of the patient's illness. For both internal and external care management teams, the cost of caring for a population of individuals with a clinical condition will depend heavily on the degree to which the individuals are affected by the disease. Stratification of patient groups can be performed using severity of illness indicators, with differential capitation or cost allocation rates assigned to each level of severity. For example, patients with breast cancer can be stratified with the stage of disease serving as a surrogate for severity, and progressively larger capitation rates or cost allocation amounts can be assigned based on the stage of the disease. If patients change from one level to another, then the reimbursement rate may change as well. Although the incentive to improve a patient's health may seem compromised by this approach, it also provides some degree of protection for the care management vendor and, if implemented properly, cost savings for the payer.

Another way of limiting financial risk for a vendor involves setting limits on the utilization of services by the patient population. If those limits are exceeded, then the capitation payment would increase. Although this approach is favorable to the vendor, payers tend to avoid such arrangements because they dampen the incentive of the care manager to decrease utilization of services. In a few cases, however, the utilization of a new service or product may be difficult to predict at the time that a contract is executed, making a utilization threshold provision more equitable for the vendor. For internal care management teams, adjustments in the budget and savings calculations should be made to ensure a fair analysis of the program.

Nearly any care management program will be constrained by a budget, particularly those that are managed internally. Most organizations will allocate resources annually, assuming a certain level of services, and when the volume of services exceeds that level, no contingency plans are available to deal with the budgetary impact. A care management program will usually be staffed by the organization to care for a specific number of individuals with specified degrees of a clinical condition. If the number of patients referred to the program surpasses those estimates, then the program will be over-whelmed and lose effectiveness. Thus, the program's financial planning must provide for adequate staffing should demand outstrip allocated resources. For external vendors, the best protection against this type of risk is to place a limit in the contract on the maximum number of clients that will be served during the contract period.

Finally, to prevent financial losses in the early phases of the project when staff members are still learning how to implement an effective care management program, a gradual implementation plan can provide a cushion of time to move down the learning curve. Although many programs must be rapidly deployed, if the team is less experienced at the mechanics of care management, then a phase-in period can prove highly cost effective. Some organizations will perform a pilot program to work out any problems before opening the system to the entire population of eligible patients.

◆ Provider Involvement in Care Management

Unfortunately, some care management programs tend to view providers as part of an "evil empire." The earlier section, "Barriers to Implementation," touched on some of the provider behaviors that result from this attitude, and the point has been made repeatedly that providers are key to making a care management program successful. A number of reporting techniques can enhance providers' understanding of the program and their relationship to the care management team.

Physicians are trained in patient care, not population health. Thus, one of the first tasks of a care management project is to help providers understand the need for a population health approach and how that approach can enhance the care of individual patients. Most physicians see care management programs as imposing on their time or on their office staff because they rarely see any kind of output demonstrating the effectiveness of the program. Care management projects collect an enormous amount of data, produce sophisticated analyses, and base decisions on this information; providers should see similar data so that they can understand the approaches taken by the care management team. One way of achieving this objective is through the use of provider profiling. Although some of these reports are labeled report cards, that term has been perceived as too pejorative by providers, leading to an accepted terminology of "profiles." These reports are designed to give providers a thumbnail sketch of their performance relative to their peers on a particular set of measures that are germane to their specialty. For example, a pediatrician may receive a profile with such parameters as

- ◆ immunization rates
- ◆ well-child visit rates
- ◆ parent satisfaction scores
- ◆ antibiotic utilization rates
- ◆ inpatient admission rates for asthma patients

Often these rates are reported as *Z*-scores (see Chapter 7) or percentiles relative to their peers and reported graphically. Any comparisons in profiles should always be among providers within a specialty or subspecialty. An example of a graphic provider profile can be found in Figure 10.6. This portion of the profile usually captures the provider's attention, but most physicians will also want to know about the source of the data and the method of analysis. Thus, most profiles will also contain a short description that includes this information.

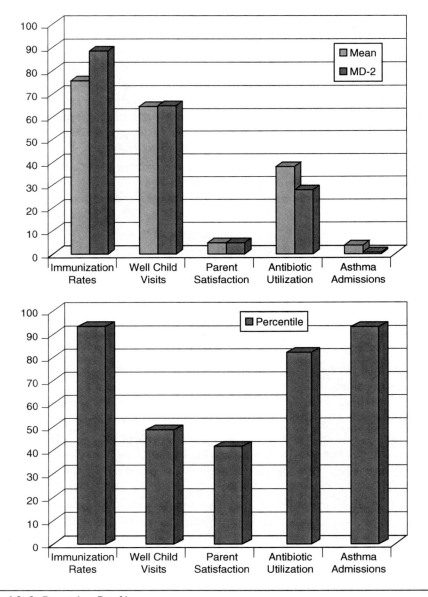

Figure 10.6 Provider Profile

Obvious problems can occur with provider profiles. If the data sources are inaccurate or the comparison base includes physicians who are substantially different in some way, then providers will quickly discount the profiles and ignore the program. When profiles leave the care management office, they must be accurate. Some providers may respond best to a personal introduction of the profile, allowing for questions and discussion of the expectations of the care management team for the provider's performance on the profile measures. A medical director or well-respected care management staff member may personally deliver the profile to these physicians to help improve acceptance of the concept. In most cases, providers will understand the profiles and accompanying explanation, but some will need the extra effort of the human touch.

Some physicians may actually use the profiles to justify complacency, especially if the profiles indicate that they are performing well. Profiles include only a few measures, so providers may be performing well in these few areas but poorly otherwise. Providers may use the profile as justification to resist other QI programs or cost containment initiatives. Practitioners who have relatively low scores on the profile measures often explain the discrepancy by asserting that their patients are different somehow. The team must be ready with data that demonstrate that the patients used in the profile have similar characteristics across all providers.

Any quality management effort made by an organization that involves clinical improvement must include providers. Teams of providers, composed of representatives of every provider group that might be affected by the new process of care, should be convened to help design and implement any QI project, especially one that deals with their areas of expertise, such as a care management program. Any program that does not consider this important input will find success difficult, if not impossible, to achieve.

◆ Partnerships Within the Industry

The health care industry is replete with opportunities for partnerships in care management programs. Nearly every segment of the industry is working feverishly on one or more components of these innovative approaches to health care delivery, and perhaps the greatest possibility of failure exists in the disjointed implementation of program fragments by various stakeholders in the delivery system. Managed care organizations, focused on cost and financial results with a 1-year time horizon, will target their high-priced procedures, without proper regard for long-term ramifications of their interventions. Physician groups will implement programs that optimize patient comfort and provider convenience but ignore the cost of care. Hospitals will find ways to cut costs and optimize their financial return, disregarding the effects on physicians and payers. Pharmaceutical companies will direct programs that increase the use of their products, whether appropriate or not. This jaded view of the health care delivery system is only partially correct, but it is widely held by payers and government officials. During the industrialization of the health care delivery system, discussed in Chapter 1, each segment of the system has worked hard to maintain its position, with devastating effects on the continuity of care. The time has come for the health care delivery system to move to the next stage of development, i.e., integration of products and services into a cohesive whole.

Pharmaceutical companies have been at the forefront of care management since the early 1990s. Large pharmacy benefit management companies suddenly began to foist huge price discounts on pharmaceutical manufacturers to satisfy the need of managed care organizations to lower costs. In an effort to increase sales volume to compensate for the price reductions, the pharmaceutical industry, led by Pfizer, codified the concepts of disease management in 1993 (Boston Consulting Group, 1993). Using concepts from finance, QI, and accounting, the paradigm of disease management organized the care of clinical conditions in a manner that was different from the traditional medical approach. Rather than look at care of a disease or risk factor as a series of independent transactions, the disease management approach viewed these transactions as contact points along a broad continuum. Most important, the approach emphasized that actions in one area of management of a clinical condition had implications in other areas, in terms both of cost and of morbidity and mortality. No longer could multiple providers justify specialized interventions without regard for the long-term well-being of the patient, and the benefits of continuity of care by primary care providers were suddenly recognized by payers. Pharmaceutical manufacturers also had substantial clinical data regarding the use of, abuse of, and adverse reactions to drug therapy. Providers often received highly sanitized versions of the data through product inserts and marketing materials, but the pharmaceutical manufacturers were finally determined to turn this information into useful tools for managing patients across the continuum of care.

Physicians generally embraced the concept of disease management as long as it did not contradict traditional practice patterns. Much of the care provided in the United States has little foundation in science, either because the evidence does not exist or because physicians have not been informed of newer patterns of care. Medical practice tends to dominate a practitioner's life, leaving little time for continuing education. Educational programs have tended to be relatively inaccessible, requiring either travel away from home for several days at a time or exhaustive reading after a hard day's work. Some specialties have multiple journals, making the acquisition of new knowledge difficult and time consuming. Considering the massive volume of medical information being promulgated each year, the probability that a practitioner will be current with all the new literature in a specialty is very small. Newer modes of "just-in-time" education may help ameliorate the problem, but these new modalities are only now gaining acceptance. Physicians are expected to serve as the purveyors of health information in the system, but because information does not yet flow smoothly through the system, they cannot realize their potential. In spite of these shortcomings, however, practitioners bring a wealth of experience about what solutions might be viable in a QI system. As the only stakeholder in the system that makes contact with every other sector, physicians can serve as the linchpin for a more effective industry.

Hospitals and other institutions also bring a great deal to the process of care management. Dealing with the most serious manifestations of disease processes, hospitals have developed expertise in managing resources for critically ill people. Like any business, however, hospitals survive by having sufficient funds to provide services and grow. Through the vagaries of the reimbursement system, hospitals have become focused on the volume of services, rather than on continuously improving quality. Of course, accrediting agencies require QI efforts for certification, but only rarely will an institution actually inculcate the QI paradigm into its operations. In spite of these fiscal pressures, however, hospitals have exceptional skill in managing the very sick patient, as well as having amassed a huge amount of clinical information over the years. This information can be of vital importance to a care management program.

Payers take a number of forms, from government agencies to managed care organizations to self-funded employer programs. The many variations in methods of reimbursing providers have added significantly to the administrative costs of providers. Not only has this lack of uniformity led to increased costs, but it has also caused discrepancies in access to care because some providers will not see patients with certain types of insurance coverage. Although a few large payers have emerged to set some standards, the system remains fundamentally inequitable. Payers are particularly interested in care management programs as a means of cutting costs, primarily by reducing variation in the delivery of services, and many managed care organizations have initiated their own programs for important diseases like diabetes, asthma, heart disease, and cancer. The problem that these organizations will face relates to the fact that they maintain ownership of the care management programs. Providers, institutions, and consumers will continue to view these efforts as a means of reducing managed care organization costs, rather than making care of patients better, and most of these stakeholders will resist the managed care organizations' autonomous efforts.

Employers, who foot the majority of the bills for health care in the United States, also must be involved in care management programs. Most people visit their providers' offices only once or twice a year at most, but they are available at work every day. Employers are interested in maintaining a healthy workforce to improve productivity, and incorporating care management preventive interventions into the workday can have significant value for many companies. Additionally, many screening tests and procedures can be done at the work site, reducing time away from work and the attendant lost productivity. A care management program can prove highly useful in improving worker health and productivity, so employers have a natural stake in the process. Employers have another function, however. By expecting more from the health care delivery system and insurers, employers have changed the way that the system conducts business. These expectations must continually be raised. Continuous QI requires an ongoing effort to improve, and once goals are met, new ones must be set. Employers can provide the impetus for the health care delivery system to move forward.

Although consumers of health care are usually mentioned as stakeholders in the system, it is important to remember that they are the reason that the system exists in the first place. Over the past few decades, consumers have become more vocal about their needs and what they desire in a health care delivery system. In some cases, misleading information has led to unreasonable expectations, but for the most part consumers are reasonable. Care management programs benefit tremendously from consumer input. They bring pragmatism to the process by discerning how people with a clinical condition will respond emotionally to diagnostic and therapeutic interventions and the cost of care. Consumers can prove worthy partners in this process.

The fact that all of these stakeholders have unique contributions to make to a care management program suggests that partnerships between all sectors of the health care system will lead to a more successful end result. No one in the system will accept a program that appears to benefit another group at their expense, but all must compromise to help these efforts reach fruition. Partnerships can take a number of forms, but they must be all-inclusive, or some element of the system will feel disenfranchised and sabotage the programs. Through a productive partnership, incentives can be aligned for all parties, improving the probability that the care management process will succeed. Partnerships require more effort, and usually more time, but the work that goes into making a partnership work will be reflected in the long-term success of the care management process in the health care delivery system.

◆ Future of Care Management

In a very short period of time, care management has evolved from the concept of disease management, and further evolution is expected. In many ways, the future of care management will parallel the future of QI in health care. Society is intent on reducing the cost of health care in the United States, but the need to maintain access to quality care remains inviolate. Thus, although care management is presently being touted as a measure for cutting costs by reducing variation in the delivery of services, the effect of this approach on costs will plateau, as did concurrent review and other medical management techniques. The longer term effect of care management, however, will come from the integration of services within the health care delivery system and the opportunity for partnerships within the delivery system that will reduce inappropriate care, measure performance, and incorporate the principles and procedures of continuous QI into the health care delivery system. The need for information will move providers into automated data collection and storage systems that will make the industry more efficient and effective. The need for process and outcome measures will advance the science of performance measurement in health care. The need for accountability throughout the system will improve the industry's attention to these issues of importance to consumers. In short, the effect of care management comes not in the short-term cost improvements that will be realized through these efforts but rather through the reengineering of the health care industry that will be necessary to achieve these goals.

◆ Discussion Points

1. Define care management. What differentiates the care management process from traditional approaches to health care?
2. Describe the basic elements of a care management program. What steps should an organization take to design a program?
3. List some of the barriers to implementation that organizations face. Describe some approaches to overcoming each barrier.
4. What important principles must be observed in selecting and validating performance measures for a care management program? Describe data sources that may be used to track process and outcome measures in a care management program.
5. Why is financial analysis of the care management program important? Describe the basic elements of cost and savings in a program analysis.
6. What sources of direct and indirect costs do the following types of health care organizations have: (1) medical practice, (2) hospital, (3) managed care organization, (4) disease management company?
7. What risks are associated with care management? Describe one or two tactics to ameliorate each type of risk.
8. List the steps that an organization should take when analyzing an administrative database. How can organizations ensure that these steps are accomplished?
9. A medical practice wishes to determine the activity-based cost for a laboratory test that it performs. The test requires an average of 10 minutes of nursing time to collect and process the blood sample, 15 minutes of laboratory technician time to process the sample and generate a report, and 5 minutes of time on a machine that cost the practice $1000 and is amortized over five years. The physician time required for the test averages 15 minutes, including time for explaining the test to the patient, analyzing the results, recording the analysis in the patient chart, and then discussing the results with the patient. Calculate the activity-based cost of the test using the cost information in the following table

and the problem description. Assume that the overhead cost includes all other costs for the practice.

	RESOURCE COST PER YEAR	AVAILABLE HOURS/YEAR
Physician	$140,000	2000
Nurse	$32,000	2000
Lab technician	$28,000	2000
Overhead	$150,000	2000

10. Describe four methods of risk sharing in care management programs. How do each of these methods compare in terms of degree of risk sharing, potential problems for providers and payers, and consumer perception of the program?
11. Discuss three methods of attenuating financial risk in a care management program. What financial risks are of greatest significance in (1) a managed care organization, (2) a medical practice, and (3) a home health agency?
12. Describe the typical elements of a provider profile. How can providers misuse the profile?
13. Discuss how each of the following stakeholders can participate in a partnership for developing and implementing a care management program: (1) providers, (2) payers, (3) pharmaceutical companies, (4) hospitals, (5) consumers.
14. What factors will lead to the success of care management in the future? When the cost containment from care management is realized, what will keep the care management process viable?

◆ Notes

American Academy of Family Physicians. (1998). AAFP *performance measure criteria and implementation plan.* Retrieved May 1999, from *http://home.aafp.org/quality/pmcip.html*

Austin E. (1997). Profile—John E. Wennberg. *Advances: The Quarterly Newsletter of the Robert Wood Johnson Foundation, 3.* Retrieved May 1999, from *http://www.rwjf.org/library/97-3-16.htm*

Balestracci D., and Barlow J. (1996). *Quality improvement: Practical applications for medical group practice.* Englewood, CO: Center for Research in Ambulatory Health Care Administration.

Bernard S., and Frist W. H. (1998). The healthcare quality debate: The case for disease management. *Disease Management, 1*(2), 91–98.

Boland P. (Ed.) (1993). *Making managed healthcare work.* Gaithersburg, MD: Aspen.

Boult C., Dowd B., McCaffrey D., Boult L., Hernandez R., Krulewitch H. (1993). Screening elders for risk of hospital admission. *Journal of the American Geriatric Society, 41*(8), 811–817.

Brunelli A., Fianchini A., Gesuita R., Carle F. (1999). POSSUM scoring system as an instrument of audit in lung resection surgery: Physiological and operative severity score for the enumeration of mortality and morbidity. *Annals of Thoracic Surgery, 67*(2), 329–331.

Byrnes J. (1998a). An interview with Dr. John Lucas, president and chief executive officer, St. Francis Health System, Tulsa, Oklahoma. *Disease Management, 1*(2), 85–89.

Byrnes J. (1998b). Does disease management really work? The Lovelace health systems experience. *Disease Management, 1*(1), 39–53.

Chassin M. R., and Galvin R. W. (1998). The urgent need to improve health care quality: Institute of Medicine national roundtable on health care quality. *Journal of the American Medical Association, 230*(11), 1000–1005.

Cokins G. (1999). *If ABC is the question, what is the answer?* Retrieved May 1999, from *http://www.abctech.com/univ/abcanswer.htm*

Court J. (1998, December). HMO malpractice liability would deter care denials. *Between Rounds, 2*(5). Retrieved May 1999, from *http://www.betweenrounds.com/ volume2/issue5/erisa/court.htm*

De Vreugd W. (1997). The need for information-based practice in case management. *Nursing Case Management, 2*(5), 192–195.

Doody R. S., Strehlow S. L., Massman P. J., Feher E. P., Clark C., Roy J. R. (1999). Baylor profound mental status examination: A brief staging measure for profoundly demented Alzheimer disease patients. *Alzheimer Disease Association Disorders, 13*(1), 53–59.

Doxtator R. F., and Rodriguez D. J. (1998). Evaluating costs, benefits, and return on investment for disease management programs. *Disease Management, 1*(4).

Drea E. J. (1998). Evaluation of outcomes achieved through peptic ulcer disease state management. *American Journal of Managed Care, 4*(4), S272–S279.

eHealth. (1999). *Ten tips for negotiating managed care and capitation contracts.* Retrieved May 1999, from *http://www.medsource.com/providers/pro5.html*

Foundation for Accountability. (1999). *Measuring quality.* Retrieved September 2003, from *http://www.facct.org*

Friedman N., Gleeson J. M., Kent M. J., Foris M., Rodriguez D. J., Cypress M. (1998). Management of diabetes mellitus in the Lovelace health systems' Episodes of Care program. *Effective Clinical Practice, 1*(1), 5–11.

Goetzel R. Z., Anderson D. R., Whitmer R. W., Ozminkowski R. J., Dunn R. L., Wasserman J. (1998). The relationship between modifiable health risks and health care expenditures: An analysis of the multi-employer HERO health risk and cost database. *Journal of Occupational and Environmental Medicine, 40*(10), 843–854.

Gonzalez E. R. (1998). The pharmacoeconomic benefits of cholesterol reduction. *American Journal of Managed Care, 4*(2), 223–230.

Hornsby P. P., Reeve R. H., Gwaltney J. M. Jr, Parsons B. D., Morse R. M. (1997). The University of Virginia health promotion and disease prevention program. *American Journal of Preventive Medicine, 13*(1), 36–44.

Institute of Medicine (Ed.) (2001). *Crossing the quality chasm: A new health system for the 21st century.* Washington, DC: National Academy Press (p. 12).

Joint Commission on Accreditation of Healthcare Organizations. (1999). *ORYX: The next evolution in accreditation.* Retrieved May 1999, from *http://wwwb.jcaho.org/ perfmeas/oryx/oryx_qa.html*

Juhn P., Solomon N., Pettay H. (1998, Spring). Care management: The next level of innovation for Kaiser Permanente. *Permanente Journal*. Retrieved November 2003, from *http://www.kpnw.org/permjournal/spring98pj/cmi.html*

Kilbourne P. T. (1998, February 16). In managed care, "consumer" laws benefit doctors. *New York Times*.

Lamberts H., and Hofmans-Okkes I. (1996). Episode of care: A core concept in family practice. *Journal of Family Practice, 42*(2), 161–169.

Lassere M., et al. (1999). Smallest detectable difference in radiological progression. *Journal of Rheumatology, 26*(3), 731–739.

Liptak G. S., Burns C. M., Davidson P. W., McAnarney E. R. (1998). Effects of providing comprehensive ambulatory services to children with chronic conditions. *Archives of Pediatric and Adolescent Medicine, 152*(10), 1003–1008.

Luke D. A., Mowbray C. T., Klump K., Herman S. E., BootsMiller B. (1996). Exploring the diversity of dual diagnosis: Utility of cluster analysis for program planning. *Journal of Mental Health Administration, 23*(3), 298–316.

McDowell K. M., Chatburn R. L., Myers T. R., O'Riordan M. A., Kercsmar C. M. (1998). A cost-saving algorithm for children hospitalized for status asthmaticus. *Archives of Pediatric and Adolescent Medicine, 152*(10), 977–984.

Miller A. (1998, May 10). Survey on managed care finds satisfaction, confusion: Majority says that health care overhaul is needed; women, minorities tend to be less pleased. *Atlanta Journal and Constitution*.

Moler F. W., and Ohmit S. E. (1999). Severity of illness models for respiratory syncytial virus-associated hospitalization. *American Journal of Respiratory and Critical Care Medicine, 159*(4), 1234–1240.

Morgan A. I. (1998). Evaluating the economic impact of member attitudes on managed care disease management programs. *Disease Management, 1*(5), 247–254.

National Committee for Quality Assurance. (1999). *HEDIS 1999*. Retrieved May 1999, from *http://www.ncqa.org/pages/policy/hedis/newhedis.htm*

Nyman J. A., Manning W. G., Samuels S., Morrey B. F. (1998). Making continuous quality improvement work—care management 373. Can specialists reduce costs? The case of referrals to orthopaedic surgeons. *Clinical Orthopedics, 350*(5), 257–267.

Physician Insurers Association of America. (1998). *Elimination of ERISA malpractice preemption not the right fix for HMO problems: Lawsuits against health plans will ultimately hurt patients, doctors*. Retrieved May 1999, from *http://www.phyins.org/erisa.htm*

Powell A. J., et al. (1996). Health risk appraisal and serum cholesterol nutrition education: An outcome study. *Military Medicine, 161*(2), 70–74.

Redford L. J., and Parkins L. G. (1997). Interactive televideo and the Internet in rural case management. *Journal of Case Management, 6*(4), 151–157.

Rooney E. M., Studenski S. A., Roman L. L. (1997). A model for nurse case-managed home care using televideo. *Journal of the American Geriatric Society, 45*(12), 1523–1528.

Schuster M. A., McGlynn E. A., Brook R. H. (1998). How good is the quality of health care in the United States? *The Milbank Quarterly, 76*(4), 517–563.

Sedgwick Detert, Moran, and Arnold. (1999). *Recent legislation regarding managed care*. Retrieved May 1999, from *http://www.sdma.com/images/kerns.html*

Self T., and Demirkan K. (1999). Maintenance drug therapy of chronic obstructive pulmonary disease. *American Journal of Managed Care, 5*(1), 91–97.

Smith A. (1999). *Insurer accountability and responsibility*. Retrieved May 1999, from *http://www.monttla.com/KUFM/3-30-99%20comm.html*

Smith P. (1998). *HMOs immunity challenged*. Retrieved May 1999, from *http://www.seamless.com/glk/hmoart.htm*

Swanson S. (1999, March 14). Patients' rights movement targets HMO liability [Internet edition]. *Chicago Tribune*. Retrieved May 1999, from *http://chicagotribune.com/news/nationworld/article/0,1051,ART-25035,00.html*

Boston Consulting Group, Inc. (1993). *The contribution of pharmaceutical companies: What's at stake for America?* Boston: Boston Consulting Group.

Thomas P. W., and Budetti J. L. (1998). *Patient protections and managed care reform: The political and policy hot topic of 1998*. Retrieved November, 2003, from *http://www.oandp.com/organiza/naaop/081098.htm*

Weaver M. T., Forrester B. G., Brown K. C., Phillips J. A., Hilyer J. C., Capilouto E. I. (1998). Health risk influence on medical care costs and utilization among 2,898 municipal employees. *American Journal of Preventive Medicine, 15*(3), 250–253.

Westerhof H. (1998, September). *Episodes of care in the new dutch GP systems*. Retrieved May 1999, from *http://www.schin.ncl.ac.uk/phcsg/conferences/cambridge1998/westerhof.htm*

◆ Additional Reading

Institute of Medicine (Eds.). (2001). *Crossing the quality chasm: A new health system for the 21st century*. Washington, DC, National Academy Press.

Bowling A. (2001). *Measuring disease: A review of disease specific quality of life measurement scales*. Philadelphia: Open University Press.

Bowling A. (1997). *Measuring health: A review of quality of life measurement scales*. Philadelphia: Open University Press.

Todd W., and Nash D. (1996). Disease management: A systems approach. Chicago: American Hospital Publishing.

Appendix 10.A

Table 10A.1 Quality Improvement and Health Statistics Data Sources

DATA SET	URL	SOURCE	DESCRIPTION
Atlas of US Mortality	http://www.cdc.gov/nchswww/products/pubs/pubd/other/atlas/atlas.htm	NCHS	Text and graphical data on mortality rates and causes by state and county; copy only
National Ambulatory Medical Care Survey	http://www.cdc.gov/nchs/about/major/ahcd/ahcd1.htm	NCHS	Longitudinal data file from 1973 to present with information on office visits from systematic random sample of office visits in the US
National Hospital Ambulatory Medical Care Survey	http://www.cdc.gov/nchs/about/major/ahcd/ahcd1.htm	NCHS	Hospital outpatient and emergency department data collected by systematic survey from 1992 to present
Natality Data, Detail	http://www.cdc.gov/nchs/births.htm	NCHS	Birth certificate data from 1968 to present
Linked Birth and Death Perinatal Mortality Data	http://www.cdc.gov/nchs/about/major/lfetaldth/abfetal.htm	NCHS	Linked birth and death certificate data for neonates from 1983 to present
Mortality Data, Multiple Cause of Death	http://www.cdc.gov/nchs/about/major/dvs/mortdata.htm	NCHS	Mortality data, all causes, 1968 to present
National Health Interview Survey	http://www.cdc.gov/nchs/nhis.htm	NCHS	Ongoing survey of US households, conducted weekly, probability sample; health status and function of household members, including physician and hospital utilization; several subsets by disability and geographic location
National Hospital Discharge Survey	http://www.cdc.gov/nchs/about/major/hdasd/nhds.htm	NCHS	Survey of hospital discharges in US from 1970 to present with discharge diagnosis, procedure codes, patient demographics, and basic hospital information

continues

Table 10A.1 *continued*

DATA SET	SOURCE	URL	DESCRIPTION
National Nursing Home Survey	NCHS	http://www.cdc.gov/nchs/about/major/nnhsd/nnhsd.htm	Survey of US nursing home clients and staff four times between 1977 and 1995; data on facility, residents, and staff characteristics
National Health and Nutrition Survey	NCHS	http://www.cdc.gov/nchs/nhanes.htm	Nutritional and health utilization data from annual surveys of probability sample from each state; three surveys were conducted with somewhat different selection criteria and labeled National Health and Nutritional Examination Survey (NHANES I), NHANES II, and NHANES III; very complete data set that includes physician exam and laboratory data for ages ≥2 months
National Health Examination Survey	NCHS	http://www.cdc.gov/nchs/under_contr/Burgess/Catalog/nhes2.htm	Very complete series of files with interview and physical examination data for various age categories: Cycle I is ages 18–79 years, Cycle II is ages 6–11 years, and Cycle III is ages 12–17 years
National Survey of Personal Health Practices and Consequences	NCHS	http://www.cdc.gov/nchs/products/elec_prods/subject/nsphpc.htm	National probability sample, random-digit dialing techniques, conducted in two waves of interviews among a panel of US citizens 20–64 years of age in 1979 and 1980; data include information about personal health habits and preventive care
National Maternal and Infant Health Survey	NCHS	http://www.cdc.gov/nchs/products/elec_prods/subject/mihs.htm	Follow-up survey in 1991 to the 1988 survey of maternal and child health; includes information about child health, provider types, hospital utilization in children in cohort
National Survey of Ambulatory Surgery	NCHS	http://www.cdc.gov/nchs/about/major/hdasd/nhds.htm	Diagnosis and procedure codes from ambulatory surgery centers from 1994 to present
National Hospital Ambulatory Medical Care Survey	NCHS	http://www.cdc.gov/nchs/about/major/ahcd/ahcd1.htm	National sample of visits to hospital emergency departments and outpatient departments 1992 to present; very thorough data including drugs and procedures used

Name	URL	Source	Description
Safety and Health Statistics	http://www.bls.gov/data/home.htm	Bureau of Labor Statistics	Comprehensive data on accident rates, employment, and types of injuries from national surveys from 1989 to present
Healthcare Cost and Utilization Project—National Inpatient Sample	http://www.ahcpr.gov/data/hcup/hcupnis.htm	AHRQ	National stratified sample of 900 hospitals in 19 states from 1988 to present; administrative data from hospital record
Healthcare Cost and Utilization Project—State Inpatient Database	http://www.ahcpr.gov/data/hcup/hcupsid.htm	AHCPR (now AHRQ)	Uniform data for all inpatient stays in 19 states, listed on the Web site, from 1988 to present
CDC Wonder	http://wonder.cdc.gov/	CDC	Query system for CDC data sets; allows inquiries into databases
Combined Health Information Database	http://chid.nih.gov/subfile/subfile.html	NIH	Listing of disease and clinical condition specific databases available from government agencies
Healthy People 2000 Health Status Indicators	ftp://ftp.cdc.gov/pub/Health_Statistics/NCHS/Datasets/Healthy_People_2000/Health_Status_Indicators/	CDC	State specific data on the 18 health status indicators for the Healthy People 2000 objectives in spreadsheet format
Cancer Statistics	http://www.nci.nih.gov/hpage/public.htm	NCI	National statistics on cancer incidence by disease type from 1993 to present
WHO Statistical Information System	http://www.who.int/whosis/#topics	WHO	International databases for specific disease entities, including incidence by country, basic health indicators, mortality, and other indicators
US Census Bureau Statistics	http://www.census.gov/	US Census Bureau	Demographic statistics and economic data of the US population
Statistical Abstract of the US	http://www.census.gov/statab/www/	US Census Bureau	Compendium of statistical information, including health data
Office of Population Research	http://opr.princeton.edu/archive/	Princeton University	Population statistics, demographics, and fertility data

continues

Table 10A.1 *continued*

DATA SET	URL	SOURCE	DESCRIPTION
MEDPAR—Medicare Provider Analysis and Review	*http://www.cms.hhs.gov/data/ requests/directory.asp*	CMS	Total charges, covered charges, Medicare reimbursement, total days, number of discharges and average total days for 100% of Medicare beneficiaries using hospital inpatient services by state and then by DRG for all short stay and inpatient hospitals for fiscal years 1990 to present
National Health Care Expenditures	*http://www.cms.hhs.gov/ statistics/nhe*	CMS	National spending for health care for a number of categories
Medicare State and County Enrollment	*http://www.cms.hhs.gov/statistics/ more_statistics.asp*	CMS	Enrollment by state and county of Medicare recipients by type of insurance coverage
HEDIS Data for Medicare Managed Care Plans	*http://www.cms.hhs.gov/ healthplans/hedis/*	CMS	HEDIS results for Medicare managed care plans
Medicaid Statistics	*http://www.cms.hhs.gov/medicaid/ mcaidsad.asp*	CMS	Master site for a number of Medicaid databases, including enrollment information, utilization statistics, and summary statistics
Medicare and Medicaid Data Resources	*http://cms.hhs.gov/researchers/ default.asp*	CMS	Master site for all Medicare and Medicaid data resources, with listing of databases and other data management tools available from CMS

NCHS, National Center for Health Statistics; AHRQ, Agency for Healthcare Research and Quality; AHCPR, Agency for Health Care Policy and Research; CDC, Centers for Disease Control; NIH, National Institutes of Health; NCI, National Cancer Institute; WHO, World Health Organization; CMS, Centers for Medicare and Medicaid Services; DRG, diagnosis-related group; HEDIS, Health Plan Employer Data and Information Set.

Chapter 11

Legal and Regulatory Issues in Quality Improvement

DONALD E. LIGHTER
SALLY A. LIGHTER

◆ Introduction

Improving quality should reduce legal liability because the risk of adverse events in a higher quality environment should be reduced. Quality improvement efforts by hospitals, physicians, managed care organizations, and other providers, such as home health agencies and skilled nursing facilities, have generally been directed at enhancing the quality of health care. These initiatives have been prompted not only by market demand but also by legislative and regulatory mandates. Nearly all health care organizations now have some type of quality directive that requires improvement efforts, either for certification or to comply with federal and state legislation. For example, managed care organizations must comply with standards from state and federal regulatory agencies, and if they participate in Medicare or Medicaid programs, they must comply with a rigid set of standards (the Quality Improvement System for Managed Care). For private managed care plans, the National Committee for Quality Assurance and the Utilization Review Accreditation Commission serve as accrediting bodies. In addition to state and federal regulations, hospitals must be accredited by the Joint Commission for Accreditation of Healthcare Organizations to qualify for reimbursement by Medicare and Medicaid. Physicians must be regularly relicensed by their state boards, as well as recertified by their specialty boards, but the process is quite different from hospital and managed care organization accreditation.

All of these accrediting organizations have produced a huge industry for the certification of quality in health care. Health care organizations maintain significant staff components and incur the associated costs to comply with these different oversight bodies, but few studies have examined the return on the investment made to satisfy the requirements of these various accreditation organizations (Barry and Kline, 2002). This chapter will not only examine the predominant regulatory organizations, but it will also present information about selected organizations that promote quality in health care without the regulatory "hammer." The first accrediting entity examined will be the federal government's effort to monitor and improve the quality of care for Medicare beneficiaries, the Quality Improvement System for Managed Care. Because this framework is quite involved, it will serve as the basis for subsequent discussions and so will be discussed in detail.

◆ Federal Legislation and Regulation

The federal government's Medicare program, managed by the Centers for Medicare and Medicaid Services (CMS), has grown to immense size, with expenditures of nearly $426 billion in 2000 (CMS, 2000). Because the program has become so overwhelmingly large and costly, CMS began in 1999 to offer a managed care option for Medicaid beneficiaries, dubbed Medicare+Choice, with the goal of decreasing costs and improving benefits (McDermott, Will, and Emery, 1999). Because managed care systems involve capitation of providers, i.e., a fixed payment for all of a patient's care over a specified time period, these plans could stabilize costs by capping reimbursements and controlling access to care. Combined with the concern that quality of care may deteriorate as the federal government relinquished control of the benefit structure for Medicaid beneficiaries, these issues led to the development of a quality oversight system known as the Quality Improvement System for Managed Care or QISMC, which is a complex set of standards for managed care organizations produced by CMS in response to the Balanced Budget Act of 1997 (CMS, 2003). For Medicare+Choice plans, the CMS has equated the QISMC standards and guidelines with a program manual representing the CMS's administrative interpretation of the requirements relating to an organization's operation and performance in the areas of quality measurement and improvement and the delivery of health care and enrollee services. These standards include provisions for the following four domains.

- ◆ Domain 1: Quality Assessment and Performance Improvement (QAPI) Program
- ◆ Domain 2: Enrollee Rights
- ◆ Domain 3: Health Services Management
- ◆ Domain 4: Delegation

Managed care organizations with Medicare+Choice plans must conform to these standards or risk financial penalties or termination of contracts. Because Medicaid programs are managed by each state and use federal funding, CMS has recommended that states may choose to use QISMC standards to ensure that Medicaid managed care organizations meet the comparable quality assurance requirements established by the Balanced Budget Act and associated regulations.

QISMC Domain 1 Standards: QAPI Program

Domain 1 standards relate to ongoing efforts for quality improvement (quality improvement) and are outlined on the CMS Web site at *http://www.cms .hhs.gov/cop/2d1.asp* and included as Appendix 11A. The standards first note that managed care organizations must perform quality improvement activities and monitor performance measures defined by the CMS or state Medicaid agencies, depending on the population. The standards require a specific number of projects for each year of review on topics specified by CMS and the state Medicaid agency. CMS will name a new project topic each year in which every Medicare+Choice managed care organization will participate, providing a basis for national benchmarks. The agency may also mandate a special project in an area of concern identified by CMS or the state Medicaid agency. For example, if the oversight body for QISMC determines that a particular managed care organization has problems with access to specialty services, that managed care organization may be required to initiate a special project to remedy that shortcoming. The projects in which a managed care organization may participate use the traditional quality improvement approach of high-volume and high-risk conditions, as well as those that involve acute and chronic conditions and continuity of care.

Section 1.4 of the domain denotes the criteria for improvement. CMS emphasizes the importance of selecting projects and measures for which benchmarks exist, allowing comparison of the performance of the managed care organization with other organizations. Measures must be related to outcomes and have national or local benchmarks available for comparisons and targets. Each measure requires an operational definition that allows consistent data collection and analysis over a period of several years to ensure longitudinal comparison of the organization's performance. The managed care organization is required to demonstrate minimum levels of improvement amounting to 10% of the nonconforming subjects, i.e., those that do not meet the criteria for inclusion in the count of "successes." For example, if the population immunization rate is 63%, indicating that 37% of children were incompletely immunized, then the managed care organization would be required to increase the immunization rate by 10% of the 37% or 3.7%. The managed care organization must demonstrate an effort to adjust for confounding variables that may change the data unrelated to the quality improvement efforts of the organization. This section also includes parameters for statistical sampling of the population.

The final sections in Domain 1 mandate data collection methods and capabilities that will ensure validity of the information used in the QAPI program, as well as a properly defined structure for the effort in the organization. Data collection, storage, and analysis are of critical importance to any quality improvement effort, and minimum requirements include organizational oversight of the data collection and analysis process to ensure that the data used in the analyses are valid. Each organization must have a well-defined structure for oversight of all quality improvement efforts to properly analyze, interpret, and use data for making substantive changes.

QISMC Domain 2 Standards: Enrollee Rights

Domain 2 regulations, relating to enrollee rights, are included as Appendix 11B. CMS considers this section to be of utmost importance because the rights of enrollees in managed care programs have concerned the agency since the beginning of Medicare+Choice. Additionally, CMS must meet stringent criteria established by Congress in the Balanced Budget Act of 1997 for ensuring access to quality care for Medicare beneficiaries. The fundamental rights of enrollees must be guaranteed by the managed care organization and include

- ◆ equal access to all services
- ◆ confidentiality
- ◆ right to refuse care
- ◆ access to all providers accepting patients
- ◆ right to be treated with dignity

In addition to these rights, the standard requires managed care organizations to promote advance directives so that individuals may be treated according to their wishes when terminally ill. All of these policies and procedures must be made explicit in the operational manuals of the organization.

Enrollees also have the right to obtain information about the health plan through plan literature, which is written at the fifth-grade level. Managed care organizations in areas of the country with non–English-speaking populations must accommodate the needs of these populations with literature in a language appropriate for each individual. This information must include information about covered services, providers, and appeals procedures, so that each enrollee has an extensive, understandable reference to all plan benefits and procedures. The standard describes the extensive store of information that must be contained in enrollee manuals and includes the following:

- ◆ enrollee rights and responsibilities
- ◆ listing of providers, with their addresses
- ◆ benefit schedule
- ◆ policies and procedures for obtaining services, both in- and out-of-plan
- ◆ access to emergency services
- ◆ any charges to enrollees, e.g., copayments and coinsurance
- ◆ procedures for making complaints and grievances
- ◆ procedures for changing doctors or making suggestions for improved service

All of these items are usually found in health plan literature, but the QISMC extends this typical information with requirements to add descriptions of other plan characteristics, including (1) the number of complaints and grievances and their resolution, (2) methods of compensating providers, and (3) the financial condition of the health plan. This information is designed to inform enrollees of the nature of the plan's operations so that they can make a better decision about which plan would provide the best coverage.

An important provision of this standard concerns the resolution of complaints and grievances. In nearly all managed care arrangements, disagreements occur between the provider and the plan regarding services needed by members. To ameliorate these problems, the QISMC requires health plans to have policies and procedures for handling disagreements, including appeals processes that allow disagreements to be evaluated appropriately. Managed care organizations often differentiate between complaints and grievances, based on the level of formality and importance of the member disagreement. Complaints are often handled quickly during a single enrollee contact with the plan, whereas grievances usually require a more formal process that may take more time to resolve. The advantage of tracking grievances cannot be underestimated because they often can be grouped into patterns and trends that can direct quality improvement efforts. Problems that can be handled by making a single change to the system are much less costly than those that must be handled individually. Disenrollment problems are also often handled through the grievance process and are subject to the provisions of this standard. The standard requires a method of tracking grievances throughout the process, as well as a method of rapidly resolving grievances that must be adjudicated to ensure necessary care. The health plan must also ensure that members and providers are quickly notified of decisions made by health plan staff through the resolution process.

QISMC Domain 3 Standards: Health Services Management

The third domain subsumed by the QISMC involves health services management, as detailed in Appendix 11C. This section includes the medical management standards for managed care organizations, setting criteria for the most important cost-containment functions. Medical management affects the quality of care significantly, so the QISMC contains substantial detail regarding the manner in which these functions are conducted. The first standard outlines the methods by which managed care organizations ensure that covered services are available to enrollees—by appropriate actuarial and geoaccess studies—and the standard makes clear that even in point-of-service plans, covered services must be available at no extra charge to members. Members must have direct access to primary care providers and not be unreasonably restricted from access to specialists. Additionally, the standard extends typical accessibility standards by compelling managed care organizations to have a plan approved by CMS (or state Medicaid agency) for meeting the needs of patients who are chronically ill or have special medical requirements. Health plans must also inform members of their rights to continue to access specialty care in the event of the plan's loss of its Medicaid contract.

The standards in this domain provide for verifying physician qualifications through a strict credentialing process and also obligate the managed care organization to ensure that covered services are available at all times (24 hours a day, 7 days a week). Services by providers must be nondiscriminatory and reasonably convenient for members, including after-hours access for medically urgent problems. Additionally, because of the nature of the Medicare and Medicaid populations, the standard requires managed care organizations to ensure that non–English-speaking and poorly served individuals such as the homeless are appropriately managed and have opportunities to access care.

Similar to the requirements of Medicaid managed care systems, the QISMC mandates that health plans establish standards regarding access to care for members. Such standards generally list the maximum waiting time for routine office visits, emergency visits, and urgent care visits. The QISMC also stipulates that managed care organizations must monitor performance and take corrective action when providers are not compliant with the requirements. Other specific requirements in this standard for health plan policies include proscription of any plan regulation that inhibits members from obtaining needed care and encouragement of input from enrollees regarding treatment plans.

The standards in Domain 3 also enjoin health plans to create a system for a primary care case manager for each beneficiary. CMS has left the method for satisfying this requirement to the health plans, but if the plan decides on a different mechanism than assigning each enrollee to a primary care physician, the enrollee must be assured access to a physician upon request. Managed care organizations must also coordinate care with community service organizations in the plan's service area and enable communications among all of the members' providers. As part of this overall health supervision, plans are expected to make certain that beneficiaries receive appropriate follow-up for clinical conditions, as well as training in self-care and health promotion. Noncompliant patients must also have counseling services available to improve adherence to treatment regimens.

The next section of this important domain requires managed care organizations to maintain written policies guaranteeing that any decisions regarding denial of health care services are based on contemporary health care science and that all such requests and adjudications are recorded and tracked. Health plans must have policies that establish time frames for responding to requests for medical services, based on the urgency of the request. In some cases, state insurance law establishes these time frames, but when left to the discretion of the plans, the time frames must be defensible and reasonable. A physician must review any denials that are deemed medically inappropriate before the service is finally disallowed. Notice of denial of services must be communicated to the physician and enrollee in a timely manner as defined by CMS. The standard also specifies that managed care organizations may neither provide incentives for reviewers to deny services nor prevent practitioners from helping the patient through the appeals process to obtain services. Perhaps most importantly in a managed care environment, the health plan is required to establish mechanisms to detect both overutilization and underutilization.

QISMC standards also require health plans to use evidence-based clinical practice guidelines (CPGs). The CPGs must be disseminated in usable form to both providers and enrollees, and the plan must ensure that medical decisions made by utilization review personnel follow the guidelines. This approach is consistent with the recommendations of the Institute of Medicine regarding the use of CPGs in health care, as described in detail in Chapter 8.

New technologies are constantly appearing in health care. QISMC regulations require managed care organizations to address these innovations systematically, using written policies and procedures that ensure a rational approach to determining coverage. Written policies must drive all deliberations, and CMS requires that decisions for coverage parallel those of Medicare and Medicaid.

Provider credentialing involves collecting and verifying all of the information that demonstrates the competence of a provider. Numerous sources must be consulted for verification, including state licensure bureaus, malpractice carriers, health institutions and training programs, the National Data Bank for medical malpractice cases, and other sources of information regarding each provider. This domain codifies these requirements, with specific recommendations on credentialing and recredentialing as well as verification that the provider is eligible for participating in Medicare or Medicaid. The standard also requires health plans to include practitioners in the process of credentials review and the establishment of standards for accepting or denying a provider's participation based on credentials. To ensure access to due process, the managed care organization must also have written policies and procedures for terminating provider contracts or initiating sanctions against a provider. The QISMC additionally requires that managed care organization sanctions and suspensions of providers be reported to state licensing boards and other regulatory authorities with provider licensure or certification responsibilities.

Minimum standards for the care of enrollee clinical records and dissemination of information to and between providers comprise the remainder of Domain 3. Unique to Medicaid, the standard requires a health risk appraisal within 90 days of each member's enrollment in the plan. Additionally, the health plan must ensure that provider records meet minimum standards for completeness. The standard also addresses the responsibilities of the plan to expedite information flow between the health plan and providers, as well as between providers caring for the same patient. For plans with point-of-service benefits, the managed care organization must periodically update each member's primary care physician with information about the services that each patient has used, allowing the primary care provider to contact any other physicians or institutions for more detailed information. Finally, the plan must make certain that information flows between referring providers and specialists and during record transfers for members who change providers or health plans.

QISMC Domain 4 Standards: Delegation

Because many managed care organizations subcontract some of their functions to outside vendors—a process called delegation—QISMC standards also address issues that arise in these situations. (Domain 4 standards are listed in Appendix 11D.) The most important aspect of this standard, however, is the first section, which firmly assigns responsibility for compliance with QISMC standards to the entity holding the contract with Medicare or Medicaid. The remaining standards in this domain relate to particulars of delegation, e.g., frequency of review, right to override the decisions of the delegate, due diligence to ensure the qualifications of the delegate before completion of the contract, and specification in the contract of reasons and procedures for revoking delegation.

Effect of the QISMC on Quality of Care

QISMC standards detail a level of organization and structure that should be required of any managed health care plan, not just those that care for Medicare or Medicaid beneficiaries. The QISMC mimics the standards of established organizations such as the National Committee for Quality Assurance (NCQA) and the American Accreditation Health Care Commission/Utilization Review Accreditation Commission, with a few additional nuances for the special needs of the Medicare and Medicaid populations. As discussed in Chapter 9, however, no studies have yet demonstrated improvements in health outcomes when managed care organizations improve compliance with standards, and some evidence suggests that the opposite may be true (Beaulieu and Epstein, 2002).

Most QISMC standards relate to the structure and functioning of the health plan, rather than improved quality of care. Although health plans must be properly structured to perform the necessary services for the health care market, those that are not properly organized will fail. The QISMC seeks to reduce the chance of failure because it can have serious repercussions for Medicare beneficiaries with complex health needs. On the other hand, incentives in the system must also be formulated to reinforce these structural elements and reward superior performance. The QISMC may serve as an interim step in this process.

◆ The NCQA

The NCQA was started in 1979 but did not develop a mandate to improve the quality of services provided by managed care organizations until 1990. The federal government and the public had become increasingly disenchanted with managed care organizations, and the NCQA was the organization selected to make health maintenance organizations (HMOs) accountable for their activities. These efforts were funded initially by grants from the Robert Wood Johnson Foundation, large employers, and the Group Health Association of America. The two major missions of the organization were accreditation and design of performance measures for HMOs. Gaining credibility through a structured approach to HMO accreditation, the NCQA created an evaluation system that improved public confidence in the industry. NCQA staff began conducting accreditation surveys in 1991, and by 1992 the organization assumed responsibility for the Health Plan Employer Data and Information Set (HEDIS), a group of performance measures for HMOs. In 1995, HEDIS became the task of the Performance Measurement Committee, a group of providers, consumers, and payers that evaluates possible measures for inclusion in the HEDIS measurements. By 1996, over half of the HMOs in the United States participated in NCQA certification. The organization initiated the Quality Compass in 1996, which consists of a database of HEDIS measures for managed care organizations that submit data to the NCQA (National Committee for Quality Assurance, 2000). The Quality Compass has evolved into the Health Plan Report Card, which is accessible through the NCQA Web site.

NCQA Accreditation

The NCQA has developed many accreditation programs, including those for

◆ managed care organizations,
◆ managed behavioral health organizations,
◆ physician organizations,
◆ credentials verification organizations
◆ disease management programs, and
◆ preferred provider organizations (PPOs);

as well as those for

◆ new health plans,
◆ the Veterans Administration Human Research Protection Accreditation Program, and
◆ the Partnership for Human Research Protection Accreditation Program.

The managed care organization certification process has generally been widely accepted by the health care industry, and some large employers now require HMOs to be certified by the NCQA in order to be offered to employees (National Committee for Quality Assurance, 2000).

NCQA reviews are conducted on-site at the health care institution after extensive off-site review of the structure and policies of the organization. Preparation for the review often consumes substantial organizational resources. All of the appropriate documentation must be assembled and organized in a form that can be expeditiously evaluated by NCQA reviewers. Additionally, the organization must ensure that all policies are in accordance with standards, and with the inclusion of HEDIS measures in the review, substantial data analysis must also be performed. Because the entire organization is evaluated, every department in the company must be involved with the preparation and on-site review. The NCQA review team includes physicians and other managed care professionals who usually spend at least 3 days at a managed care organization during the on-site phase of the evaluation. The team generates a report, which is evaluated by the Review Oversight Committee of the NCQA, which then makes a final determination of the plan's accreditation status. Health plans can receive any one of several designations: excellent, commendable, accredited, provisional, denied, appealed by plan, in process, revoked, scheduled, suspended, or under review by NCQA.

The designations relate to the duration of the accreditation, from 1 to 3 years, and the frequency of return reviews by the NCQA on-site team. In some instances, the NCQA will require more information to ensure that a health plan is performing at expected levels, so a review may be delayed until all information can be collected.

Just as with QISMC, NCQA standards for health plans are segregated into domains, and reviewers generally examine six different areas of organizational function:

◆ quality management and improvement
◆ utilization management
◆ credentialing and recredentialing
◆ member rights and responsibilities
◆ preventive health services
◆ medical records

In 1999, HEDIS scores were added to the scoring mix and now represent up to 25% of a health plan's review score. Although the structure of the organization and its policies are an important part of the evaluation, the health plan's performance in each of the domains is also measured to determine if the organization is implementing policies effectively.

The design of standards and measures in all of the domains is similar, consisting of the following sections:

◆ program structure
◆ program operations
◆ relationship and effects on providers

◆ relationship and effects on members
◆ performance measurement
◆ delegation

Specific standards within each of the categories above vary according to the area of review, and much of the content in QISMC standards was derived from the NCQA accreditation framework.

The NCQA has expanded its reach to other types of organizations, as noted previously. The advantage of this extension of the NCQA into other areas is that health plans may delegate functions to NCQA-accredited organizations and not perform the extensive oversight functions required if the delegate were not accredited by the NCQA. For example, health plans that delegate credentialing functions to subcontractors must perform extensive NCQA-like reviews of the subcontractor each year to satisfy the credentialing and recredentialing standard for the plan's NCQA accreditation. If the health plan delegates credentialing and recredentialing to a credentials verification organization certified by NCQA, then the plan is not required to perform a yearly review of the subcontractor to maintain accreditation. The advantage to the health plan in administrative and cost savings can be substantial.

The process for review of managed behavioral health organizations is similar to that for managed care organizations, with the addition of a domain for access, availability, and triage, which includes standards for ensuring access to behavioral health services. This domain adds extra standards for response time and availability of triage services and appropriate providers. Just as with the managed care organization standards, the NCQA requires a study of the plan's population to determine the needs for specific providers and looks for indications that the plan has made adequate arrangements to meet those needs. The medical records domain in the managed care organization standards is termed "treatment records" in the managed behavioral health organizations' standards, and the provisions are very similar with regard to confidentiality and minimum content of patient records.

Accreditation of physician organizations is substantially more complex and includes the same functional domains as those for managed care organizations: (1) quality management and improvement, (2) utilization management, (3) credentialing and recredentialing, (4) member rights and responsibilities, (5) preventive health services, and (6) medical records.

The organization must meet the same standards as the managed care organization, and the advantage for the physician organization is elimination of multiple annual audits by health plans for delegated services. The physician organization may be certified for any one of or a combination of the domains, and according to the NCQA Web site listing of certified physician organizations (National Committee for Quality Assurance, 2003–2), the most commonly completed certification is for credentialing and recredentialing.

Some organizations seek to perform services related to verifying physician credentials. These services are particularly valuable to physicians, health plans, hospitals, and other organizations because they can reduce redundancy and cost within the system. Because credentialing is such an important part of the activities of nearly every health care organization, and because it is often one of the most frequently delegated functions for managed care organizations, the NCQA has created a credentials verification organization certification process that examines several attributes of a credentials verification organization, including (1) policies and procedures for credentials verification and confidentiality, (2) data collection and updating of methods, (3) quality improvement initiatives, (4) content and information in physician credentialing applications, and (5) management of physician disciplinary actions.

Credentials verification organizations can be certified for any or all of 10 different elements of credentialing, and the credentialing process involves review of the following areas:

◆ licensure
◆ hospital privileges
◆ Drug Enforcement Administration registration
◆ medical education and/or board certification
◆ malpractice insurance
◆ liability claims history
◆ national practitioner data bank queries
◆ medical board sanctions
◆ Medicare and/or Medicaid sanctions
◆ provider application

The NCQA maintains a current credentials certification status list on its Web site (National Committee for Quality Assurance, 2003).

The NCQA has worked to make the certification process useful for consumers. Over 50% of managed care plans in the United States now participate in the certification process, and the NCQA maintains a current accreditation list on its Web site at *http://www.ncqa.org*. The list is updated monthly with the most recent information about health plan, behavioral health plan, physician organization, and credentials verification organization certifications.

HEDIS Measures

HEDIS measures are operational definitions or precise definitions of the data required for analysis (and the specific analytic techniques to apply to the data) of over 50 measures of health plan performance. Since the NCQA introduced HEDIS in 1993, the measures have undergone extensive revision with the goal of improving the validity and usefulness of the measures. The current list of HEDIS 2004 measures is included as Table 11.1. The measures are divided into six categories: (1) access and availability, (2) effectiveness of care, (3) utilization of services, (4) member satisfaction, (5) cost of care, and (6) health plan stability.

Table 11.1 HEDIS 2004 Measures

DOMAIN	MEASURES
Effectiveness of Care	◆ Childhood immunization status
	◆ Adolescent immunization status
	◆ Appropriate treatment for children with upper respiratory infection
	◆ Appropriate testing for children with pharyngitis
	◆ Colorectal cancer screening
	◆ Breast cancer screening
	◆ Cervical cancer screening
	◆ Chlamydia screening in women
	◆ Osteoporosis management in women who had a fracture
	◆ Controlling high blood pressure
	◆ Beta blocker treatment after a heart attack
	◆ Cholesterol management after acute cardiovascular events
	◆ Comprehensive diabetes care
	◆ Use of appropriate medications for people with asthma
	◆ Follow-up after hospitalization for mental illness
	◆ Antidepressant medication management
	◆ Medical assistance with smoking cessation
	◆ Flu shots for adults aged 50–64 years
	◆ Flu shots for older adults
	◆ Pneumonia vaccination for older adults
	◆ Medicare health outcomes survey
	◆ Management of urinary incontinence in older adults
Access/Availability of Care	◆ Adults' access to preventive/ambulatory health services
	◆ Children's and adolescents' access to primary care practitioners
	◆ Prenatal and postpartum care
	◆ Annual dental visit
	◆ Initiation and engagement of alcohol and other drug dependence treatment
	◆ Claims timeliness
	◆ Call answer timeliness
	◆ Call abandonment
Satisfaction with the Experience of Care	◆ HEDIS/CAHPS 3.0H (adult; Medicaid and commercial)
	◆ HEDIS/CAHPS 3.0H (child; Medicaid and commercial)
	◆ ECHO Survey 3.0H for MBHOs
	◆ HEDIS/CAHPS Medicare

continues

Table 11.1 *continued*

DOMAIN	MEASURES
Health Plan Stability	◆ Practitioner turnover
	◆ Years in business/total membership
Use of Services	◆ Frequency of ongoing prenatal care
	◆ Well-child visits in the first 15 months of life
	◆ Well-child visits in the 3rd, 4th, 5th, and 6th years of life
	◆ Adolescent well-care visits
	◆ Frequency of selected procedures
	◆ Inpatient utilization: general hospital/acute care
	◆ Ambulatory care
	◆ Inpatient utilization: nonacute care
	◆ Discharge and average length of stay: maternity care
	◆ Cesarean section rate
	◆ Vaginal birth after Cesarean rate
	◆ Births and average length of stay: newborns
	◆ Mental health utilization: inpatient discharges and average length of stay
	◆ Mental health utilization: percentage of members receiving inpatient, day/night, and ambulatory care services
	◆ Chemical dependency utilization: inpatient discharges and average length of stay
	◆ Chemical dependency utilization: percentage of members receiving inpatient, day/night, and ambulatory care services
	◆ Identification of alcohol and other drug services
	◆ Outpatient drug utilization
Cost of Care	◆ Rate trends
	◆ High-occurrence/high-cost DRGs
Health Plan Descriptive Information	◆ Board certification
	◆ Total enrollment by percentage
	◆ Enrollment by product line
	◆ Unduplicated count of Medicaid members
	◆ Cultural diversity of Medicaid membership
	◆ Weeks of pregnancy at time of enrollment in the health plan

HEDIS, Health Plan Employer Data and Information Set; CAHPS, Consumer Assessment of Health Plans Survey; ECHO, Experience of Care and Health Outcomes; MBHO, managed behavioral health organization; DRG, diagnosis-related group.

The measures in each of these categories have been validated by the NCQA and are continually reviewed by the Performance Measurement Committee, among others. Revisions to the measures are disseminated publicly for comment before they are finalized.

Prior to 1999, health plans calculated their own HEDIS measures and reported them to the NCQA; however, the NCQA began requiring audited HEDIS reports from health plans in 1999 to increase confidence in the measures and improve comparisons between plans. Audits must be performed by organizations that have been certified by the NCQA to perform the analyses. Additionally, HEDIS measures were incorporated into the health plan review process beginning in 1999, with nearly 25% of the plan's score depending on their performance on HEDIS measures.

Consumer Assessment of Health Plans Surveys

The Consumer Assessment of Health Plans Survey (CAHPS) was originally designed by the Agency for Healthcare Research and Quality (AHRQ), formerly known as the Agency for Health Care Policy and Research (AHCPR), in conjunction with Harvard Medical School, the RAND Institute, and the Research Triangle Institute, and it too figures into the accreditation process. The quality management and improvement domain includes a requirement for a consumer survey of health plan performance on a number of issues. Prior to 1999, the survey was specially designed as an extension of the HEDIS measures, but starting in that year, the NCQA combined its HEDIS Member Satisfaction Survey with the CAHPS of the AHRQ to update the survey to the CAHPS 2.0H version instrument that was adopted as the standard metric for health plans. To ensure validity and comparability between plans, health plans must employ NCQA-certified vendors to perform and analyze the surveys. The results of the surveys can then be included with the data in the Quality Compass to provide a better comparison between plans. Table 11.2 lists the topic and subject areas of the standard CAHPS developed by the AHRQ. The current version—CAHPS 3.0H—is very similar but contains a few specific questions related to NCQA requirements.

Over the past 3 years, additional CAHPSs have been included for specific population groups, including the consumers of Medicaid managed care and Medicare managed care and children. The surveys are divided into core and supplemental questions, with the core questions covering the issues listed in Table 11.2. Supplemental questionnaires add inquiries about transportation, dental care, pregnancy, and other issues that are not common to all respondents. The AHRQ has also developed a telephone survey script for use when respondents have not completed the written surveys or if the managed care organization prefers direct contact with members. All of the surveys are available on the AHRQ Web site (Agency for Healthcare Research and Quality, 2003).

Table 11.2 CAHPS Domains and Topics

TOPIC	QUESTION DESCRIPTION
Getting needed care	◆ Problems finding doctor
	◆ Problems getting referral
	◆ Problems getting tests or treatment
	◆ Problem with care being delayed due to approval by health plan
Getting care quickly	◆ Getting medical help by phone
	◆ Waiting time to make an urgent appointment
	◆ Waiting time to get care
	◆ Waiting time over 15 minutes in doctor's office
Doctors who communicate well	◆ Provider listens
	◆ Provider explains care
	◆ Provider shows respect
	◆ Provider spends enough time
Office staff	◆ Office staff shows respect
	◆ Office staff helpful
Health plan customer service	◆ Written materials
	◆ Customer service phone line
	◆ Paperwork
Rating of personal doctors	0–10 scale
Rating of specialists	0–10 scale
Rating of health care	0–10 scale
Rating of health plan	0–10 scale

These instruments have been developed and validated to provide a reproducible set of consumer responses on satisfaction with services provided by health plans and physicians. The standardization of the questionnaires allows comparable results that can allow consumers to evaluate health plan performance in accordance with individual needs while maintaining anonymity. Additionally, health plans and purchasers can perform population studies using survey information to determine which features of health plans and provider performance are most valuable to consumers. The goal of the AHRQ and the NCQA in promoting these surveys is to standardize the information gathered on consumer surveys and to ensure that the survey scientifically measures consumer sentiment.

The CAHPS kits can be obtained from the federal government free of charge. The kits consist of handbooks with information on conducting the surveys, as well as information on interpreting and analyzing results. The reporting kit also includes methods of disseminating the information to consumers and informational brochures and letters to inform consumers about the need to assess the quality of a health care insurer. The system is designed for direct application or for use when engaging survey vendors to conduct the actual poll. The AHRQ provides free technical support for the publicly available surveys.

◆ Utilization Review Accreditation Commission

Starting in 1990, the Utilization Review Accreditation Commission (URAC), became the leader in accreditation of PPOs and continues to offer multiple accreditation programs for managed care organizations in the following areas:

- case management
- claims processing
- core accreditation
- credentials verification organizations
- disease management organizations
- health call centers
- health networks
- health plans
- health provider credentialing
- health Web sites
- health utilization management
- Health Insurance Portability and Accountability Act (HIPAA) privacy
- HIPAA security
- independent review
- workers' compensation utilization management

A managed care organization may become accredited in any of a number of these areas, depending on the business structure of the organization. As indicated by the list above, managed care organizations can be accredited for provider network management operations, utilization management operations, or special functions such as telephone triage or credentialing.

Several states require URAC certification as part of the regulatory process of licensure by the state insurance commission. By settling on a national set of standards for organizational functions, the state can reduce regulatory burdens on the managed care organization as well as on the state bureaucracy. Additionally, many contemporary health plans operate in many states, and compliance with a nationally recognized set of standards allows the companies to implement uniform systems throughout their service areas. States usually either require (mandated status) or recommend (deemed status) URAC accreditation for specific functions such as credentialing, and many simply require adherence to the standards without accreditation. A listing of the states requiring AAHCC/URAC accreditation can be found on the organization's Web site (URAC, 2003).

URAC Accreditation Programs

URAC's accreditation programs have evolved into substantive reviews of organizational prowess in conducting managed care operations. Full health network accreditation standards were formulated in 1996 and apply to PPOs, HMOs, and point of service (POS) plans. The standards address five areas: (1) network management, (2) utilization management, (3) quality improvement, (4) credentialing, and (5) member protection.

Network management standards subsume all of the issues surrounding interactions with provider networks: contracts, rules and regulations for providers, quality management, etc. This set of standards provides a comprehensive approach to managed care and is especially suited to PPOs that rely on utilization and quality management systems for organizational success. Credentialing accreditation is available for less stringently managed networks that require only verification of proper credentialing procedures.

URAC also offers basic network accreditation, involving standards for provider network management, quality improvement, credentialing, and member protection standards. Some network-based health care systems do not provide utilization management, so the basic network accreditation reviews all of the usual standards except for utilization management. For organizations that provide only utilization management services, the URAC has a category of certification termed "health utilization management accreditation." These standards relate to typical utilization management activities, such as

◆ confidentiality
◆ staff qualifications and credentials
◆ program qualifications
◆ quality improvement programs
◆ accessibility and on-site review procedures
◆ information requirements
◆ utilization review procedures
◆ appeals

Organizations seeking utilization management accreditation often serve as subcontractors to managed care organizations, and the accreditation designation allows the organization to serve as a delegate without continued review by the managed care organizations. Finally, the AAHCC/URAC also provides accreditation programs for workers' compensation networks and utilization management, as well as accreditation for call centers that are offered by many managed care organizations.

◆ Joint Commission on Accreditation of Healthcare Organizations

The Joint Commission on Accreditation of Healthcare Organizations (JCAHO or Joint Commission) is very well known in the health care industry for its work in accrediting hospitals for over 70 years. It evaluates and accredits more than 16,000 health care organizations in the United States and around the world, including hospitals, health care networks, managed care organizations, and health care organizations that provide home care, long-term care, behavioral health care, laboratory, and ambulatory care services. The organization was formalized in 1951, when the hospital accreditation function of the American College of Surgeons was joined by the American College of Physicians, the American Hospital Association, the American Medical Association, and the Canadian Medical Association in the predecessor to the Joint Commission, the Joint Commission on Accreditation of Hospitals (JCAH). In the years since the JCAH was formed, the organization gradually assumed responsibility for certifying other types of health care organizations, and in 1987 the organization's name was changed to the Joint Commission on Accreditation of Healthcare Organizations to reflect the broadening scope of organizational activities.

Review Process

The review process entails a site visit by trained surveyors who evaluate the facility according to standards maintained by the Joint Commission. Surveyors spend several days at the health care organization, during which time they examine documents, check the facility and physical plant, and talk with staff members regarding operations and compliance with standards. Although the review process is voluntary, it is required by states for hospital licensure, by many payers (including Medicare and Medicaid) to be eligible for payment, and many liability insurance companies to qualify for insurance. Because the accreditation reviews occur in 3-year cycles, hospital staff members often found that the site visit was a difficult task involving a year of preparation and 2 years of waiting. Thus, in 2004, the JCAHO will change the process to one that provides more continuity through the Shared Visions–New Pathways program, which consists of the following approach.

- ◆ **Self-assessment.** The health care organization assesses its own compliance with standards using an automated system on the JCAHO's extranet site, then enters a plan to bring the organization into compliance.
- ◆ **Priority focus process.** This process refers to the use of presurvey information to focus the site visit survey on areas of quality improvement and patient safety that are specific to the unique characteristics of the health care organization.

◆ **Priority focus tool.** This tool is an automated instrument that enhances the priority focus process by identifying areas of importance for the organization's survey by analyzing data that profiles the institution prior to the site visit.

The goal of the new survey process is to create a continuous improvement process that avoids the cycles of compliance activity associated with the current process.

Performance Measurement: ORYX

As part of the accreditation process, the Joint Commission added a method of assessing performance in 1997. With public demand for greater performance measurement in health care, the Joint Commission added a performance-measure component called ORYX to the accreditation process. Although much more flexible, the ORYX system was also more complex than other systems such as HEDIS. ORYX allowed health care organizations to determine which measures were most germane to organizational needs and report those metrics as part of the accreditation process for the Joint Commission. For hospitals and long-term care, home care, and behavioral health care organizations, the total number of measures that organizations are required to identify, collect, and submit has been set at a minimum of six. Originally, the ORYX measurement sets were linked to a certain percentage of an institution's patient volume, but those requirements were dropped. The Joint Commission has recently added a requirement to report four core measures, but in those cases for which the core measures are not applicable to a particular institution, they can be supplanted by non-core metrics that are agreed upon by the JCAHO and the institution.

Core measures fall into four categories that are related to those required by the federal government for evaluating Medicare patients in hospitals: acute myocardial infarction, heart failure, community-acquired pneumonia, and pregnancy and related conditions. The overlap of these measures with other accrediting organization measures provides health care organizations with the ability to track one set of measures for several accrediting bodies. This coordination of effort has resulted from the collaboration of the JCAHO with the NCQA and the American Medical Association through the Performance Measurement Coordinating Council.

The objective of the Joint Commission in this approach is to preserve the ability of the institution to choose which performance measures are most relevant for quality improvement. Performance measurement systems must be process and/or outcome measures that can be tracked over time and used for internal benchmarking and external comparisons. The Joint Commission plans to use the collected data to monitor the progress of each institution in improving quality and directing the priority focus process to make site visit reviews more helpful for health care organizations trying to improve their performance.

Performance Measurement Coordinating Council

With all of the potential measures that can be used for evaluating the performance of health care organizations, the amount of data and analysis could easily become overwhelming. For this reason, the Joint Commission joined the American Medical Association and the NCQA to create the Performance Measurement Coordinating Council to coordinate measurement systems and minimize redundancy and confusion. The organization began meeting in May 1998, and although each of the organizations intends to continue its own measurement systems, greater efforts will be made to coordinate measures to provide a better indication of the quality of care over the continuum. The JCAHO core measures in the ORYX system represent one example of the results of these efforts. Presently, the Council meets and makes recommendations annually.

◆ ## Foundation for Accountability

The Foundation for Accountability (FACCT) is a not-for-profit organization governed by a board of trustees from consumer organizations and purchasers of health care services and insurance. The FACCT creates tools that help people understand and use quality information, develops consumer-focused quality measures, supports public education about health care quality, supports efforts to gather and provide quality information, and encourages health policy to empower and inform consumers. Although the FACCT does not currently perform accreditation reviews, the organization is included in this chapter because it has helped produce performance measures that are used by other accrediting bodies. The organization was formed through the efforts of the Jackson Hole Group, a health policy think tank in Jackson Hole, Wyoming, in 1996 and published a set of performance measures later that year.

In 1997, FACCT introduced the FACCT consumer information framework in response to a request from CMS for a method of helping Medicare beneficiaries understand the flood of quality data that is being released by Medicare+Choice plans. The FACCT consumer information framework guides the creation of information resources for consumers to improve their understanding of health care quality, allowing comparison of the performance of health plans and providers. To create the framework, the FACCT worked with hundreds of consumers to discern issues of importance and then created performance measures for these parameters. The framework has three key components: (1) messages, (2) a model, and (3) measures.

Messages help people think about quality and the health care system in a new way. The messages are designed to (1) emphasize facts and eliminate misunderstandings; (2) educate and motivate consumers to consider quality in health care decisions; and (3) make comparative quality information useful and informative. The FACCT is developing educational language and approaches to convey these messages effectively in print, interactive settings, and live workshops. In addition, the FACCT has developed display formats and explanations that make comparative information easy for consumers to understand and use.

The model of the framework organizes comparative information about quality performance into five categories based on how consumers think about their care.

- ◆ **The Basics** deals with relationships with physicians, rules for getting care, information and service, and consumer satisfaction.
- ◆ **Staying Healthy** involves preventive care, reduction of health risks, early detection of illness, and education.
- ◆ **Getting Better** means recovery through appropriate treatment and follow-up.
- ◆ **Living With Illness** is about self-care for chronic illness, controlling symptoms, and avoiding complications.
- ◆ **Changing Needs** deals with catastrophic changes in health status through the use of comprehensive services, caregiver support, and hospice care.

The FACCT developed an eight-step process for standardizing quality measures for each of the five categories and subcategories, and the process can be used to create scores to measure performance for specific clinical conditions. Measures have been derived from a number of sources, including HEDIS and the CAHPS, as well as measures previously developed by the FACCT.

FACCT Measures

The first measurement sets were released by the FACCT shortly after the creation of the organization in 1996. Since that time, the FACCT has published measures and surveys for a number of clinical conditions, including

- ◆ adult arthritis
- ◆ adult and pediatric asthma
- ◆ adolescent care
- ◆ alcohol misuse
- ◆ breast cancer
- ◆ cardiovascular disease
- ◆ diabetes
- ◆ major depressive disorders
- ◆ health status
- ◆ health risks
- ◆ human immunodeficiency virus (HIV) infection
- ◆ adults and children with special health care needs

All of these measurement sets and surveys are available on the organization's Web site (Foundation for Accountability, 2003), and examples of several FACCT measures are included as Table 11.3.

The FACCT completed development of new measures for early childhood development, children with chronic illness, adolescent health, HIV/AIDS care, and end-of-life care in 2000. These measures became part of the organization's Internet site and part of the evolution of online tools for consumers to use to evaluate their care. As part of these efforts, the Child and Adolescent Health Measurement Initiative was launched, and the measures that resulted are now being used in over 25 states. In 2002, the organization launched a consumer-oriented Web site, the Clearinghouse, for materials for consumers to use in evaluating health care.

Table 11.3 Sample FACCT Measures

DISORDER	MEASURE
Adult asthma	◆ Patient education
	◆ Peak flow meter possession and use
	◆ Correct inhaler use
	◆ Experience and satisfaction with care
	◆ Patient functional status (SF-36)
	◆ Patient-reported symptom level
	◆ Patient self-management knowledge and behavior
	◆ Ability to maintain daily activities
Alcohol misuse	◆ Performance of population health screening for alcohol misuse
	◆ Routine alcohol misuse screening
	◆ Accessibility of provider and adequacy of information on alcohol use
	◆ Quality of alcohol risk reduction information and education from provider
	◆ Quality of alcohol risk reduction information from health plan
Breast cancer	◆ Mammography rate
	◆ Early stage (0 or 1) detection
	◆ Proportion of patients informed about radiation therapy options
	◆ Proportion of patients informed about breast conserving surgery
	◆ Radiation therapy following breast conserving surgery
	◆ Patient satisfaction with care
	◆ Experience of disease on CYC survey
	◆ Five-year disease-free survival (cancer treatment center measure)

continues

Table 11.3 *continued*

DISORDER	MEASURE
Diabetes	◆ Proportion of patients with foot exams on annual physical examination
	◆ Frequency of HbA1c testing
	◆ Retinal exams
	◆ Advice to quit smoking
	◆ Patient satisfaction
	◆ Patient functional status (SF-36)
	◆ HbA1c control
	◆ Lipid levels
	◆ Smoking cessation
	◆ Patient ability to maintain daily activities
Major depressive disorder	◆ Percentage of patients lost to follow-up
	◆ Patient satisfaction
	◆ Patient functional status (SF-36)
	◆ Proportion of patients in remittance in six months
	◆ Patient ability to maintain daily activities
Health status	◆ Improving or maintaining the physical and mental health of adults aged 18–64 years (SF-36)
Health risk	◆ Advice to quit smoking
	◆ Awareness of health habits
	◆ Completion of smoking cessation
Customer satisfaction	◆ Getting needed care
	◆ Skill of providers
	◆ Choice of providers
	◆ Good results from treatment
	◆ Recommend health plan to others
	◆ Relationships and communications with providers
	◆ Overall quality of health plan

CYC, Compare Your Care.

◆ Malcolm Baldrige National Quality Award

The Malcolm Baldrige National Quality Award was established in 1987 when Congress passed P.L. 100-107. The Baldrige award has many purposes, including

◆   promotion of awareness of the importance of quality improvement to the national economy

◆ recognition of organizations that have made substantial improvements in products, services, and overall competitive performance
◆ fostering sharing of best practices information among US organizations

Managed by the National Institute of Standards and Technology through the board of overseers of the Malcolm Baldrige National Quality Award, the program has become a factor in the health care industry through the prestige that can be garnered from winning the award.

The Baldrige award program promotes both conceptual and institutional strategies. The conceptual part of the strategy includes the creation of consensus criteria that project clear values, set high standards, focus on key requirements for organizational excellence, and create means for assessing progress relative to these requirements. The institutional part of the strategy then applies the consensus criteria for consistent communications within and among organizations of all types. Such communications stimulate broad involvement and cooperation and create an environment conducive to sharing information. Baldrige award recipients are expected to share their experiences and knowledge to advance the quality efforts of American organizations. Since the inception of the Award in 1987, health care professionals have served on the organization's board of examiners. By 1993, the Baldrige award foundation decided to establish a health care award and began studying the issue in 1994. Criteria for the health care industry were adopted by 1997, and reviews for the Award were first conducted in 1999.

The Baldrige program is based on core values established by the governance board for the award. The values are embedded in the criteria used to benchmark and evaluate organizations, and they represent the foundation for integrating organizational processes and results into a continually improving, learning organization. The core values include

◆ visionary leadership
◆ patient-focused excellence
◆ organizational and personal learning
◆ valuing staff and partners
◆ agility
◆ focus on the future
◆ managing for innovation
◆ management by fact
◆ social responsibility and community health
◆ focus on results and creating value
◆ systems perspective

These values represent the practices of the best-in-class organizations in the United States and have evolved since the inception of the Baldrige program. The health care criteria evolved from these core values with the use of the business criteria that had been established for American industry, and include the following categories:

- leadership
- strategic planning
- focus on patients, other customers, and markets
- information and analysis
- staff focus
- process management
- organizational performance results

Each category includes specific items for evaluating an organization's performance, and volunteer examiners for the Baldrige Award use specific criteria within each of these categories (National Institute for Standards and Technology, 2003). The review process involves three stages: (1) submission of an application by an organization, review of the application by several examiners, and assignment of a score to the application; (2) consensus teleconferences among the examiners and assignment of a consensus score; and (3) a site visit for successful applicants. At each stage, trained examiners from many industries review an application using the Baldrige criteria. Successful applicants receive the award from the President of the United States in the spring of each year. The criteria for the Baldrige Award are in many ways similar to those used by the Joint Commission (Fisher and Simmons, 1996), but they emphasize the business organizational aspects to a much greater extent.

The Baldrige criteria can be used as a self-assessment mechanism for institutions trying to achieve organizational excellence. The items within each one of the criteria specify the parameters for meeting the goal of excellent performance, and a health care organization can use these items as an evaluation method for a self-assessment. The self assessment can be the basis for continuous improvement efforts throughout the enterprise.

The first Baldrige Award recipient in health care was named in 2003. SSM Healthcare in St. Louis, MO, received the award and has shared a great deal of its expertise with the industry through its Web site (SSM Healthcare, 2003).

◆ International Organization for Standardization 9000

The International Organization for Standardization (ISO) is composed of national standards organizations from over 130 countries (Simmons, 1998). Established in 1947, the ISO seeks to promote the development of standardization and related activities to facilitate international trade and to foster cooperation throughout the business community by improving communications. ISO standards are promulgated by a number of industry-specific committees that focus on issues of quality and standardization. The goal of these committees is to facilitate trade, exchange, and technology transfer through standardization, with the following effects:

◆ improved product quality and reliability at a reasonable price
◆ adherence to health, safety, and environmental protection standards
◆ reduction of waste
◆ greater compatibility of goods and services from different companies and countries
◆ simplification for improved usability and cost-effectiveness
◆ reduction in cost through reduction in the number of models
◆ increased distribution, efficiency, and ease of maintenance

These goals closely follow those of total quality management systems, and the international focus of the ISO is designed to provide the impetus for improvements across the continuum of goods and services. ISO standards have been promulgated in numerous industries as diverse as automobile manufacturing and oil rigs. The ISO 9000 series of standards relating to quality management are considered most germane to health care.

Representation in the ISO is limited to only one organization in each country, chosen because it is the most representative of standardization in its country. The United States representative is the American National Standards Institute in New York. Over 2850 committees with over 30,000 members meet throughout the world to conduct the business of the ISO (International Organization for Standardization, 1999), and all of these activities are coordinated by a general secretariat in Geneva, Switzerland. Each member organization may have a representative on any committee. These committees develop voluntary, industrywide ISO standards by consensus, and after an exhaustive review and comment period by member organizations, the standard is added to the ISO catalog of standards, which currently contains over 12,000 standards.

The ISO 9000 standards were first published in 1987 as generic management system standards. These criteria were designed to help companies systematize the flow of goods and services through the firm, with the goal of improving value by improving quality and lowering cost. The standardized definition of quality in ISO 9000 refers to all those features of a product (or service) that are required by the customer. "Quality management" means what the organization does to ensure that its products conform to the requirements of the customer. In contrast to the reviews performed by the NCQA, the Joint Commission, and the URAC, ISO 9000 relates only to a company's processes, not its outcomes. For companies that have successfully implemented ISO 9000 standards, the outcomes (products or services) have usually improved, but, again, the focus of the intervention was on the process, not the outcome. ISO certification, therefore, is not a product or service validation but rather a sign that an organization has effective processes for producing quality output. In 2000, a new set of standards were published (International Organization for Standardization, 1999), consisting of ISO 9000 (definitions and concepts), ISO 9001 (quality systems requirements), and ISO 9004 (guidance for quality improvement).

ISO 9001 and 9004 standards have been created to provide consistency between the standards for demonstrating the ability to meet customer needs (ISO 9001) and the methods for developing a comprehensive quality management system (ISO 9004). These new standards are based on the following quality improvement principles (International Organization for Standardization, 1999):

◆ customer-focused organization
◆ leadership
◆ involvement of people
◆ process approach
◆ system approach to management
◆ continual improvement
◆ factual approach to decision making
◆ mutually beneficial supplier relationship

The new version of ISO 9001 combines several standards into a single set of criteria addressing four main areas: (1) management responsibility, (2) resource management, (3) product and/or service realization, and (4) measurement, analysis, and improvement.

One deviation from the ISO concentration on process is the new requirement for customer satisfaction measurement, which in health care systems would be considered one type of outcome measurement. Resource allocation includes intangible resources, such as information and communication, as well as the usual equipment and monetary resource requirements.

Use of ISO 9000 in Health Care

ISO 9001 are useful frameworks to evaluate and improve quality and operations within an organization. The standards are directed at the following objectives:

◆ a better understanding of quality practices throughout the organization
◆ to ensure continued use of the quality system required by the ISO
◆ improved documentation of quality activities
◆ improved awareness of quality improvement efforts
◆ enhancement of both supplier and customer confidence and relationships
◆ increased profitability and reduced costs
◆ to provide a foundation for improvement activities and compliance with other accrediting agencies

ISO 9000 compliance does not necessarily indicate that every service meets the requirements of the customer, only that the quality system that is deployed is capable of meeting standards. Like the Baldrige criteria, ISO 9001 requirements describe what must be done to make up a quality system, not how to set it up.

The ISO is not intended to replace the JCAHO, URAC, NCQA, or College of American Pathologists (CAP) accreditation processes but it does make the compliance demonstration process much easier to manage, less time-consuming, and less costly. A particular benefit can be realized for blood banking organizations because the American Association of Blood Banking standards are based on the same principles and concepts as the ISO 9001 standards.

The registration process is made up of three primary activities: 1) a document review that assesses whether all of the requirements of the standard have been addressed; 2) the onsite audit that determines whether all of the processes have been implemented; and 3) annual follow-up visits to ensure that the system is maintained. A qualified registrar selects an audit team based on their knowledge and experience in the health care industry and expertise in QI principles and methods. The audit team submits a flexible time schedule prior to the audit so that the organization can prepare. During the site visit, the audit team interviews staff members, reviews policies and procedures, observes operations, and assesses results to ensure compliance with ISO standards. In contrast to many review processes, the audit team discusses issues as they arise during the site visit, instead of creating a report at the end of the on-site activity. At the end of the site visit, the audit team conducts an exit conference to discuss the findings of the review.

Any issues that arise during the audit are openly discussed as they occur. In this way, there will be no surprises, and the organization will know exactly where it stands during the entire process. A short debriefing will take place at the end of each day as an overall review. After the assessment is completed, the audit team will have a closing meeting to officially discuss the audit findings and determine whether or not the organization is being recommended for registration.

Although not widely used in the health care industry at this point, the ISO 9000 standards can prove useful in a number of ways. First, the standards provide a generic, internationally accepted method of approaching QI. Although there might be some nuances of application to health care, the specifics of these applications should not be difficult to customize. Because the standards are generic and so widely accepted, payers who are familiar with the standards could conceivably begin to require health care organizations to comply with the standards and undergo registration with a certified ISO 9000 registrar, much as credentials verification organizations, physician organizations, and managed behavioral health organizations now can be certified by NCQA to satisfy contractual requirements for managed care organizations. A few health care organizations have begun to realize this potential and have undergone registration with an ISO 9000 registrar (Pulaski Community Hospital, 2003).

Second, the effect of working to comply with ISO 9000 standards will provide focus for the QI efforts of an organization. Nothing focuses employees on an issue better than the drive for achievement of a goal. NCQA and Joint Commission reviews require employees to organize information and implement policies to achieve certification, and working toward ISO 9000 can have the same effect, except that it is purely directed toward improving organizational processes.

Finally, achievement of ISO 9000 certification can make an organization more competitive because the international imprimatur of quality bestows substantial credibility. Payers may be more willing to relent on price issues if ISO 9000 quality mechanisms are in place, and payers may even contract preferentially with the organization that has achieved ISO 9000 registration. As the merits of the ISO 9000 system become well understood in the health care sector, registration through this source could reduce the regulatory burden in the industry. The advent of the ISO 9000:2000 series of standards could provide the impetus for broader adoption of the standards for health care.

◆ QI and Reducing Risk

Health care organizations will come under increasing pressure to implement QI programs over the next few years, and failure to properly introduce effective plans could increase an organization's medical–legal liability. Care plans and CPGs with best practices identified by national organizations are becoming increasingly widespread, and failure to comply with a well-publicized care plan has been used as a theory for liability in a number of cases (Forkner, 1996; Jacobson, 1997; King, 1997). Additionally, government regulatory agencies will demand adherence to internally and externally developed QI policies as a means of preventing fraud and abuse as well as ensuring quality (Mills, 1999; National Senior Citizens' Law Center, 1997; Sage, et al., 1994).

On the other hand, QI interventions can also do harm (Applebaum, 1993; Lo and Groman, 2003), and practitioners must be prepared to override interventions that are detrimental to patient care in some situations (Beerworth and Tiller, 1998; Manuel, 1996). When providers are proscribed from performing certain procedures or even excluded from hospital staffs due to quality issues, restraint-of-trade actions by physicians against institutions may result (Brown vs. Presbyterian Health Care Services, 1996). Although the Health Care Quality Improvement Act of 1986 provided physicians immunity for peer review activities, cases such as Brown have demonstrated that such QI efforts can still be overturned.

QI efforts often result from risk management interventions (Scott, et al., 1996; Spoon, et al., 1996), and one of the underlying benefits of a QI program should be to reduce risk in the institution (Reeves, et al., 1995). In most cases, interventions for QI should reduce liability to providers and institutions because the interventions should increase the quality of care, thus reducing errors and adverse outcomes. The QI approach was identified as a method of reducing medical errors by the Institute of Medicine in the 2001 book *Crossing the Quality Chasm*. Inherent in this assumption is the need for continually monitoring the results of interventions to ensure that the outcomes that were predicted actually occur.

◆ Regulatory Agencies and the Growth of QI in Health Care

Although the health care industry has been slow (in societal terms) to adopt QI methodologies as a means of improving care and reducing costs, a number of government and regulatory bodies are imposing these techniques on the industry through the regulatory and accreditation systems. The next chapter examines the future of QI in health care, with emphasis on society's escalating demand for increased value in health care and increasing consumerism in the care delivery system.

◆ Discussion Points

1. What is the function of the Quality Improvement System for Managed Care (QISMC)? For which sector(s) in the health care delivery system was QISMC designed and why?
2. Provisions of Domain 1 of the QISMC relate to quality improvement. Discuss quality improvement methods implicit in the regulations within the domain.
3. Give a brief description of the National Committee for Quality Assurance (NCQA). How are reviews by the NCQA designed to improve quality?
4. Discuss the role of the Health Plan Employer Data and Information Set (HEDIS) measures in measuring the quality of care in managed care organizations. Do managed care organizations have control over all of the variables that are measured by HEDIS?
5. The Consumer Assessment of Health Plans Survey (CAHPS) was created by the Agency for Healthcare Research and Quality (AHRQ) to assess consumer satisfaction with health plans. How does the CAHPS measure satisfaction? Could a managed care organization add a few questions and improve the survey?
6. The Utilization Review Accreditation Committee (URAC) was created to review what types of organizations? What types of reviews does URAC perform at the present time?
7. The ORYX initiative of the Joint Commission on Accreditation of Healthcare Organizations (JCAHO) is designed to measure performance

in health care organizations. Discuss how the ORYX approach differs from those of the QISMC and HEDIS.

8. What is the function of the Performance Measurement Coordinating Council? How will it improve quality in health care organizations?

9. The Foundation for Accountability has designed a number of measures for disease entities of interest to the health care industry. Discuss how these measures differ from the clinical measures in HEDIS.

10. The Malcolm Baldrige National Quality Award has been available since 1987. Why have health care organizations not pursued the award more actively? How do the Baldrige criteria promote quality improvement in health care organizations?

11. International Organization for Standardization (ISO) 9000 standards are internationally accepted and based on sound quality improvement science. How might they be influential in the future of quality improvement in health care?

12. How can health care organizations reduce their risk with quality improvement approaches?

◆ Notes

Agency for Healthcare Research and Quality. (1999, December). *Consumer assessment of health plans survey (CAHPS). Fact sheet* (AHCPR Pub. No. 97-R079). Rockville, MD: Agency for Health Care Policy and Research. Available from *http://www.ahcpr.gov/qual/cahpfact.htm*

Applebaum P. S. (1993). Legal liability and managed care. *American Psychologist, 48,* 251–257.

Beerworth E. E., and Tiller J. W. (1998). Liability in prescribing choice: The example of the antidepressants. *Australia / New Zealand Journal of Psychiatry, 32*(4), 560–566.

Beaulieu D., and Epstein A. (2002). National Committee for Quality Assurance health-plan accreditation: predictors, correlates of performance, and market impact. *Medical Care, 40*(4), 325–337.

Brown v. Presbyterian Health Care Services, No. 96-2013 (10th Cir. 1996). Retrieved September 2003, from *http://www.law.emory.edu/10circuit/nov96/95-2293.wpd.html*

Centers for Medicare and Medicaid Services. (2002). *National health care by type of expenditure: Calendar year 2000.* Retrieved September 2003, from *http://cms.hhs.gov/researchers/pubs/datacompendium/2002/02pg12.pdf*

Centers for Medicare and Medicaid Services. (2003). *Quality Improvement system for managed care (QISMC).* Retrieved September 2003, from *http://cms.hhs.gov/cop/2d.asp*

The Commonwealth Fund. (2002, April). *Medicare managed care: Medicare+Choice at five years* (Issue Brief No. 537). Barry C., and Kline J. Available from *http://www.cmwf.org/programs/medfutur/barry_fiveyears_ib_537.pdf*

Fisher D. C., and Simmons B. P. (1996). *The Baldrige workbook for healthcare.* New York: Quality Resources.

Forkner D. J. (1996). Clinical pathways: Benefits and liabilities [Electronic version]. *Nursing Management,* 30:8 Retrieved August 1999, from *http://www.springnet.com/ce/m611a.htm*

Foundation for Accountability. (2003). *Measuring quality*. Retrieved September 2003, from *http://www.facct.org*

International Organization for Standardization. (1999, January 8). *The Magical Demystifying Tour of ISO 9000 and ISO 14000*. Retrieved November 2003, from *http://www.iso.ch/iso/en/iso9000-14000/basics/general/basics_1.html*

International Organization for Standardization. (May 1999). *The year 2000 revision of ISO 9000 quality management standards*. Retrieved May 1999, from *http://www.iso.ch/9000e/execabstract.htm*

International Organization for Standardization. (30 June 1999). *Quality management principles and guidelines on their application*. Retrieved June 1999, from *http//www.bsi.org.uk/iso-tc176-sc2/N376.doc*

Jacobson P. (1997). Legal and policy considerations in using clinical practice guidelines. *American Journal of Cardiology, 80*(8B), 74H–79H.

King J. (1997). Practice guidelines and medical malpractice litigation. *Med Law., 16*(1):29–39.

Lo B., and Groman M. (2003). Oversight of quality improvement: Focusing on benefits and risks. *Archives of Internal Medicine, 163*(12), 1481–1486.

Manuel B. M. (1996). Physician liability under managed care. *Journal of the American College of Surgeons, 182*(6), 537–546.

McDermott W., and Emery W. M. (1999). *Medicare+Choice interim final rules*. Retrieved August 1999, from *http://www.mwe.com/news/hlu1509.htm*

Mills G. (1999). *Preventing fraud and abuse allegations when furnishing services performed by home health aides*. Retrieved March 1999, from *http://www.aahha.org/actiongram.html*

National Committee for Quality Assurance. *NCQA's state of health care quality—2003*. Retrieved September 2003, from *http://www.ncqa.org/Communications/News/sohc2003.htm*

National Committee for Quality Assurance. (2003–2). *Physician organization certification status list*. Retrieved September 2003, from *http://hprc.ncqa.org/pocresult.asp*

National Committee for Quality Assurance. (2003). *CVO certification status list*. Retrieved September 2003, from *http://hprc.ncqa.org/cvoResult.asp*

National Institute for Standards and Technology. (2003). Retrieved September 2003, from *http://www.baldrige.gov*

National Senior Citizens' Law Center. (1997, November 7). HCFA retreats from regulatory role. *Nursing Home Law Newsletter.*

Pulaski Community Hospital. (2003). *Pulaski Community Hospital meets ISO quality standards yet again*. Retrieved September 2003, from *http://www.pch-va.com/CustomPage.asp?guidCustomContentID={18DC6BE5-40A2-11D4-A2E1-00508B62BE1F}*

Reeves S., Matney K., Crane V. (1995). Continuous QI as an ideal in hospital practice. *Health Care Supervisor, 13*(4), 1–12.

Sage W. M., Hastings K. E., Berenson R. A. (1994). Enterprise liability for medical malpractice and health care QI. *American Journal of Law and Medicine, 20*(1–2), 1–28.

Scott F. F., Levitsky M. E., Smith J. A., Flannery K., Agesen S. (1996). Organizational risk management: A case study. *Caring, 15*(9), 40–47.

Simmons D. (1998). Examining ISO 9000 in health care. *Quality Digest, 18*(3), 26–30.

Spoon B. D., Hamlin A., Lowry J., Reimels E. (1996). CQI applications in a community hospital. *Nursing Connections, 9*(2), 35–42.

SSM Healthcare. (2003). Retrieved September 2003, from *http://www.ssmhc.com/internet/home/ssmcorp.nsf/documents/our+quality+journey*

Utilization Review Accreditation Commission. (2003). *States that recognize URAC/American Accreditation Health Care Commission Accreditation.* Retrieved September 2003, from *http://www.urac.org/govrecognition_main.asp?navid=govrecognition&pagename=govrecognition_main*

Appendix 11.A

QISMC Domain 1

DOMAIN 1: Quality Assessment and Performance Improvement (QAPI) Program

STANDARD NUMBER	DESCRIPTION OF STANDARD

1.1   *Basic Requirements. The organization:*

1.1.1   *Achieves required minimum performance levels, as established by CMS (for Medicare) or by the State Medicaid agency (for Medicaid), on standardized quality measures;*

1.1.2   *Conducts performance improvement projects that achieve, through ongoing measurement and intervention, demonstrable and sustained improvement in significant aspects of clinical care and non-clinical services that can be expected to have a beneficial effect on health outcomes and enrollee satisfaction; and*

1.1.3   *Corrects significant systemic problems that come to its attention through internal surveillance, complaints, or other mechanisms.*

The basic requirements for this domain establish three distinct, but related, strategies for promoting high quality health care in organizations serving Medicare or Medicaid enrollees. First, each managed care organization must meet certain required levels of performance when providing specific health care and related services to enrollees. These required levels of performance will be established by CMS (for Medicare) or the State Medicaid agency (for Medicaid). For example, a State agency might require all organizations with Medicaid enrollees to achieve, at a minimum, a specific numerical rate (e.g., 80 percent) of immunization of Medicaid children. The minimum performance level would be established by examining historical performance levels, as well as benchmarks (best practices), of managed care organizations and other delivery systems with respect to immunizing children.

Second, managed care organizations must conduct performance improvement projects that are outcome-oriented and that achieve demonstrable and sustained improvement in care and services. The standards expect that an organization will continuously monitor its own performance on a variety of dimensions of care and services for enrollees, identify its own areas for potential improvement, carry out individual projects to undertake system interventions to improve care, and monitor the effectiveness of those interventions.

Third, the organization must take timely action to correct significant systemic problems that come to its attention through internal surveillance, complaints, or other mechanisms. For instance, if an external quality review organization discovers a systemic problem pertaining to an aspect of care delivery as a result of performing an analysis of quality of care on a different aspect of health care, the organization is expected to address the problem promptly.

The succeeding standards in this domain elaborate on the basic requirements set forth in standard 1.1 (standards 1.2, 1.3, and 1.4) and specify requirements pertaining to the infrastructure necessary in a managed care organization to carry out the activities required in this domain (standards 1.5 and 1.6):

◆ Standard 1.2, *Performance Levels*, specifies that organizations must report their performance on standardized measures and achieve established performance levels for specified measures.

◆ Standard 1.3, *Performance Improvement Projects*, requires that an organization's individual improvement projects, in the aggregate, address a broad spectrum of key aspects of enrollee care and services. It also includes specifications for phase-in of these requirements.

◆ Standard 1.4, *Attributes of Performance Improvement Projects*, establishes criteria for promoting the validity, methodologic soundness and effectiveness of each performance improvement project carried out by an organization. In addition to the guidelines contained in this document for implementing and assessing quality improvement projects, readers are directed to "Health Care Quality Improvement Studies in Managed Care Settings—Design and Assessment" a technical assistance manual developed by and available from the National Committee for Quality Assurance under CMS contract CMS-92-1279.

◆ Standard 1.5, *Health Information System*, specifies the characteristics of an organization's information systems needed to support its QAPI program.

◆ Standard 1.6, *Administration of the QAPI Program*, specifies basic structural and procedural requirements for the organization's QAPI program, including a requirement that the organization routinely assess the effectiveness of its QAPI program.

1.2   *Performance Levels.*

1.2.1   *The organization measures its performance, using standard measures established or adopted by CMS (for Medicare) or by the State Medicaid agency (for Medicaid), and reports its performance to the applicable agency.*

1.2.2   *The organization achieves any minimum performance levels that may be established by CMS (for Medicare) or by the State Medicaid agency (for Medicaid) with respect to the standard measures.*

1.2.3   *The organization meets any goals for performance improvement on specific measures that may be established for that particular organization by CMS (for Medicare) or by the State Medicaid agency (for Medicaid).*

The particular measures for which reporting is required are not specified in these standards, so as not to limit CMS's and State Medicaid agencies' ability to adapt to new developments in the measurement of health care quality. Performance measures typically required by CMS and State Medicaid agencies address: how well the care provided by an organization meets established standards for preventive care or the care and treatment of certain health conditions, how well an organization assures access and appropriate utilization of services, and measures of beneficiaries' experience with the care provided. Performance measures specified by State Medicaid agencies and CMS may be contained in standardized national data collection and reporting instruments such as HEDIS and CAHPS. They may also be standardized measures unique to a State or specified solely by CMS. CMS and each State Medicaid agency, in advance of each contract year, will decide on the measures for which reporting will be required and will notify organizations of those measures. *(Note: Minimum performance level reporting and compliance activities regarding assessment of M+CO performance on this standard will not be implemented before 2002.)*

1.3 *Performance Improvement Projects. Projects conducted under the organization's QAPI program address and achieve improvement in major focus areas of clinical care and nonclinical services.*

1.3.1 *Definitions*

1.3.1.1 *A project is an initiative by the organization to measure its own performance in one or more of the focus areas described in standards 1.3.4 and 1.3.5, undertake system interventions to improve its performance, and follow-up on the effectiveness of those interventions.*

Assessment of the effectiveness of an organization's QAPI program will include review of individual performance improvement projects. In the first two years, review will focus on whether an organization has initiated performance improvement projects. In all subsequent years, reviews will focus on whether or not projects have achieved demonstrable improvement in quality indicators. For each project, the organization will be required to supply documentation sufficient to assess the extent to which the project has met all relevant Domain I standards, most especially standard 1.4 regarding achievement of demonstrable and sustained improvement.

1.3.1.2 *Project topics and the quality indicators used to assess each project are chosen either by the organization itself, or by CMS (for Medicare) or by the State Medicaid agency (for Medicaid) either for an individual organization or on a national or Statewide basis.*

The organization will be required to conduct projects relating to certain topics selected by CMS or the State Medicaid agency, as well as projects relating to topics of its own choosing, as outlined in standards 1.3.2 and 1.3.3.

1.3.1.3 *A project will be considered to have achieved demonstrable improvement in a focus area during any review year in which an improvement meeting the minimum thresholds of standard 1.4.4 is attained.*

It is not expected that a project initiated in a given year will necessarily achieve improvement in that same year. Some—for example, a project focusing on improving health outcomes for patients with a given condition—might continue for several years before it would be possible to measure the effect of the organization's interventions. Such a project would not be counted as achieving improvement until the year in which the necessary level of improvement is demonstrated. (An exception for certain multi-year projects is provided under standard 1.3.7.2.)

1.3.1.4 *The first review year begins on a date established by CMS (for Medicare) or by the State Medicaid agency (for Medicaid).*

All subsequent review years begin on the anniversary of the beginning of the first review year. Note that review years are not defined in terms of the dates on which reviews by CMS or States are actually conducted. There may be instances in which an organization completes a project after the end of a review year but before the review for that year is conducted. In this case, the organization may ask that the project be considered in the review for the past review year, provided that all necessary documentation is available at the time of the review.

1.3.2 *Phase-in Requirements. An organization has a two-year phase-in period during which its projects are not required to achieve demonstrable improvement assuming a three-year project cycle.*

1.3.2.1 *Phase-in requirements for an organization contracting with Medicare or Medicaid but not both:*

1.3.2.1.1 *By the end of the first review year, the organization has initiated at least two projects addressing two of the focus areas specified under standard 1.3.4 and/or 1.3.5. For an organization contracting with Medicare, one of those projects relates to a topic and involves quality indicators chosen by CMS. For an organization contracting with Medicaid, one of those projects may relate to a topic and involve quality indicators chosen by the State Medicaid agency.*

1.3.2.1.2 *By the end of the second review year, the organization has initiated at least two additional projects addressing two of the focus areas specified under standard 1.3.4 and/or 1.3.5 but which were not addressed by the projects initiated in the first review year. For an organization contracting with Medicare, one of those projects relates to a topic and involves quality indicators chosen by CMS. For an organization contracting with Medicaid, one of those projects may relate to a topic and involve quality indicators chosen by the State Medicaid agency.*

1.3.2.2 *Phase-in requirements for an organization contracting with both Medicare and Medicaid:*

1.3.2.2.1 *By the end of the first review year, the organization has initiated at least three projects addressing three of the focus areas specified under standard 1.3.4 and/or 1.3.5. One of those projects relates to a topic and involves quality indicators chosen by CMS. The second project relates to a topic and involves quality indicators chosen by the organization itself. The third project relates to a topic and involves quality indicators chosen either by the State Medicaid agency or the organization.*

1.3.2.2.2 *By the end of the second review year, the organization has initiated at least three additional projects addressing three of the focus areas specified under standard 1.3.4 and/or
1.3.5 but which were not addressed by the projects initiated in the first review year. One
of those projects relates to a topic and involves quality indicators chosen by CMS. The
second project relates to a topic and involves quality indicators chosen by the organization itself. The third project relates to a topic and involves quality indicators chosen either
by the State Medicaid agency or the organization.*

A project is considered to have been initiated when it has proceeded at least to
the point of baseline data collection. That is, the organization has selected a particular aspect of care for study, has identified the statistical indicator or indicators
that will be used, and has begun the process of collecting the data needed for an
initial assessment of its performance on the indicator(s). Review for the first year
will therefore focus on compliance with standards 1.4.1 through 1.4.3.

1.3.3 *Ongoing Requirements.*

1.3.3.1 *Requirement for an organization contracting with Medicare or Medicaid but not both: By
the end of the first review year after the two-year phase-in period, and each subsequent
review year, at least two of the organization's projects have achieved demonstrable improvement in two of the focus areas specified in 1.3.4 and/or 1.3.5. For an organization
contracting with Medicare, one of those projects has related to a topic and involved quality indicators chosen by CMS. For an organization contracting with Medicaid, one of those
projects may have related to a topic and involved quality indicators chosen by the State
Medicaid agency.*

1.3.3.2 *Requirement for an organization contracting with both Medicare and Medicaid: By the
end of the first review year after the two-year phase-in period, and each subsequent review year, at least three of the organization's projects have achieved demonstrable improvement in three of the focus areas specified in 1.3.4 and/or 1.3.5. One of those projects has related to a topic and involved quality indicators chosen by CMS. The second
project has related to a topic and involved quality indicators chosen by the organization
itself. The third project has related to a topic and involved quality indicators chosen either
by the State Medicaid agency or the organization.*

The purpose of performance improvement projects is to actually improve the
quality of care and services provided to Medicare and Medicaid beneficiaries. After the phase-in (start up) period described in standard 1.3.2.2, each plan that
contracts with either Medicare or Medicaid (but not both) will have to demonstrate every 12 months (beginning in the third review year) that it has improved
care or beneficiary health outcomes in at least two focus areas. These focus areas
may be in either clinical or non-clinical areas, as specified in 1.3.4 and 1.3.5. For an
organization contracting with both Medicare and Medicaid, this requirement is not
doubled—such an organization must show that it has achieved improvement in
three areas (again, in any combination of clinical and non-clinical areas) every
12 months.

1.3.3.3 *Requirements for all organizations.*

For Medicare, managed care organizations may use an existing on-going project for either of their required annual QAPI projects if that existing project meets certain requirements as defined annually by CMS. They must, however, conduct a remeasurement on the relevant quality indicators during this initiation year to establish a new baseline against which demonstrable improvement may be determined at the end of a three-year project period. M+C organizations are encouraged to contact CMS Regional Offices regarding the specific conditions under which such credit may be afforded for monitoring purposes. For Medicaid, it is at the discretion of the State to determine criteria for compliance with this standard.

1.3.3.3.1 *Before the organization initiates another project in a previously addressed focus area, it has initiated projects that achieve demonstrable improvement in all of the focus areas specified in 1.3.4 and 1.3.5, unless CMS (for Medicare) or the State Medicaid agency (for Medicaid) grants prior approval.*

1.3.3.3.2 *The project topics include both physical health and mental health/substance abuse, unless, in the case of an organization contracting with Medicaid, the organization's benefit structure doesn't permit this breadth.*

Although it is not possible for any organization to measure all aspects of health care provided to every beneficiary, it is possible for it to measure diverse aspects of care, and care provided to diverse populations of enrollees. By undertaking a variety of quality improvement projects, an organization can improve the quality of care provided to the greatest number of its enrollees and to those enrollees who, while perhaps not great in number, are those in greatest need; e.g., specially vulnerable populations such as the mentally ill, children with special health care needs. For this reason, the managed care organization will be required to assure that the chosen topic areas for quality improvement projects are not limited to only recurring, easily measured subsets of the health care needs of its enrolled population; e.g., primary preventive care of adults, high cost care of adults.

Quality improvement projects additionally must focus both on mental and physical conditions and their care, and on all ten clinical and non-clinical areas addressed in standards 1.3.4 and 1.3.5, before it can return to one of these focus areas. Because of the requirement that two areas be completed every year, a managed care organization should have covered all clinical and non-clinical focus areas every five years. At the end of the five-year cycle, CMS (for Medicare) or the State Medicaid agency (for Medicaid) will determine whether a managed care organization has included mental health and substance abuse topics among its performance improvement projects; if the managed care organization has not, CMS (for Medicare) or the State Medicaid agency (for Medicaid) will direct the organization to do so.

Because this standard creates a "distributive requirement" in that an organization may not repeat a project in a previously addressed focus area until all have been studied, managed care organizations must conduct studies which focus on a broad array of enrollee health issues.

1.3.4 *Clinical Focus Areas: Clinical focus areas applicable to all enrollees are as follows:*

CMS recognizes that it is possible to achieve improvement in multiple focus areas within the context of a single project. If an organization implements projects which achieve demonstrable improvement in several focus areas within a given year, these will not count as separate projects to meet the annual QAPI study initiation requirement (two for Medicare, three for dual eligible Medicare and Medicaid organizations).

Instead, in each focus area for which improvement is achieved, organizations will be given credit under the distributive requirement.

In addition, standard 1.3.1.2 allows CMS (for Medicare) and State Medicaid agencies (for Medicaid) to specify project topics and quality indicators to be used by a particular plan, if CMS or a State determines that the managed care organization has not achieved sufficient diversity in its quality improvement projects, such that important populations or health care services are not receiving sufficient attention within the managed care organization.

1.3.4.1 *Primary, secondary, and/or tertiary prevention of acute conditions;*

1.3.4.2 *Primary, secondary, and/or tertiary prevention of chronic conditions;*

1.3.4.3 *Care of acute conditions;*

1.3.4.4 *Care of chronic conditions;*

1.3.4.5 *High-volume services;*

1.3.4.6 *High-risk services; and*

1.3.4.7 *Continuity and coordination of care.*

Primary prevention consists of preventing a disease from occurring by reducing an individual's susceptibility to an illness; e.g., immunizations are a form of primary prevention. Secondary prevention takes place once an individual is already afflicted with a condition (e.g., hypertension, asthma, uterine cancer) but through secondary prevention (e.g., taking of medications, use of a peak flow meter, early detection) the effects of the condition can be controlled or prevented. Tertiary prevention is applicable when an illness has already caused disability, but the disability can be reduced or prevented from worsening; e.g., early treatment and rehabilitation of stroke victims.

Sometimes, however, quality improvement projects can focus not on a clinical condition, per se, but on a service, particularly a high-volume service, and how it can be improved. A managed care organization may target quality improvement in its labor and delivery services, in a frequently performed surgical procedure, or across different surgical or invasive procedures. In such cases, the managed care organization would be targeting the service, as opposed to a clinical condition.

A managed care organization also must target high-risk procedures even if they may sometimes be low in frequency. A managed care organization may assess experiences with care received from specialized centers inside or outside of the organization's network; e.g., burn centers, transplant centers, cardiac surgery centers. It could assess and improve the way in which it detects which of its members have functional disabilities and assess these members' satisfaction with the care received from the organization. It could also analyze high-risk conditions such as invasive procedures in ambulatory settings.

Finally, an organization must also improve continuity and coordination of care. Both of these characteristics of good quality health care address the manner in which care is provided when a patient receives care from multiple providers and across multiple episodes of care. Such studies may be disease or condition-specific or may target continuity and coordination across multiple conditions. For example, an organization could assess the extent to which care is coordinated across primary care providers and mental health providers subsequent to a discharge from an inpatient psychiatric facility.

1.3.5   *Non-clinical focus areas. Non-clinical focus areas applicable to all enrollees are as follows:*

1.3.5.1   *Availability, accessibility and cultural competency of services;*

Projects in this area should focus on assessing and improving the accessibility of specific services or services for specific conditions, including reducing disparities between services to minorities and services to other members (see also standard 1.4.4.1.4) as well as addressing barriers due to low health literacy. Projects may also focus on improving the effectiveness of communications with enrollees, targeting areas of improvement identified as a result of the evaluation conducted under standard 2.3.4.

This standard works in conjunction with standard 3.1.7.1 which requires the organization to develop and monitor its own standards of timely access to all services and continuously monitor its own compliance with these standards. This standard requires that the plan go beyond examining how it evaluates compliance with its own standards, but requires the plan to identify ways to exceed its own standards and continue to identify ways to improve the ability of consumers to receive the services that they need in a timely manner. For example, a project might focus on reduction of inpatient admissions for ambulatory sensitive conditions (those for which timely ambulatory care may prevent inpatient admissions). A project might address the promptness with which referral services are furnished in response to a positive result on a given diagnostic test.

For detailed guidance regarding definition and implementation of cultural competency requirements, see standard 3.1.5.

1.3.5.2   *Interpersonal aspects of care, e.g., quality of provider/patient encounters; and*

Donabedian defines the interpersonal components of health care as "... the management of the social and psychological interaction between client and practitioner." They include the milieu, manner, and behavior of the provider in delivering care to and communicating with the patient, and address such concerns as:

◆   Does a practitioner take sufficient time with the patient to explain an illness and answer questions?

◆   Is the patient examining room/physician office clean, comfortable, and easily accessible?

◆ Does the patient have to wait a long time in the office before seeing a provider?

Assessment of interpersonal aspects of care can be addressed through use of consumer surveys such as the CAHPS survey.

1.3.5.3 *Appeals, grievances, and other complaints.*

Projects related to the grievance and coverage determination processes may aim either to improve the processes themselves or to address an underlying issue in care or services identified through analysis of grievances or appeals. For example, an organization with a high rate of grievances not resolved until the third or fourth step in its grievance procedure might focus on how grievances are addressed in the initial phases of the process. An organization with a high rate of grievances related to one particular type of service might instead focus on improvements in access to or delivery of that service. Similarly, an organization with a high rate of adverse determinations overturned by the Medicare independent reconsideration contractor, or by the State agency administering the State fair hearing process, might aim to reduce this rate by improving its procedures for initial review of authorization requests. An organization with a high rate of sustained adverse determinations (for example, denials of inappropriate emergency room care) might instead focus on measures to improve provider and enrollee understanding of its procedures for obtaining covered services.

1.3.6 *Special projects.*

1.3.6.1 *CMS (for Medicare) or the State Medicaid agency (for Medicaid) may require an organization to conduct particular projects that are specific to the organization and that relate to topics and involve quality indicators of CMS's or the State Medicaid agency's choosing.*

The focus areas specified in standards 1.3.4 and 1.3.5 are intended to highlight key components of care and services for organizations serving a typical Medicare or Medicaid population. There may be instances in which CMS or the Medicaid agency believes that some aspects of care require greater emphasis, either because of the organization's relationship to populations with special health care needs or because the organization's performance is in need of greater improvement in some areas than in others. In this case, it may be appropriate for an organization to conduct more work in a specific area identified by CMS (for Medicare) or the State Medicaid agency (for Medicaid).

1.3.6.2 *Collaborative projects. Organizations may satisfy the requirements of standards 1.3.2 and 1.3.3 by collaborating with one another, subject to the approval of CMS or the State Medicaid agency.*

Some State Medicaid agencies, as well as CMS, have encouraged collaborative efforts, under which several contracting organizations undertake a joint quality improvement project addressing a common topic. For Medicare, PROs are not only the convening structure for national performance improvement projects, but they are also a regional presence for convening local collaborative performance improvement projects. These standards would not preclude such collaborative efforts under either Medicare or Medicaid. However, any such initiative would need to be individually evaluated and approved, and CMS or the State agency would establish criteria for assessing the extent to which each organization's participation constituted compliance with these standards. For example, if several organizations conducted a joint project to improve childhood immunization rates, the State might determine that all participating organizations would be considered as having addressed the focus area that is the subject of the project. However, the State would also need to decide how improvement should be measured. If aggregate immunization rates for the entire target population improved, would all participating organizations be considered as having achieved improvement, or would the improvement for each participant have to meet the minimum thresholds specified in standard 1.4.4? These guidelines do not establish a uniform principle for this kind of question; the appropriate answer will depend on features of each particular project (such as whether interventions involve administrative changes in each individual organization or changes in the practice patterns of practitioners who serve enrollees of multiple organizations).

1.3.7 *Multi-year projects. If a project is conducted over a period of more than one review year—*

1.3.7.1 *The project will be considered as achieving improvement in each year for which it achieves an improvement meeting the requirements specified in standard 1.4.4; or*

An organization may continue a project that has already been determined to have achieved demonstrable improvement. If further improvement occurs, the project may again be considered to have achieved demonstrable improvement. However, the improvement will not be measured relative to the original baseline, but relative to the improved performance level previously scored. For example, an organization could meet standard 1.4.4 in Year One by reducing its percentage of non-immunized children from a baseline of 20 percent to a level of 18 percent. It could continue the project for an additional year, and could meet the standard again in Year Two by reducing the percentage of non-immunized children to 16.2 percent. It is not necessary that the improvements be achieved in successive years for a project to be counted in this way. For example, a four-year project might achieve the 18 percent level in its second year, 17 percent in its third year, and 16 percent in its fourth year. It would then be considered as having achieved demonstrable improvement in the second and fourth years; the improvement in the third year would not be counted because it did not represent a 10 percent reduction from the previously scored level of 18 percent.

1.3.7.2 *A project may be considered as achieving improvement in each year for which it achieves an improvement that does not meet the requirements specified in standard 1.4.4, but that constitutes an intermediate target specified in a project work plan developed in consultation with CMS or the State Medicaid agency.*

An organization may undertake a particularly complex or difficult project that is not expected to achieve demonstrable improvement, as defined under standard 1.4.4, for several years (i.e., more than three years). This might occur because:

◆ Improvement in the targeted outcome cannot be measured for a long period; for example, the organization wishes to improve five-year survival rates for breast cancer.

◆ Improvement in outcomes can come only after process improvements that are not closely enough related to outcomes to meet the requirement of standard 1.4.3.2.

◆ Improvement will require multiple system interventions that cannot be implemented over a short period.

Such a project would not ordinarily be counted as achieving improvement until an improvement meeting the thresholds of standard 1.4.4 could be documented. The organization would then need to conduct other projects in the same focus area that achieve improvement more rapidly, because of the requirement that improvement be achieved in two areas during each twelve-month review period after the initial two-year phase-in period. This standard creates an exception for certain multi-year projects (more than three years) with measurable interim goals.

Prior approval is required for such a project. An organization that anticipates that it will meet the minimum requirements of this standard for a review year only if a multi-year project is counted must request advance review of the project plan at the time the project is initiated. A multi-year project may be approved under the following circumstances:

1. The timetable for the project is reasonably related to the complexity of the project or the length of time that must elapse before the outcomes of the project can be assessed. There must be a clear and defensible reason for defining a project as a multi-year project.

2. There must be significant ongoing activity related to the project during each of the review years for which the project is to be counted. For example, while a project that involves a one-time system change that is expected to affect five-year survival rates cannot measure its success until five years have elapsed, it will not necessarily be considered as an ongoing project during each of the intervening years. It would be treated as ongoing only if it provided for continuous data collection throughout the project period, along with ongoing efforts to identify and implement system changes aimed at improving the long-term outcome.

3. The project must specify some form of quantifiable interim goals or intermediate outcomes for each project year, so that it is possible to monitor the continuing progress of the project. For example, an organization conducting a project on breast cancer survival rates might track a process of care (such as mammography screening rates) or an intermediate outcome (such as stage of breast cancer at detection) and set goals for each year of the project.

1.4 *Attributes of Performance Improvement Projects*

An individual project involves: (1) identification of an aspect of clinical care or non-clinical services to be studied, (2) specification of quality indicators to measure performance in the selected area, (3) collection of baseline data, (4) identification and implementation of appropriate system interventions to improve performance, and (5) repeated data collection to assess the immediate and continuing effect of the interventions and determine the need for further action.

◆ Standard 1.4.1 addresses the relevance and importance of each project conducted by an organization.

◆ Standards 1.4.2 and 1.4.3 assess the meaningfulness of the specific performance indicators selected for measurement in an individual project and the validity and reliability of the measurement.

◆ Standards 1.4.4 and 1.4.5 evaluate the extent to which a project resulted in demonstrable and sustained improvement.

An individual project is regarded as successfully completed only if it meets each of these standards, 1.4.1 through 1.4.4. Because the key project components identified in those standards are interdependent, failure on any one of them invalidates the entire project. For example, if the organization chooses to measure its performance on quality indicators that have no likely relation to outcomes, improvement in the indicators cannot be expected to improve health or functional status. If the organization cannot collect reliable data, it cannot demonstrate improvement, and so on. The organization's documentation of a completed project must provide evidence of compliance with each standard.

1.4.1   *Selection of topics. Within each required focus area, the organization selects a specific topic or topics to be addressed by a project.*

1.4.1.1   *Topics are identified through continuous data collection and analysis by the organization of comprehensive aspects of patient care and member services.*

1.4.1.2   *Topics are systematically selected and prioritized to achieve the greatest practical benefit for enrollees.*

1.4.1.3   *Selection of topics takes into account: the prevalence of a condition among, or need for a specific service by, the organization's enrollees; enrollee demographic characteristics and health risks; and the interest of consumers in the aspect of care or services to be addressed.*

These standards relate to focus areas for projects selected by the organization itself. Projects conducted at the specific direction of CMS or the Medicaid agency will be deemed to have met this standard.

Documentation of completed projects must show the basis on which the organization selected project topics; i.e., continuing monitoring of population needs and preferences and organizational performance; identification of areas of concern; and clear criteria, identified by the organization, for prioritizing the areas to be addressed.

As standards 1.4.1.4 and 1.6.1.3 indicate, the organization's affiliated providers and enrollees must have formal opportunities to participate in the selection and prioritization of QAPI projects.

Sources of Information

The QAPI program must routinely collect and interpret information from all parts of the organization, to identify areas of clinical concern, health delivery system issues, and issues in member services. Types of information to be reviewed include:

◆ Population information. Data on enrollee characteristics relevant to health risks or utilization of clinical and non-clinical services, including age, sex, race/ethnicity/language, and disability or functional status.

◆ Performance measures. Data on the organization's performance as reflected in standardized measures, including, when possible: local, state, or national information on performance of comparable organizations.

◆ Other utilization, diagnostic, and outcome information. Data on utilization of services, procedures, medications, and devices; admitting and encounter diagnoses; adverse incidents (such as deaths, avoidable admissions, or readmissions); and patterns of referrals or authorization requests.

◆ External data sources. Data from outside organizations, including Medicare or Medicaid fee-for-service data, data from other managed care organizations, and local or national public health reports on conditions or risks for specified populations. (In newly formed organizations, or organizations serving a new population, external data may be the major source of potential project topics.)

◆ Enrollee information on their experiences with care. Data from surveys (such as the Consumer Assessment of Health Plans Study, or CAHPS), information from the grievance and appeals processes, and information on disenrollments and requests to change providers. (Note that general population surveys may under-represent populations who may have special needs, such as linguistic minorities or the disabled. Assessment of satisfaction for these groups may require over sampling or other methods, such as focus groups or enrollee interviews.) The QAPI program should assess, in addition to information generated within the organization, information supplied by purchasers, such as data on complaints and disenrollments processed by the Medicaid agency.

The QAPI program's project selection process must explicitly take into account quality of care concerns identified by a peer review organization (PRO) or external quality review organization (EQRO). While it is not expected that each such concern will be addressed through a formal QAPI project meeting the requirements of these standards, the organization should be able to show that issues raised by these organizations were considered in the formulation of its QAPI program agenda and that alternative remedial action is taken in cases for which a QAPI project is not initiated.

Prioritizing Topics

In general, a clinical or non-clinical issue selected for study should affect a significant portion of the organization's Medicare or Medicaid enrollees (or a specified subpopulation of enrollees) and have a potentially significant impact on enrollee health, functional status, or satisfaction. There may be instances in which infrequent conditions or services warrant study, as when data show a pattern of unexpected adverse outcomes; however, the prevalence of a condition or volume of services involved must be sufficient to permit meaningful study.

A project topic may be suggested by patterns of inappropriate utilization—for example, frequent use of the emergency room by enrollees with a specific diagnosis. However, the project must be clearly focused on identifying and correcting deficiencies in care or services that might have led to this pattern, such as inadequate access to primary care, rather than on utilization and cost issues alone. This is not to say that the organization may not make efforts to address overutilization, but only that such efforts might not be considered QAPI activities for the purpose of assessing compliance with these standards, unless the primary objective is to improve health outcomes. Thus it would be acceptable for a project to focus on patterns of overutilization that present a clear threat to health or functional status, for example because of a high risk of iatrogenic problems or other adverse outcomes.

Because the achievement of demonstrable improvement is a central criterion in the evaluation of QAPI projects, projects must necessarily focus on areas in which meaningful improvement can be effected through system interventions by the organization. Most organizations are likely to give priority to areas in which there is significant variation in practice and resulting outcomes within the organization, or in which the organization's performance as a whole falls below acceptable benchmarks or norms.

It is recognized that the requirement for demonstrable improvement creates incentives for organizations to focus their QAPI activities on aspects of care in which rapid and measurable improvement is possible through simple interventions. It is not the intention of these standards to discourage organizations from undertaking more complex projects or innovative projects that have a high risk of failure but that offer some offsetting potential for making a significant difference in the health or functional status of enrollees. Organizations considering such projects should avail themselves of the opportunity, under standard 1.3.7.2, to work in consultation with CMS or the State agency to develop long-range goals for projects and establish agreed-upon criteria for evaluation of the organization's progress in implementing its project.

Organizations Using Physician Incentive Plans

An organization that adopts a physician incentive plan that places physicians at substantial financial risk (as defined in 42 CFR 422.208(d)) for the care of Medicare or Medicaid enrollees must include in its QAPI program continuous monitoring of the potential effects of the incentive plan on access or quality of care. This monitoring should include assessment of the results of surveys of enrollees and former enrollees required under 42 CFR 422.479(h). In addition, the organization should review utilization data to identify patterns of possible underutilization of services that may be related to the incentive plan (such as low rates of referral services ordered by physicians at risk for the cost of such services).

Concerns identified as a result of this monitoring should be considered in development of the organization's focus areas for QAPI projects.

1.4.1.4   The QAPI program provides opportunities for enrollees to participate in the selection of project topics and the formulation of project goals.

The organization must establish some mechanism for obtaining enrollee input into the priorities for its QAPI program. Possibilities could include enrollee representation on a quality assurance committee or subcommittees or routine inclusion of QAPI issues on the agenda for a general enrollee advisory committee. To the extent feasible, input should be obtained from enrollees who are users of or concerned with specific focus areas; for example, priorities in the area of mental health or substance abuse services should be developed in consultation with users of these services or their families.

1.4.2   Quality indicators. Assessment of the organization's performance for each selected topic is measured using one or more quality indicators.

1.4.2.1   Quality indicators are objective, clearly and unambiguously defined, and based on current clinical knowledge or health services research. When indicators exist that are generally used within the public health community or the managed care industry and are applicable to the topic, use of those measures is preferred.

Each QAPI project must establish one or more quality indicators that will be used to track performance and improvement over time. An indicator is a variable reflecting either a discrete event (an older adult has/has not received a flu shot in the last 12 months) or a status (an enrollee's hypertension is/is not under control). In either case, an indicator must be clearly defined and subject to objective measurement.

An organization may adopt standard indicators from outside sources, such as the National Committee for Quality Assurance (NCQA)'s Health plan Employer Data and Information Set (HEDIS) or the Foundation for Accountability (FACCT)'s measures, or develop its own indicators on the basis of clinical literature or findings of expert consensus panels. When the organization develops its own indicators, it must be able to document the basis on which it adopted an indicator. It also should be able to show that the process included consultation with affiliated providers and enrollees to assure that measures are meaningful, relevant to the organization's enrolled population, and reflective of accepted standards of practice.

An organization is not required to select specific indicators at the outset of a QAPI project. There may be instances in which a project would begin with more general collection and analysis of baseline data on a topic, and then narrow its focus to more specific indicators for measurement, intervention, and reevaluation. The success of the project will be assessed in terms of the indicators ultimately selected.

1.4.2.2   All indicators measure changes in health status, functional status, or enrollee satisfaction, or valid proxies of these outcomes. Measures of processes are used as a proxy for out-

comes only when those processes have been established through published studies or a consensus of relevant practitioners to be significantly related to outcomes.

The object of the QAPI program is to improve outcomes, defined as objective measures of patient health, functional status, or satisfaction following the receipt of care or services. Under this definition, measures of costs, or other administrative results do not constitute outcomes. It is recognized, however, that relatively few standardized performance measures actually address outcomes. For example, of the 12 effectiveness measures in HEDIS 3.0-1998 in active use, only one (health of seniors) is truly outcome-related. Even when outcome measures are available, their utility as quality indicators for QAPI projects may be limited because outcomes can be significantly influenced by factors outside the organization's control; e.g., poverty, genetics, environment. In other instances, improvement is possible, but the resources and sophistication needed to analyze the complex factors involved in the outcome and develop meaningful interventions might be beyond the reach of many organizations.

This standard therefore does not require that quality indicators always be outcome measures. Process measures are acceptable so long as the organization can show that there is strong clinical evidence that the process being measured is meaningfully associated with outcomes. To the extent possible, this determination should be based on published guidelines that support the association and that cite evidence from randomized clinical trials, case control studies, or cohort studies. A plan may furnish its own similar evidence of association between a process and an outcome so long as this association is not actually contradicted by a published guideline. Although published evidence is generally required, there may be certain areas of practice for which empirical evidence of process/outcome linkage is limited. At a minimum, the organization must be able to demonstrate that there is a consensus among relevant practitioners with expertise in the defined area as to the importance of a given process.

1.4.2.3   *Indicators selected for a topic in a clinical focus area (under standard 1.3.4) include at least some measure of change in health status or functional status or process of care proxies for these outcomes. Indicators may also include measures of the enrollee's experience of and satisfaction with care.*

While organizations are encouraged to consider enrollee satisfaction as an important aspect of care in any of the clinical areas listed in standard 1.3.4, improvement in satisfaction must not be the sole demonstrable outcome of a project in any of these areas. Some improvement in health or functional status must also be measured. (Note that this measurement can rely on enrollee surveys that address topics in addition to satisfaction. For example, self-reported health status may be an acceptable indicator, or reduction in reported school absences could be used as an indicator of functional status in children.) For projects in the non-clinical areas, use of health or functional status indicators is generally preferred, particularly for projects addressing access and availability. However, there may be some non-clinical projects for which enrollee satisfaction indicators alone are sufficient.

1.4.2.4   *The organization selects some indicators for which data are available that allow comparison of the organization's performance to that of similar organizations or to local, state, or national benchmarks.*

As is discussed under standard 1.4.4, demonstrable improvement may be defined either as reaching a prospectively set benchmark or as improving performance by a fixed percentage amount. While the latter form of improvement is acceptable for the purpose of standard 1.4.4, an organization that works only toward incremental improvements relative to its own past performance can never determine that its performance is optimal—or even minimally acceptable relative to prevailing standards in the community. Whenever possible then, an organization should select indicators for which data are available on the performance of other comparable organizations (or other components of the same organization), or for which there exist local or national data for a similar population in the fee-for-service sector. Because the availability of such data will vary by topic and by population, this standard does not set a fixed number of focus areas for which benchmarks must be adopted. However, every organization should be able to establish benchmarks for at least some project topics (e.g., immunizations or initiation of prenatal care).

1.4.3   *Data collection and methodology. Assessment of the organization's performance on the selected indicators is based on systematic, ongoing collection and analysis of valid and reliable data.*

Assessment of compliance with this standard will be coordinated with review of the organization's information systems under standard 1.5.

1.4.3.1   *The organization establishes a baseline measure of its performance on each indicator, measures changes in performance, and continues measurement for at least one year after a desired level of performance is achieved.*

Documentation of completed QAPI projects must include a detailed account of the data collection methodology used and the procedures through which the organization has assured that the data are valid and reliable.

Methodology

Most quality indicators are reported in terms of percentages or ratios; for example, the percentage of pregnant women who begin prenatal care in the first 13 weeks of the pregnancy. An organization adopting this measure must show that it can accurately compute the relevant denominator or population at risk (all pregnant women) and the numerator or indicator (pregnant women beginning prenatal care in the specified time frame).

Identification of the population at risk requires particular scrutiny. For some indicators, the population can be identified in readily available administrative data (all children under age 2, or all inpatient discharges with a diagnosis of heart attack). For others, needed data may be more difficult to obtain. For example, even in an organization that collects individual encounter data, this data might not be able to identify all enrollees with diabetes, because physicians may not report ongoing conditions at every encounter. Instead, the organization must identify the population at risk through a patient disease registry, if present, or through a pharmacy data base.

Therefore, the organization must clearly specify what data are used to identify the population at risk and show that these data can reliably and validly capture the entire population; i.e., without systematically excluding a subset or subsets of the population. The organization may study a sample of the relevant population. If so, it must show that the sample size is sufficient to achieve an appropriate level of confidence in the estimates of the incidence of the indicator under study, and that pre- and post-sample sizes are sufficiently large and representative to allow tests of statistical significance to be performed on any apparent change (improvement in the rate of occurrence of selected indicators) (see standard 1.4.4.2). The organization also must show that the sampling method is such that all members of the population are equally likely to be selected. (This will generally mean random sampling, although stratified random sampling may be appropriate when the intent is to compare care by different practitioners or at different sites.)

In addition to assuring that data collection is complete and free from bias, the study methodology may need to address other issues in the computation of the indicator. For example, when an indicator relates to receipt of a specific service, the denominator may need to be adjusted to reflect instances in which the patient refuses the service or the service is contraindicated. Similar problems may affect the numerator. For example, in a study of immunization rates, the organization would need to establish how it would detect and account for instances in which immunizations were received at school or at a health department, rather than through the primary care practitioner.

Validation

Data most commonly will be derived from administrative data generated by the organization's health information system or from review of medical records. In assessing non-clinical services, other sources such as enrollee or provider surveys may be appropriate. When data are derived from the health information system, their reliability is obviously a function of the general integrity of the system. In this case, assessment of compliance with this standard will be coordinated with review of compliance with the information system requirements in standard 1.5.

When data are derived from direct review of medical records or other primary source documents, steps must be taken to assure that the data are uniformly extracted and recorded. Appropriately qualified personnel must be used; this will vary with the nature of the data being collected and the degree of professional judgment required. There must be clear guidelines or protocols for obtaining and entering the data; this is especially important if multiple reviewers are used or if data is collected by multiple subcontractors. Inter-reviewer reliability should be assured through, for example, repeat reviews of a sample of records.

NOTE: If the indicator selected for a QAPI project is a performance measure that the organization is required to report routinely to CMS or a State Medicaid agency, review of compliance in this area might be coordinated with whatever validation process CMS or the State establishes for such reporting. Furthermore, note that all data collection for QAPI projects is subject to the confidentiality requirements of standard 2.2.1.

1.4.3.2   *When sampling is used, sampling methodology for assessment of the organization's performance shall be such as to ensure that the data collected validly reflect:*

1.4.3.2.1   *the performance of all practitioners and providers who serve Medicare or Medicaid enrollees and whose activities are the subject of the indicator; and*

Once a topic has been selected, the organization must assure that its measurement and improvement efforts are system-wide. Each project must, to the extent feasible, reach all providers in its network who are involved in the aspect of care or services to be studied. This standard does **not** establish a requirement that an organization review the performance of each and every provider who furnishes the services that are the subject of the project. Sampling is acceptable so long as the organization assures that its samples are genuinely random. The organization must be able to show that:

◆   Each relevant provider has a chance of being selected; no provider is systematically excluded from the sampling;

◆   Each provider serving a given number of enrollees has the same probability of being selected as any other provider serving the same number of enrollees; and

◆   Providers who were not included in the sample for the baseline measurement have the same chance of being selected for the follow-up measurement as providers who were included in the baseline.

This is, of course, easier to meet if the organization selects for study a condition that affects relatively few of its enrollees or is treated by a limited number of providers. However, the organization might then be unable to show that its selection of topics meets the criteria in standard 1.4.1, including the core requirement that topics be selected so as to achieve the greatest practical benefit for enrollees.

A Medicare organization may use a single sample that combines Medicare members with other members if it is authorized to do so by the Medicare project officer. A combined sample will only be authorized when there is substantial empirical evidence that performance has been similar for the groups that are combined in the single sample. However, because States have to report to CMS the results of performance improvement projects relative to the Medicaid population, States typically will require when organizations conduct a study that includes multiple populations (e.g., Medicaid, Medicare, and commercial) that Medicaid organizations use a stratified sample that can show demonstrable improvement for the Medicaid population separately. However, this does not prohibit States from permitting Medicaid organizations to use other approaches. States and their Medicaid organizations are free to collaborate to develop ways to supply the States with the information they need while minimizing the burden imposed upon Medicaid organizations.

1.4.3.2.2 The care given to the entire population (including populations with special health care needs and populations with serious and complex health care needs) to which the indicator is relevant.

Similar to the equal treatment of all providers and practitioners by the sampling methodology, a sampling methodology should not exclude any population subgroups to which the topic area and indicators are applicable. For example, when studying well child care, a managed care organization should not exclude children with special care needs whose primary care provider is a specialist other than a pediatrician or family medicine practitioner. When studying use of preventive services an organization needs to design its study to include all persons who are in need of the service (e.g., routine health screening) as opposed to including only those individuals who have already made a visit to a managed care organization's providers.

1.4.4 Demonstrable improvement. The organization's interventions result in significant demonstrable improvement in its performance as evidenced in repeat measurements of the quality indicators specified for each performance improvement project undertaken by the organization.

The organization must demonstrate, through repeated measurement of the quality indicators selected for the project, meaningful change in performance relative to the performance observed during baseline measurement. The repeat measurement should use the same methodology as the baseline measurement, except that, when baseline data was collected for the entire population at risk, the repeat may instead use a reliable sample. When an organization measures its performance using the identified indicators, it can do so by collecting information on all individuals, encounters or episodes of care to which the indicator is applicable (a census) or by collecting information on a representative subset of individuals, encounters, providers of care, etc. Standards 1.4.4.1 and 1.4.4.2 address requirements for achieving "demonstrable" improvement when using a census and a sample, respectively.

1.4.4.1 When a project measures performance on quality indicators by collecting data on all units of analysis in the population to be studied (i.e., a census), significant improvement is demonstrated by achieving:

1.4.4.1.1 in the case of a national Medicare project, a benchmark level of performance defined in advance by CMS;

1.4.4.1.2 in the case of a statewide Medicaid project, a benchmark level of performance defined in advance by the State Medicaid agency; or

1.4.4.1.3 in the case of a project developed by the organization itself, a benchmark level of performance that is defined in advance by the organization. The organization's benchmark must reduce the performance gap (the percent of cases in which the measure is failed) by at least 10 percent.

1.4.4.1.4 in the case of a project developed by the organization to reduce disparities between minorities and other members, a reduction of at least 10 percent in the number of minor-

ity enrollees (or the specified unit of analysis) that do not achieve the desired outcome as defined by the quality indicators.

Benchmarks

Benchmarks will be established by CMS for national projects that the organization participates in. Similarly, State Medicaid agencies will establish benchmarks for Statewide quality improvement projects that the organization participates in. When the project is one determined by the managed care organization, the organization's benchmark must represent at least a ten percent reduction in enrollees not receiving the care or services under study. Benchmarks must also reflect performance in other organizations, local or national norms as established through comparative data, or reasonable expectations of optimum performance. The organization must be able to document the basis on which its benchmark was determined.

Percent Change

An organization meets this if, for example, its child immunization rate is 80 percent in the baseline and increases to 82 percent, because the percentage of children **not** immunized has dropped from 20 percent to 18 percent, a 10 percent reduction. An organization whose baseline rate was 60 percent would have to reach 64 percent—a reduction in non-immunized children from 40 percent to 36 percent. (Note that, to assure uniform computation of improvement across indicators, all indicators must first be stated in the form of a positive outcome, and improvement measured as a reduction in its inverse.)

The requirement for a 10 percent reduction in adverse outcomes is based on two considerations. First, the use of a constant percentage reflects the likelihood that change is harder to achieve when an organization's baseline performance is already superior. Thus the organization with an 80 percent immunization rate is only expected to achieve a 2 percent improvement, while the organization with a 60 percent rate must achieve a 4 percent improvement. Second, the 10 percent level is consistent with results CMS has observed in successful improvement projects sponsored by the agency.

1.4.4.2 *When a project measures performance on quality indicators by collecting data on a subset (sample) of the units of analysis in the population to be studied, significant improvement is demonstrated by achieving the benchmarks specified under 1.4.4.1, using a sample that is sufficiently large to detect the targeted amount of improvement.*

Managed care organizations must provide documentation that the sampling procedure actually implemented was random, valid, and unbiased. Organizations should be aware that using a sample creates a risk of underestimating actual improvement because of a statistical phenomenon called sampling error. If an organization demonstrates an inadequate amount of improvement based on an estimate that is derived from a sample, CMS will not assume that the inadequate amount of improvement is attributable to sampling error. Organizations therefore face a tradeoff between the cost of using a larger sample to minimize the sampling error, and the risk that their actual improvement will be underestimated if they use a smaller sample. Organizations should consult with a statistician about this tradeoff before making a decision regarding sample size.

1.4.4.2.1 *The sample or subset of the study population shall be obtained through random sampling.*

1.4.4.2.2 *The samples used for the baseline and repeat measurements of the performance indicators shall be chosen using the same sampling frame and methodology.*

In order to accurately measure improvement, it is essential that the measures of performance before and after the organization's interventions be comparable. The same methods for identifying the target population and for selecting individual cases for review must be used for both measurements. For example, in a project to improve care of diabetes, it would not be acceptable to draw the baseline sample from a population identified on the basis of diagnoses reported in ambulatory encounter data, and draw the follow-up sample from a population identified on the basis of pharmacy data. In a project to address follow-up after hospitalization for mental illness, it would not be acceptable to shift from a sampling method under which an individual with multiple admissions could be chosen more than once to a method under which the individual could be chosen only once.

1.4.4.3 *The improvement is reasonably attributable to interventions undertaken by the organization (i.e., a project and its results have face validity).*

It is expected that interventions associated with improvements on quality indicators will be system interventions; i.e., educational efforts, changes in policies, targeting of additional resources, or other organization-wide initiatives to improve performance. Interventions that might have some short-term effect but that are unlikely to induce permanent change (such as a one-time reminder letter to physicians or beneficiaries) are insufficient.

The organization is not required to demonstrate conclusively (for example, through controlled studies) that a change in an indicator is the effect of its intervention; it is sufficient to show that an intervention occurred that might reasonably be expected to affect the results. Nor is the organization required to undertake data analysis to correct for secular trends (changes that reflect continuing growth or decline in a measure as a result of external forces over an extended period of time). To the extent feasible, however, the organization should be able to demonstrate that its data have been corrected for any major confounding variables with an obvious impact on the outcomes. (For example, an organization should not use a baseline measure of asthma admissions during pollen season and then measure an improvement during another season.)

To the extent feasible, interventions should be designed to address underlying system problems uncovered in the analysis, rather than simply to improve performance on a specific indicator. For example, the organization might determine that one factor in poor outcomes for a given condition was an access problem: too few providers in a given specialty or in a given part of the service area. While the immediate intervention might be to recruit additional providers, the finding should also trigger a review of the organization's policies and procedures for ongoing monitoring of network adequacy.

The expectation of system-level intervention is in contrast to that expressed in some earlier Medicare guidelines on quality assurance activities, that intervention would occur at a provider-specific or patient-specific level. This does not mean that individual instances of substandard care observed in the course of QAPI projects should merely be recorded for statistical purposes and then forgotten. For example, if reviewers identify a specific case in which an enrollee's health is in jeopardy because a given test result has never been followed up, there is clearly an ethical and professional responsibility to assure that the specific needs of that enrollee are promptly addressed. In other instances, findings of QAPI studies may trigger intensive review of the practice patterns of an individual provider, leading to interventions in the form of counseling, possible contract sanctions, or reporting to appropriate professional disciplinary bodies.

1.4.5 *Sustained improvement. The organization sustains the improvements in performance described in 1.4.4 for at least one year after the improvement in performance is first achieved. Sustained improvement is documented through the continued measurement of quality indicators for at least one year after the performance improvement project described in 1.4.4 is completed.*

The organization must repeat measurement of the indicators one year after the initial indicator measurement on the basis of which demonstrable improvement was achieved. This is necessary in order to demonstrate that the improvement that was achieved has been sustained. We recognize that because of random year-to-year variation and sampling error, performance on any given individual measure may decline in the second measurement. However, when all of the repeat measurements for a given review year are taken together, this decline should not be statistically significant and should never be statistically significant in two succeeding years (that is, with all of the projects remeasured in each of the two years). Therefore, when all of the organization's repeat measurements for a given review year across all clinical and non-clinical focus studies are taken together, the combined repeat measurements in the aggregate must demonstrate that the improvement over the combined original baseline performance levels still meets the requirements of 1.4.4.

Note that a project that has achieved improvement, and under which no further system interventions are undertaken by the organization, will not be regarded as an ongoing project for the purposes of 1.3.3 during the period that elapses between the measurement of improvement and the repeat measurement. The organization must carefully distinguish between active projects and projects that have been concluded but for which the repeat measurement has not yet been conducted.

1.5 *Health Information System. The organization maintains a health information system that collects, integrates, analyzes, and reports data necessary to implement its QAPI program.*

The organization's health information system is central to its efforts to manage patient care and to assess and improve health care quality and outcomes. Every organization should be able to collect and integrate data from all components of its network, in order to develop a comprehensive picture of enrollee needs and utilization, including changes in these over time. It should be able to use these data in its quality assessment and performance improvement program, as well as in other management activities.

While there are numerous reasons for organizations to improve their information system capacities, the overarching goal for both CMS and State Medicaid agencies is to improve patient care. For this reason, standard 1.5 focuses on the system's capacity to provide the information required to conduct an effective QAPI program of performance improvement projects and reporting on standard measures that meets the requirements of other standards in this domain.

Although an encounter data system may often be the most efficient means of meeting the requirements of this standard, the organization may use any methods or procedures for data collection, so long as it can demonstrate that its system achieves the objectives of this standard. The organization must be able to document that each of its QAPI activities is based on complete and valid information, however this information is compiled.

1.5.1   *The system collects data on enrollee and provider characteristics, and on services furnished to enrollees, as needed to guide the selection of performance improvement project topics (standard 1.4.1) and to meet the data collection requirements for performance improvement projects (standard 1.4.3).*

Measurement of compliance with this standard will be an integral part of assessment of compliance with standards 1.4.1 and 1.4.3.

Topic selection. The system must provide information needed to identify priority areas for quality improvement. Ideally, an organization's system should be able to generate such information as:

I.   Longitudinal profiles of treatment or services furnished to enrollees with a specific diagnosis;

II. Profiles of referral services ordered by each primary care practitioner;

III. Statistical reports on the prevalence of different conditions or diagnoses among a specific group of enrollees, such as Medicare beneficiaries; and

IV. Prescription medication usage by type of enrollee, by diagnosis, or by prescribing practitioner.

However, review will focus not on these general system capacities, but on the specific methods adopted for prioritizing topics and on the extent to which the method was applied using valid data.

For example, an organization may indicate that it selected a given condition for a QAPI project because the condition affected 30 percent of its Medicare enrollees. If so, it must be able to show how it knows the prevalence of different conditions among its Medicare enrollees. If its administrative data set has incomplete data from half its providers, the organization cannot make this assertion, unless the information has been obtained through sampling or other means. Again, the standard does not impose a general requirement that organizations be able to report the prevalence of all conditions or diagnoses for all enrollees. It requires that the organization have the specific information it needs to carry out its own particular approach to quality measurement and improvement.

Data collection for QAPI projects. The organization must be able to collect valid baseline and follow-up measurements for quality indicators selected for QAPI projects. If, for example, the organization selects as a Medicaid indicator the HEDIS measure on prenatal care in the first trimester it must be able to:

◆ Collect and analyze data on inpatient hospital discharges for Medicaid enrollees during the study period, and be able to identify discharges in live births, with appropriate methods for validating live births under different coding schemes;

◆ Collect information on live births occurring in any other site, such as birthing centers;

◆ Link this data with enrollment information, in order to restrict the measure to women who were continuously enrolled for a period specified in HEDIS;

◆ Either obtain encounter data with sufficient procedural and diagnostic information to establish which women received prenatal care visits meeting the criteria applied by the measure, or conduct a review of a sample of medical records. (If the latter method is used, the organization must obviously be able to determine which, if any, practitioners the woman visited during the period from 6 to 44 weeks prior to delivery.)

Once again, the standard does not require that any of these processes be carried out through any specific type of information system. However, the organization must be able to show how each process was performed and be able to show that all reasonable steps have been taken to assure that the data are complete, accurate and reliable. Any project for which an organization cannot demonstrate compliance with this cannot be counted towards the requirements of standards 1.3.2 or 1.3.3 for completed projects in identified focus areas.

1.5.2 *The organization ensures that information and data received from providers are accurate, timely, and complete.*

This standard does not require that organizations receive encounter reporting. However, if the organization relies on encounter reporting or aggregate data reporting for any QAPI activity (e.g., counting enrollees who had prenatal care visits), then it must have an ongoing process for assuring the accuracy and completeness of the data, whether compiled in its own facilities or reported by outside contractors.

1.5.2.1 *The organization reviews reported data for accuracy, completeness, logic, and consistency.*

If the organization receives individual encounter data directly from providers, it must have a system for comparing reported data to a sample of medical records, to verify the accuracy of reporting or transmission. The objective is to assure that, to the extent feasible, there is a one-to-one correspondence between items included in an organization's summary data and specific services entered in medical records or equivalent source documents. (That is, no reported service was not performed, and no service performed was not reported.)

If the organization receives aggregate information, instead of individual patient encounter reporting, from any provider, the organization must approve the provider's own system for collecting, recording, aggregating, and reporting the data, and must assure that the provider has its own mechanisms for validation.

Identified deficiencies in reported data must be addressed through provider education or other corrective action. The organization's process for recredentialing or recontracting with practitioners and providers, under standard 3.5, must specify the actions to be taken in the event of ongoing failure by a contractor to meet the organization's health information standards.

The organization, or any contractor developing aggregate data from individual encounter reporting, must have mechanisms to assure that reported data contain all data elements required by the organization. Data must be subject to logic edits to assure, for example, that reported services are consistent with the place of service or type of provider; that the number of services performed is consistent with the span of time (e.g., 20 physician hospital visits in a 2-day span of time is a potential inconsistency); or that procedures or diagnoses applicable only to enrollees of a particular age or sex are not reported for other enrollees. Finally, the integrity of data entry must be assured, through double keying or other recognized methods.

1.5.2.2 *Service data are collected in standardized formats to the extent feasible and appropriate.*

Standard formats are needed to assure that data elements are reported uniformly by all providers, and that reports from multiple sources are comparable and can be reliably merged into more comprehensive reports. Verification of conformity to the organization should be included in the validation required under standard 1.5.2.1.

The Health Insurance Portability and Accountability Act of 1996 includes data utilization provisions that will apply to managed care organizations and providers. Until these requirements take effect, each organization remains free to specify its own formats. However, because national standardization is forthcoming, an organization should have a plan for progressing toward commonly accepted data formats as rapidly as possible. In the interim, the use of organization-specific formats has a bearing on evaluation of the organization's compliance with other standards in this section. For example, an organization may need to validate data from contractors more carefully than it would if contractors could use the coding they routinely use in reporting to other payers. In addition, the organization may have difficulty calculating and reporting standardized performance measures that are keyed to non-standard coding.

1.6 *Administration of the QAPI Program.*

1.6.1 *The organization's QAPI program is administered through clear and appropriate administrative arrangements, such that:*

In most organizations, the QAPI program is administered by a multi-disciplinary committee that includes both clinical and administrative personnel. Other arrangements are permissible, so long as the organization can demonstrate that clearly identified individuals or organizational components are responsible for each aspect of QAPI activity and that effective organizational structures are in place to assure communication and coordination. In either case, the organization's QAPI program description must show the role, structure, staffing, and function of each participating component and the interrelations among components.

There must be evidence that the committee or other coordinating structure is effectively functioning. Meetings should be held at appropriate intervals and adequately attended. There should be evidence that issues raised are appropriately followed up in subsequent meetings or through other means, and that deliberations lead to actual directions to committee staff, other organization personnel, and/or affiliated providers.

1.6.1.1 *The policy making body oversees and is accountable for the QAPI program.*

The policy making body is defined as the governing body of the organization or a committee of senior executives that exercises general oversight over the organization's management, policies, and personnel. The policy making body as a whole may oversee the QAPI program, or it may designate a committee to perform this function. There must be evidence that the policy making body approves changes in the QAPI program description and approves the annual work plan. It must receive and review periodic reports on QAPI activities. The policy making body must review the annual evaluation required under standard 1.6.2 and take action on any resulting recommendations.

1.6.1.2 *A designated senior official is responsible for QAPI program administration.*

There must be a single official responsible for the overall functioning of the QAPI program. This may be the organization's chief executive officer, chief medical officer or director, or another senior official who has direct authority to commit organizational resources to the QAPI effort. If the responsible official is not the chief medical officer, the organization must show, through the QAPI program description or other documentation, that the chief medical officer has substantial involvement in QAPI activities, including participation in meetings of the committee or other coordinating structure. Some organizations have a separate official who performs the functions of a medical director for mental health and substance abuse services; it is acceptable for this officer to oversee QAPI activities in these areas.

1.6.1.3 *Employed or affiliated providers and consumers actively participate in the QAPI program.*

All contracts with providers must require participation in QAPI activities, including provision of access to medical records and cooperation with data collection activities. If affiliated providers are not represented on the organization's QAPI committee or other core coordinating structure, there must be a clinical subcommittee or other advisory group to assure that clinicians actively participate in key activities, including: selecting and prioritizing QAPI projects, developing indicators, analyzing study results, identifying and proposing solutions to problems, and aiding in communication of QAPI activities and results to other providers.

Note that consumer involvement in establishment of QAPI program priorities is required under standard 1.4.1.4. This does not create an additional requirement, but merely emphasizes that consumer input should be sought from the very outset of the organization's QAPI program planning.

1.6.1.4   *There is formal and ongoing communication and collaboration among the policy making body that oversees the QAPI program and the other functional areas of the organization, e.g., health services management and member services.*

Interaction with the QAPI program is specifically referred to in the following standards or related guidelines:

I. 2.4, Resolution of enrollee issues

II. 3.3.2, Service authorization process

III. 3.4.1, Development of practice guidelines

IV. 3.5.1.2, Recredentialing of practitioners.

1.6.2   *The organization formally evaluates, at least annually, the effectiveness of the QAPI program strategy, and makes necessary changes.*

The evaluation should assess both progress in implementing the QAPI strategy and the extent to which the strategy is in fact promoting the development of an effective QAPI program. It should consider whether activities in the organization's work plan are being completed on a timely basis or whether commitment of additional resources is necessary. The evaluation should include recommendations for needed changes in program strategy or administration. These recommendations must be forwarded to and considered by the policy making body of the organization (see standard 1.6.1.1).

Note that this standard does not require that an organization make major revisions in its QAPI strategy each year.

Appendix 11.B

QISMC Domain 2

DOMAIN 2: Enrollee Rights

STANDARD NUMBER	DESCRIPTION OF STANDARD

2.1   *Organization Policies.*

2.1.1   *The organization implements written policies with respect to the enrollee rights specified in standard 2.2.*

The organization must articulate enrollees' rights, promote the exercise of those rights, and ensure that its staff and affiliated providers are familiar with enrollee rights and treat enrollees accordingly. While most of the standards in this domain address basic procedural protections for enrollees, they are closely related to quality of care. Interpersonal aspects of care are highly important to most patients. Enrollees' interactions with the organization and its providers can have an important bearing on their willingness and ability to understand and comply with recommended treatments, and hence on outcomes and costs. For further technical assistance with this domain, readers are directed to the Consumer Bill of Rights and Responsibilities as promulgated in November 1997 by the President's Advisory Commission on Consumer Protection and Quality in the Health Care Industry.

2.1.1.1   *Policies are communicated to enrollees, in the enrollee statement furnished in accordance with standard 2.3, and to the organization's staff and affiliated providers, at the time of initial employment or affiliation and annually thereafter.*

Material on enrollee rights must be included in provider contracts or provider manuals and in staff handbooks or other training materials.

2.1.1.2   *The organization monitors and promotes compliance with the policies by the organization's staff and affiliated providers.*

The organization should monitor compliance through analysis of complaints or grievances, requests to change providers, enrollee satisfaction surveys, rapid disenrollment surveys, and other sources of enrollee input. Issues in compliance should be addressed through education or counseling of the staff or providers or other corrective action, and information on compliance with the policies should be considered during the recredentialing and staff evaluation process and within the QAPI program.

2.1.2   *The organization ensures compliance with Federal and State laws affecting the rights of enrollees.*

Applicable Federal laws include, but are not limited to:

1. Title VI of the Civil Rights Act;

2. Section 504 of the Rehabilitation Act of 1973;

3. The Age Discrimination Act of 1975;

4. Titles II and III of the Americans with Disabilities Act;

5. Section 542 of the Public Health Service Act (pertaining to nondiscrimination against substance abusers); and

6. Title 45, Part 46 of the Code of Federal Regulations, pertaining to research involving human subjects.

In general, these laws are enforced by agencies other than CMS or the State Medicaid agency, and reviews conducted under these standards will not include detailed assessment of an organization's compliance. However, CMS or States will report any observed violations and refer any enrollee complaints to the appropriate agency for resolution.

The organization must include provisions relating to compliance with Federal and State laws in subcontracts with providers. Assessment of compliance should be included in the organization's credentialing procedures to the extent feasible and appropriate; for example, if site visits to individual providers' offices are conducted, they should include a general assessment of physical accessibility. Compliance issues identified may be addressed through the organization's QAPI program.

2.2   *Specification of Rights. Each enrollee has a right—*

2.2.1   *to be treated with respect, dignity, and consideration for enrollee privacy;*

The organization must ensure that enrollees' dignity and privacy are respected in its own facilities and must address these issues in site visits to offices or facilities of affiliated primary care providers (see standard 3.5.1.1). Examples of privacy concerns include privacy of examining rooms and measures to ensure that enrollees are not interviewed about medical, financial, or other issues within the hearing range of other patients in ambulatory settings.

2.2.1.1   *The organization implements procedures to ensure the confidentiality of health and medical records and of other information about enrollees.*

The organization's confidentiality procedures should apply not just to medical records, but to any information in the possession of the organization or its contractors that could disclose medical conditions or the use of specific services, such as claims information or information collected in the course of QAPI, utilization or case management, or other processes. Procedures must address both written materials and information created in other formats, such as electronic records, facsimiles, or electronic mail. The organization's procedures should protect against unauthorized or inadvertent disclosure of information to any individual, including the organization's own employees or contractors, who does not have an identifiable need for the information. In addition, procedures should assure that no individual retains information after putting it to use for the purpose for which it was obtained.

The organization's confidentiality protections must extend to minors. The organization must have policies that, consistent with State and Federal law, define whether and under what circumstances treatment may be furnished to a minor without parental consent and what information will be released to a parent on request. Specific issues to be addressed should include family planning, other reproductive health services, and mental health or substance abuse services.

Review of primary care providers' own confidentiality procedures should be included as part of any site visits conducted under standard 3.5.1.1.

An organization with Medicaid enrollees must have specific procedures to ensure that information on enrollees' Medicaid eligibility status is released only when necessary (for example, when a provider must be able to identify Medicaid beneficiaries who are exempt from copayment requirements) and that recipients of this information in turn agree to maintain confidentiality.

2.2.1.1.1   *The right to privacy includes protection of any information that identifies a particular enrollee. Information from, or copies of, records may be released only to authorized individuals, and the organization must ensure that unauthorized individuals cannot gain access to or alter patient records. Original medical records must be released only in accordance with Federal or State laws, court orders, or subpoenas.*

This standard pertains to the release of information to third parties and is not meant to impede the exchange of information among the organization, its affiliated providers, and other contractors as necessary to carry out the organization's contractual responsibilities.

When a State's managed care program (e.g., by "carving out" certain services such as mental health care) or an enrollee's dual coverage by both Medicaid and Medicare creates a situation in which a Medicare or Medicaid beneficiary is enrolled in more than one managed care organization, all such Medicaid and Medicare managed care organizations in which beneficiaries are enrolled are not considered "third parties" for purposes of this standard. Individual, identifiable personal information pertaining to such enrollees' health and health care may be released, to the extent allowed under State and Federal law, without the prior consent of the beneficiary, to any other Medicare or Medicaid managed care organization so as to ensure continuity and coordination of care.

2.2.1.2   *The organization implements procedures to ensure that enrollees are not discriminated against in the delivery of health care services consistent with the benefits covered in their policy based on race, ethnicity, national origin, religion, sex, age, mental or physical disability, sexual orientation, genetic information, or source of payment.*

This standard is intended to ensure that all health care services, including specialist referrals and special medical procedures, are consistently available to all enrollees. The organization must have in place administrative procedures that describe and promote nondiscriminatory practices in the delivery of health care.

Participating providers must have practice policies that demonstrate that they accept for treatment any enrollee in need of the health care services they provide.

The organization and its providers must make public declarations (e.g., through posters, member handbooks, organizational mission statements, strategic plans) of their commitment to nondiscriminatory behavior in conducting business with all enrollees. These documents should explain that this expectation applies to all personnel, clinical and non-clinical, in their dealings with each enrollee.

2.2.2 *to accessible services, as specified in standard 3.1;*

2.2.2.1 *The organization ensures that all services, both clinical and non-clinical, are accessible to all enrollees, including those with limited English proficiency or reading skills, with diverse cultural and ethnic backgrounds, the homeless and individuals with physical and mental disabilities.*

The aim of this standard is to ensure that the organization's service planning takes into account the needs of its entire enrolled population and that the organization works to reduce barriers to access.

Standard 1.3.5.1 requires that the organization include among the focus areas for its QAPI activities issues relating to access to care and cultural competency. It is expected that an organization's activities in this area will include identification of significant sub-populations within its enrolled population that may experience special barriers to access and continued efforts to improve accessibility of both clinical and member services for these specific groups.

In addition, the organization must develop appropriate policies and administrative systems to address access barriers likely to be encountered by individual enrollees (whether or not part of a defined sub-population). The organization is expected to ensure that its facilities and those of a sufficient number of affiliated providers are readily accessible to the physically and mentally disabled, that translator services are available as needed for non-English speaking enrollees, and that interpreter services and other accommodations (such as teletypewriter or TTY connections for member services) are made available to the hearing-impaired.

2.2.2.2 *The organization instructs enrollees that they have the right to access emergency health care services without prior authorization, consistent with the enrollee's determination of the need for such services as a prudent layperson.*

Emergency health care services are covered by inpatient and outpatient services provided by contracting or non-contracting providers that are needed to evaluate or stabilize an emergency medical condition. An organization is required to instruct enrollees that they have the right to access emergency health care services without prior authorization when an enrollee's medical condition manifests acute symptoms of sufficient severity (including severe pain) such that a prudent layperson, with an average knowledge of health and medicine, could reasonably expect the absence of immediate medical attention to result in serious jeopardy to the health of the individual, serious impairment to bodily functions, or serious dysfunction of an organ or body part. An organization may enforce appropriate use of emergency services through retrospective payment denials where enrollees did not act as prudent laypersons, as described above.

2.2.3 *to choose providers from among those affiliated with the organization;*

Each enrollee must have a right to select his or her primary care provider, as provided under standard 2.2.3.1, and to change this selection at any time. Similarly, in the case of mental health and substance abuse services, although an enrollee's primary provider of these services may initially be assigned through, for example, a triage system, the enrollee must have a right to select a different primary provider. The standard does not however confer a right with respect to referral or other services: specifically, an enrollee may be referred to a specific provider designated by the referring provider or by the organization (although the enrollee must have the right, provided under standard 2.2.3.2, to refuse care from the designated provider and to request referral to a different affiliated provider).

In order to facilitate enrollee selection of providers, the organization must make available to enrollees, on request, information including education, board certification, and recertification status; names of hospitals where physicians have admitting privileges; years of practice as a physician and as a specialist, if so identified; experience with performing certain medical or surgical procedures; consumer satisfaction measures; and clinical quality performance measures.

2.2.3.1 *Each enrollee may select his or her primary care provider from among those accepting new Medicare or Medicaid enrollees.*

New enrollees must be informed of the primary care providers available and the procedures for selecting a provider. An organization that requires use of the primary care provider to obtain other services may assign a provider for enrollees who have failed to make a selection within a reasonable time period specified in the organization's procedures. In the event of assignment, the enrollee must be notified of the assignment and of the procedures for changing the designated provider.

In the event a primary care provider ceases to be affiliated with the organization, the organization must promptly assist enrollees in obtaining a new primary care provider. The organization's procedures must provide for notice to affected enrollees within 15 working days of the receipt or issuance of the notice of termination in the case of Medicare, and within as many days as the State Medicaid agency may specify in the case of Medicaid. The notice must include information on how to select a new primary care provider. In the event an affiliation is terminated because a specific provider has left a group or facility that continues to contract with the organization, the enrollee may be offered an opportunity to select from among other providers at the site who are continuing to accept new patients. However, the enrollee must also be notified of the right to select another site or provider.

2.2.3.2 *Each enrollee may refuse care from specific providers.*

An enrollee referred to a specific provider for any service other than primary care must have an opportunity to refuse care from the designated provider and to select a different affiliated provider. (Medicare enrollees requesting a second surgical opinion must also be permitted to select the affiliated provider for this service.) To the extent feasible, this means that an enrollee must never be in the position of having only one possible source of care or services. There are two exceptions:

1. The service is highly specialized and is available from only one provider within the organization's network within the service area.

2. The organization has designated a single supplier for a service that does not involve a personal encounter with a provider. Examples might include clinical laboratory services, radiology, medical supplies, or transportation.

This standard is not intended to require that an organization allow enrollees to use highly specialized providers for care that can be appropriately furnished by other affiliated providers. For example, an organization that includes a tertiary care facility among its contracting hospitals need not allow an enrollee to select that facility for a routine delivery.

Subnetworks

An organization may contract with formal subnetworks that provide a broad spectrum of care and services, or the organization may allow individual providers to establish informal subnetworks.

A formal subnetwork exists when each enrollee is required, at the time of initial selection of a primary care provider, to choose an entire subnetwork that may also include specialists, hospitals, or other providers. For example, an organization might contract with several different integrated health systems in its service area. An enrollee selecting a primary care provider affiliated with a particular health system may be required to obtain covered services through the other providers affiliated with the system. This is permissible when:

1. Enrollee information materials clearly indicate that the organization is using a subnetwork approach and the materials are in such form that the enrollee can readily identify the providers available through each subnetwork;

2. Enrollees are afforded a meaningful choice of providers within the subnetwork; and

3. The enrollee may change his or her choice of subnetwork at any time.

An informal subnetwork exists when an organization has delegated to a provider the authority to refer the enrollee for services of other providers, and the delegate limits the enrollee's choice to a subset of the providers affiliated with the organization. For example, an organization's contract with a primary care provider may hold that provider financially responsible for specialty physician services, and the provider may in turn make financial arrangements for those services with one or more of the specialists affiliated with the organization. The enrollee retains the right to refuse care from the specialist selected by the primary care provider and to request referral to a different specialist who is affiliated with the organization but is not a member of the provider's informal subnetwork. An enrollee may not be required to select a new primary care provider in order to exercise this right;

this is permitted only in the case of a formal subnetwork arrangement as defined above.

2.2.4 *to participate in decision-making regarding his or her health care;*

The organization's policies must promote enrollees' understanding of their conditions or problems and facilitate development of mutually agreed upon treatment goals. While participation in treatment planning is important for all enrollees, special emphasis should be placed on involvement of enrollees and/or their families in development of plans of care for enrollees with mental health or substance problems, with chronic diseases, or at the end of life.

2.2.4.1 *The organization provides for the enrollee's representative to facilitate care or treatment decisions when the enrollee is unable to do so.*

Written policies and procedures address the care and treatment of enrollees who are unable to exercise rational judgment or give informed consent. State law will generally govern who may act as an enrollee's representative. A representative may be (1) a person who is designated as the enrollee's representative (e.g., by a power of attorney); (2) a court appointed guardian; (3) a spouse or other family member as designated by the enrollee; or (4) another person designated by a state agency.

2.2.4.2 *The organization provides for enrollee or representative involvement in decisions to withhold resuscitative services, or to forgo or withdraw life-sustaining treatment, and complies with requirements of Federal and State law with respect to advance directives.*

With respect to advance directives, the organization is specifically required:

(1) to inform all Medicare and Medicaid enrollees at the time of enrollment of their right (under state law, whether statutory or recognized by the courts of the state) to accept or refuse treatment and to execute an advance directive, such as living wills or durable powers of attorney, and of the organization's written policies on implementation of that right (including a clear and precise statement of limitation, if the organization cannot implement an advance directive as a matter of conscience);

(2) to document in the enrollee's medical records whether or not an individual has executed an advance directive;

(3) to not make treatment conditional or otherwise discriminate on the basis of whether an individual has executed an advance directive;

(4) to comply with state law, whether statutory or recognized by the courts of the state, on advance directives; and

(5) to provide (individually or with others) for education of staff and the community on advance directives.

As a practical matter, compliance with patients' or representatives' instructions in these areas is largely in the hands of physicians, hospitals or other facilities and their attending staff. However, the organization should take at least the following steps to assure enrollees' rights:

    I. Include information on advance directives and other end-of-life issues in enrollee information;

    II. Require documentation of advance directives in medical records, verify compliance in its reviews of medical recordkeeping, and ensure that providers are educated about their responsibility to communicate enrollees' wishes to attending staff in hospitals or other facilities;

    III. Review policies of affiliated hospitals and other contracting facilities; and

    IV. Assure that practice guidelines or guidelines used in utilization management do not impede enrollees' decision making with respect to end-of-life care.

Note that requirements related to advance directives are not limited to directives concerning care at the end of life. The organization should also assure compliance with other forms of patient instructions, such as psychiatric advance directives.

2.2.5 *to receive information on available treatment options (including the option of no treatment) or alternative courses of care and other information specified in standard 2.3; health care professionals must provide information regarding treatment options in a language that the enrollee understands.*

Contracts with providers may not limit a provider's ability to counsel or advise a Medicare or Medicaid enrollee on treatment options that may be appropriate for the enrollee's condition or disease, whether or not the options are covered by the organization. Enrollees have a right to a clear explanation of: their condition; any proposed treatments or procedures and alternatives; the benefits, drawbacks, and likelihood of success of each option; and the possible consequences of refusal or non-compliance with a recommended course of care.

In ensuring that health care professionals provide information in a language that the enrollee understands, see standard 3.1.5.

2.2.6 *to have access to his or her medical records in accordance with applicable Federal and State laws; and*

The organization must have procedures through which an enrollee can obtain timely access to all medical records and health information maintained by the organization, including records maintained by subcontracting providers from whom the enrollee has received services.

2.2.7 *to obtain a prompt resolution, through the procedures established under standard 2.4, of issues raised by the enrollee, including complaints or grievances and issues relating to authorization, coverage, or payment of services.*

  2.3 *Enrollee Information*

Enrollee understanding of the workings of the organization, procedures for obtaining services, and rights and responsibilities, are essential to the provision of quality care. This standard measures the comprehensiveness of the content of enrollee information and the accessibility of this information. Review of compliance with this standard is part of a broader review of the organization's basic information for enrollees. This standard addresses only those elements of enrollee information that are directly related to the use of health services. (Guidelines are pro-

vided below only for those individual elements that are not self-explanatory.)
Note that information required to be furnished to enrollees must also be made
available to any representative designated by or on behalf of the enrollee.

2.3.1 *Each enrollee receives, at the time of enrollment and at least annually thereafter, a written statement including information on:*

2.3.1.1 *Enrollee rights;*

2.3.1.2 *Enrollee responsibilities;*

While it is advisable to include a discussion of enrollee responsibilities in enrollee
information, the discussion should clearly indicate that enrollment and subsequent
receipt of care is not conditional on the enrollee's agreement to follow a particular course of prescribed treatment.

2.3.1.3 *The names and locations of network providers, including information on which providers are accepting new Medicare or Medicaid patients and any restrictions on enrollees' ability to select from among network providers;*

Enrollees making a decision about whether to enroll in a particular organization
may rely on the organization's provider listings in making their selection and may
assume that (subject to the organization's authorization procedures) they will be
able to obtain covered services from any of the providers listed. It is essential that
the organization's informational materials emphasize any limitations on enrollees'
provider selections. If the organization contracts with formal subnetworks (see
standard 2.2.3.2) and requires enrollees selecting a particular subnetwork for primary care to use that subnetwork's affiliated providers for referral services, informational materials must clearly indicate which individual providers are available
under each subnetwork (for example, through a simple coding system or separate
provider listings for each subnetwork). If the organization's arrangements with primary care providers allow for the establishment of informal subnetworks, informational materials must so indicate and must explain the procedures under which
an enrollee may request referral to an affiliated provider not included in the informal subnetwork.

2.3.1.4 *Amount, duration and scope of all benefits and services included and excluded as a condition of enrollment, including a description of how the organization evaluates new technology for inclusion as a covered benefit;*

It is not expected that standard enrollee information will include every specific
coverage decision made by the organization, such as a listing of its entire drug formulary or its criteria for approval of specific medical procedures. However, materials must indicate how an enrollee may obtain this information.

2.3.1.5 *Procedures for obtaining services, including authorization requirements, any special procedures for obtaining mental health and substance abuse services, procedures for obtaining out-of-area coverage and, in the case of enrollees eligible for a point of service benefit, procedures for obtaining services through the benefit, including special conditions or charges that may apply;*

2.3.1.6   *In the case of Medicaid enrollees, procedures for obtaining services covered under the Medicaid state plan and not covered by the organization, and notice of the right to obtain family planning services from any Medicaid-participating provider;*

2.3.1.7   *Provisions for after-hours and emergency coverage. Materials must instruct enrollees that enrollees have the right to access emergency health care services from contracting or non-contracting providers without prior authorization, consistent with the enrollee's determination of the need for such services as a prudent layperson.*

2.3.1.8   *Policies on referrals for specialty care and other services not furnished by the enrollee's primary care provider;*

2.3.1.9   *Charges to enrollees, if applicable;*

2.3.1.10   *Procedures established under standard 2.4 for resolving enrollee issues, including complaints or grievances and issues relating to authorization of, coverage of, or payment for services;*

2.3.1.11   *Procedures for changing primary care providers;*

2.3.1.12   *Procedures for recommending changes in policies or services;*

2.3.1.13   *Information on service area; and*

2.3.1.14   *Notice of the right to obtain the following information:*

2.3.1.14.1   *The information in standards 2.3.1.1 through 2.3.1.13.*

2.3.1.14.2   *The procedures the organization uses to control utilization of services and expenditures.*

2.3.1.14.3   *The number of grievances and appeals and their disposition in the aggregate, in a manner and form specified by CMS (for Medicare) and the State Medicaid agency (for Medicaid).*

2.3.1.14.4   *A summary description of the method of compensation for physicians.*

2.3.1.14.5   *The financial condition of the organization, including the most recently audited information regarding its condition.*

2.3.2   *The organization notifies enrollees affected by termination of or changes in benefits, services, service sites, or affiliated providers. To the extent practical, enrollees are informed of such terminations or changes prior to their effective date.*

Notice of changes in benefits or in the organization's rules for obtaining benefits must be provided to affected beneficiaries at least 30 days before the change takes effect. Notice of a termination of a contracted provider must be provided within 15 working days of receipt or issuance of the notice of termination. Changes affecting enrollees generally should be communicated through bulletins, newsletters, or other plan-wide documents. Notice of the termination or withdrawal of specific providers may be furnished only to the enrollees using those providers; when the provider is a designated primary care provider, the notice should include a reminder on the procedures for changing providers.

2.3.3   *Enrollee information is—*

2.3.3.1   *readable and easily understood;*

Generally materials should be understandable to enrollees at a fifth-grade reading level (or another level established by the State Medicaid agency). Materials should use an easily readable typeface and frequent headings, and should provide short, simple explanations of key concepts. Technical or legal language should be avoided whenever possible.

2.3.3.2 *Available in the language(s) of the major population groups served and, as needed, in alternative formats for the visually impaired.*

The organization must have a procedure for ascertaining the primary language of enrollees and for making information materials available in any language that is the primary language of more than 10 percent of the geographic area. Basic enrollee information, except for the provider listing required under standard 2.3.1.3, must also be made available to the visually impaired in large print and Braille formats or through recorded cassettes.

2.3.4 *The organization evaluates the effectiveness of its communications with enrollees.*

The organization's enrollee surveys could include a focus on the extent to which Medicare and Medicaid enrollees understand key concepts of health plan enrollment and are able to use information materials. Alternatively, materials could be tested with focus groups, enrollee advisory committees, or other groups of Medicare and Medicaid enrollees.

2.4 *Resolution of Enrollee Issues. The organization has a system for resolving issues raised by enrollees, including: complaints or grievances; issues relating to authorization of, coverage of, or payment for services; and issues relating to discontinuation of a service. [NOTE: references to an enrollee in these standards include reference to an enrollee's representative.]*

Medicare and State Medicaid programs use a variety of terms for circumstances in which an enrollee voices a concern with, or requests an action by, the organization. Different processes, both for the organization and for CMS or the State Medicaid agency, govern the resolution of different types of issues raised by enrollees. This standard presents a unified structure for evaluating the organization's performance in carrying out those elements of each process for which it is responsible.

The standard distinguishes among three basic categories of enrollee issues:

1. Initial requests that the organization or its subcontractor provide or authorize a service or pay for a service already obtained.

This category includes requests made directly to a provider, requests made by an enrollee or a provider through an organization's system for prior approval of services, and requests in the form of claims for payment filed by the enrollee or a provider. Any such request results in an initial decision by the organization (or by a provider to whom the initial decision-making authority has been delegated) to approve or disapprove provision of or payment for the service. Under Medicare, this decision is known as an "organization determination." Under Medicaid, an initial decision to deny, reduce or terminate a service or to deny payment, or to not furnish a service with reasonable promptness is known as an "action."

Standard 3.3, on service authorizations, sets forth some basic rules for initial consideration by the organization or its delegate of service or payment requests that are considered through the organization's prior authorization system or claims processing system (or comparable systems operated by subcontractors). As explained under standard 3.3, those rules do not apply when an enrollee requests a service directly from a provider and the provider decides whether or not to furnish or arrange the service without referring the request to anyone else for formal approval. For example, an enrollee may ask his or her primary care physician to make a referral for a given surgical procedure. If the physician agrees to make the referral and then seeks approval through the organization's authorization system, a decision (or "organization determination") has not been made until the organization's authorization system has approved or denied the request for Medicare or Medicaid. If, on the other hand, the physician determines that a referral is inappropriate and declines to seek authorization, for Medicare only, the physician has already made an initial decision and must explain to the enrollee how to obtain a reconsideration of that decision under standard 2.4.3. The same would be true if the physician declined to perform a requested service that the physician could furnish on his or her own.

2. Requests that the organization, its subcontractor, or a government agency reconsider a decision not to provide or authorize a service or pay for a service already obtained.

When an organization or its subcontractor makes an initial decision ("organization determination" or "action") not to provide or pay for a covered service (or a service that is perceived by the enrollee as covered), the enrollee is entitled to reconsideration under Medicare. This is true both of determinations that a requested service is not covered under the Medicare contract and of decisions that a covered service is not necessary or appropriate for the particular enrollee.

Under Medicare, a request for reconsideration is initially reviewed by the organization. If the organization does not make a "fully favorable" determination—that is, agree to provide or pay for the service in whole—the request is forwarded to the "reconsideration contractor" (an entity under contract to CMS to resolve coverage disputes), and may be subject to further levels of administrative or judicial review. This process applies for basic services (services covered under the Medicare statute for all beneficiaries), "mandatory" supplemental services (services covered under a package that all Medicare enrollees must purchase as a condition of enrolling in the organization under its Medicare contract), and (as established by the BBA) optional supplemental benefits (non-Medicare services covered under a supplemental benefit package that each Medicare enrollee may choose whether or not to purchase). Standard 2.4.3 addresses the process of reconsideration by the organization itself and does not address the subsequent steps in the process.

Under Medicaid, an enrollee has a right to appeal the organization's initial decision to the State agency, through the fair hearing process established by the State agency under 42 CFR 431.200. The organization must comply with fair hearing decisions. Standard 2.4.3 thus applies only to instances in which the enrollee files a grievance with the organization.

3. Complaints or grievances on all other matters.

In Medicare, enrollee concerns on all issues not involving a request for provision of or payment for a service are treated as grievances and are subject to the procedures established under standard 2.4.2. This is not the case in Medicaid, because requests for provision of or payment for a service are considered complaints or grievances and are subject to the procedures established under 2.4.2. This standard does not distinguish between "formal" and "informal" grievances, or between "grievances" and "complaints." For the purpose of these standards a grievance is defined as:

Any communication, oral or written, from an enrollee to any employee of the organization or of its providers, expressing dissatisfaction with any aspect of the organization's or provider's operations, activities, or behavior, regardless of whether any remedial action is requested.

Examples of possible subjects of grievances include, but are not limited to, complaints about:

I. The quality of services provided (other than a refusal to furnish a requested service);

II. Interpersonal aspects of care, such as rudeness by a provider or staff member;

III. Failure to respect any of the enrollee's rights, as set forth in standard 2.2.

Under both Medicare and Medicaid, certain issues relating to disenrollment of an enrollee may also be considered through the organization's grievance process. Medicare requires that an organization seeking the involuntary disenrollment of an enrollee for cause must allow the enrollee to contest the organization's decision through the grievance process.

If the Medicaid agreement with an organization provides for "lock-in"—a fixed period during which an enrollee may disenroll only for "good cause"—enrollee requests for disenrollment for cause may at the State's option be initially processed through the organization's grievance procedure. In this case, the time frames specified in the organization's procedures must be such as to comply with the requirement that disenrollments for cause take effect no later than the first day of the second month following the month during which the enrollee requested disenrollment.

2.4.1 *Intake of Enrollee Issues. The organization follows written procedures for the receipt and initial processing of all issues raised by enrollees. The organization—*

The organization has received an issue when the enrollee directs any oral or written communication about the issue to any employee of the organization or its contracting providers, or when an enrollee concern is forwarded to the organization by another entity (for example, when a Social Security or Railroad Retirement office transmits a complaint made by a Medicare beneficiary). It is therefore essential that all personnel who may come into contact with enrollees understand the basic procedures for receiving and recording an issue and for initiating the applicable process for resolving the issue.

2.4.1.1 *documents each issue raised by an enrollee;*

When an enrollee raises an issue, the enrollee must immediately be informed of whether the issue is (a) one that the enrollee must present to the organization in writing or (b) one that the enrollee may present orally and that will be recorded by the person receiving the issue. Requests for a service or payment, or for reconsideration of an initial decision to deny a service or payment request, should be presented by the enrollee in writing. However, in the case of expedited reviews, oral requests are permitted. In Medicaid, grievances may be presented orally, although the enrollee must always be notified that he or she has the right to present a written grievance. If the person receiving the issue is uncertain of what category it falls into, the issue must be presented by the enrollee in writing.

There may be instances in which an enrollee expresses a concern orally to the staff of the organization or an affiliated provider, and the issue is resolved to the enrollee's satisfaction immediately and informally. Nevertheless, the issue and its resolution must be recorded, through a complaint log or other means, so that information on volume and nature of enrollee issues is available in the QAPI process and for other management functions.

2.4.1.2 *promptly determines whether the issue is to be resolved through: (a) the grievance process established under standard 2.4.2, (b) the process for making initial determinations on coverage and payment issues established under standard 3.3, or (c) the process for resolution of disputed initial determinations established under standard 2.4.3;*

Except in the case of grievances that are immediately resolved to the enrollee's satisfaction, the person receiving the enrollee issue must determine what type of issue it is and how it will be resolved (or must promptly forward the issue to personnel authorized to make this determination). This exception does not apply to Medicaid.

2.4.1.3 *acknowledges receipt of the issue and explains to the enrollee the process to be followed in resolving his or her issue;*

As soon as the organization has made the determination required under standard 2.4.1.2, the enrollee must receive an acknowledgment that the issue has been recorded and a clear explanation of how it will be resolved, describing each step in the process, the time frame for each step, and the enrollee's rights or responsibilities at each step. In the case of grievances, acknowledgment of receipt and explanation of the process may be made orally; however, grievances relating to quality of care issues must be acknowledged in writing, and the acknowledgment must specifically describe the issue raised by the enrollee.

2.4.1.4 *assists the enrollee as needed in completing forms or taking other necessary steps to obtain resolution of the issue; and*

2.4.1.5 *informs the enrollee of any applicable mechanism for resolving the issue external to the organization's own processes.*

The enrollee must be notified of alternative routes for resolution of his or her issue. Under Medicare, for example, an enrollee has a right to submit a quality of care complaint for investigation by the PRO, instead of pursuing it through the organization's grievance process. Under Medicaid, coverage and payment issues may

be presented to the State agency at any time. In addition, some States may have issue resolution mechanisms that are available to commercial enrollees of organizations as well as to Medicare and Medicaid enrollees, such as a hotline or other
complaints system maintained by the Insurance Commissioner or another State
agency. (Such a system would supplement, but not replace, the State Medicaid
agency's own hearing process.)

2.4.2 *Grievances. The organization implements a procedure, with clearly explained steps and
time limits for each step, for the resolution of a complaint or grievance.*

2.4.2.1 *The grievance is transmitted in a timely manner to staff who have authority to take corrective action. A grievance relating to quality of care is transmitted to appropriately qualified clinical personnel.*

2.4.2.2 *The organization investigates the grievance and notifies the concerned parties of the results of the investigation and the proposed resolution.*

The resolution must directly address the issue raised in the grievance, and the
proposed solution must be appropriate to the seriousness of the complaint.

2.4.2.3 *The organization provides an opportunity for reconsideration of the proposed resolution.*

When the enrollee is not satisfied with the proposed resolution of a grievance,
there must be an opportunity for further consideration by an individual or individuals other than the individual who initially reviewed the grievance.

2.4.2.4 *The organization tracks each grievance until its final resolution.*

The organization must have a system for monitoring its progress in reviewing and
resolving each grievance, to assure that each step is completed within the time
frame specified in the organization's grievance procedures.

2.4.2.5 *The organization has an expedited grievance process for issues requiring immediate
resolution.*

Standard 3.3.1.1 provides for expedited consideration of urgent requests for service. Under Medicare, however, there may be issues that are treated as grievances
and are therefore not subject to this process, but that may nevertheless require
rapid response. This would be true, for example, when an enrollee reports that he
or she is unable to obtain a timely appointment from a primary care provider for
a problem in need of immediate attention. Thus an expedited grievance process is
required in all organizations, regardless of the applicable procedure for obtaining
reconsideration of denials of service.

2.4.3 *Reconsideration of Coverage and Payment Determinations. The organization implements
a procedure, with clearly explained steps and time limits for each step, for reviewing requests for reconsideration of initial decisions not to provide or pay for a service.*

As noted earlier, this standard applies to all Medicaid actions and to Medicare reconsiderations related to basic or mandatory or optional supplemental services.

2.4.3.1 *The organization's notice to an enrollee and/or provider of its decision to deny, limit, or
discontinue authorization of, or payment for, a service includes information required under standard 3.3.1.5, including information about how to obtain a reconsideration of the
decision. The notice to the enrollee must be in writing.*

When a service request is made directly to a provider and the provider denies the request orally, the organization/provider must provide written notice to the enrollee of the right to obtain reconsideration and the procedure for requesting reconsideration.

2.4.3.2 *The organization's process complies with procedural requirements and time limits established by CMS (for Medicare) or the State Medicaid agency (for Medicaid), conforming with CMS requirements.*

Medicare regulations specify procedural time limits for service and payment determinations.

2.4.3.3 *Requests for reconsideration by the organization of a denial based on lack of medical necessity are reviewed by a physician (for Medicare) or health care professional (for Medicaid) who is appropriately credentialed with respect to the treatment involved and who is not the individual who made the initial determination.*

Both the physician (for Medicare) and the health care professional (for Medicaid) must be appropriately credentialed. If the organization delegates any phase of the reconsideration process to a subcontractor, the subcontractor must have its own procedures for complying with this standard. This standard means that the reconsideration function may not be delegated to a single provider.

2.4.4 *Monitoring of Issue Resolution Processes. The organization maintains, aggregates, and analyzes information on the nature of issues raised by enrollees and on their resolution.*

2.4.4.1 *The information is used to develop activities under the organization's QAPI program, both to improve the issue resolution process itself, and to make improvements that address other system issues raised in the issue resolution process.*

See standard 1.3.5.3.

2.4.4.2 *Information related to coverage and payment issues is maintained for at least three years following final resolution of the issue, and is made available to the enrollee on request.*

Appendix 11.C
QISMC Domain 3

DOMAIN 3: Health Services Management

STANDARD NUMBER	DESCRIPTION OF STANDARD

3.1   *Availability and Accessibility. The organization ensures that all covered services, including additional or supplemental services contracted for by or on behalf of Medicare or Medicaid enrollees, are available and accessible.*

The organization must ensure that all services are available: that is, that it has employed or contracted with appropriately qualified institutional and individual providers, and that these providers have sufficient capacity to make services available to the organization's enrollees. The organization must also ensure accessibility: that is, enrollees must be informed about the existence of the services and procedures for obtaining services when needed. Accessibility further requires that: services be geographically reachable, consistent with local community patterns of care; and that enrollees not experience undue waiting periods, either for obtaining an appointment or at the time of the appointment. Finally, language and cultural barriers as well as barriers to those individuals with physical or mental disabilities must also be addressed. (See standard 2.1.2 and 2.2.2 for further discussion of enrollee rights to accessible services.)

The organization's initial assessment of availability must consider, for each type of covered service and for major specialties within each type:

    I. Expected utilization of services, taking into account enrollee characteristics and health care needs.

The aggregate number of providers needed, and their distribution among different specialties, will vary according to the organization's projected population (in terms of age, disability, prevalence of certain conditions). It may also be affected by practice patterns within the organization, such as the rate of referrals for specific services.

    II. The numbers and types of providers needed to furnish these services.

Assessment of the numbers of providers needed to meet an expected level of demand for services can be based on national norms (such as physician/patient ratios) or on an organization's past experience. However, simple counts of providers, or even providers reportedly accepting new patients, are insufficient to establish capacity. Except when providers serve an organization's enrollees exclusively, assessment of capacity necessarily entails assessment of the volume of services being furnished to patients other than the organization's enrollees. The organization must therefore have a process for measuring available full-time equivalents (in the case of individual providers) or unused capacity (in the case of hospitals or other facilities).

Where more than one type of provider is qualified to furnish a particular item or service, the organization's standards must define the types of provider to be used. Some states may have laws requiring health plans to make specific types of providers available. The organization's standards should specifically define the types of mental health and substance abuse providers to be included (e.g., psychiatrists, psychologists, clinical social workers, psychiatric nurses). In addition, the organization must specify the types of providers who may serve as an enrollee's primary care provider (see standard 3.1.1.1). Note also that Medicaid rules specifying who may furnish services to pregnant women and children were repealed by the Balanced Budget Act of 1997.

An organization is expected to make specialists available to enrollees for services customarily furnished by specialists in the organization's service area. However, these standards do not require that any specific specialty service be furnished by board-certified specialists.

III. Geographic location of providers and enrollees.

The organization must ensure that providers are so distributed that no enrollee residing in the service area must travel an unreasonable distance to obtain any covered service. As a general rule, primary care services and commonly used specialty and referral services must be available within 30 minutes driving time from any point in the service area. Longer travel times for a particular service are permissible when residents in part or all of the service area customarily travel greater distances to obtain that service (e.g., in rural areas, or when there is only one provider of a given type in a broad region.)

Organizations with significant numbers of Medicare or Medicaid enrollees must consider not just driving time, but the usual means of transportation used by those enrollees. In areas where elderly, disabled, or low-income residents rely heavily on public transportation, the organization must ensure that providers are accessible through these means. (Unless, as under some Medicaid arrangements, the state or the organization makes alternative transportation available, or unless the organization ensures access through alternative means, such as home visits.)

3.1.1   *The organization maintains and monitors a network of appropriate providers, supported by written arrangements, that is sufficient to provide adequate access to covered services and to meet the needs of the population served.*

The organization's network consists of employees and facilities of the organization, if any, along with providers who have entered into written agreements to serve the organization's enrollees. Agreements must conform to applicable requirements of these standards and to other Medicare and Medicaid requirements for subcontracts. If the organization's subcontracts with providers allow those providers to enter into sub-subcontracts with other providers for services to Medicare or Medicaid enrollees, those sub-subcontracts must also meet applicable standards.

Services (other than in-area emergency care and out-of-area emergency and urgent care) must generally be available within the organization's network. Network providers must be located within the organization's approved service area, except that an organization operating solely in a non-metropolitan area may make a service (other than primary care and emergency care) available outside the area if it is unable to contract with a sufficient number of providers within the area.

An infrequently used service may be made available through providers who have not entered into a formal written agreement with the organization. If any service is to be furnished through non-contracting providers, the organization must have procedures for identifying appropriate providers, referring enrollees to the providers as needed, and assuring that the providers will accept payment from the organization as payment in full (subject to any allowable copayments or other cost-sharing).

An organization that offers a point-of-service benefit must still make all services available within its network (or through arrangements with non-contracting providers as described above). No enrollee may be required to use the point-of-service benefit, or pay any extra charges imposed under that benefit, in order to obtain any medically necessary covered service.

Because enrollee needs, the types of providers used by an organization to meet those needs, and other factors such as availability of public transportation will vary for each organization, it is impossible to develop a single set of fixed guidelines for the number and types of providers needed for all populations and all circumstances (such as prescribed primary physician/enrollee ratios or specified waiting times for appointments of different kinds). CMS or State Medicaid agencies may establish such standards for managed care organizations serving specific populations or areas. For example, a State might include specific guidelines in a request for proposals or standards may be developed in the course of the general contract negotiation process. Ultimately, however, it is the organization that must assess the needs of the population it proposes to enroll and construct a network to meet those needs. Compliance with this standard will therefore generally focus on the organization's own service planning and on the basic assumptions used by that organization in determining that its network is adequate to serve Medicare or Medicaid beneficiaries in a given area.

3.1.1.1 *Primary care providers. The organization offers a panel of primary care providers from which the enrollee may select a personal primary care provider.*

The organization must provide a listing from which enrollees may select and/or change their primary care providers without interference from the managed care organization. The listing of providers should specify: the location of the provider's practice site(s), their non-English language capabilities, board and/or advanced practice certifications, whether the provider also practices as a specialist within the plan's network, and designate if the provider's practice is open or closed to new enrollees.

The organization must also develop procedures for either ensuring that the information in the listing is updated regularly or making updated information on providers easily accessible to current and potential enrollees.

In the case of Medicare, if an M+CO requires its enrollees to obtain a referral in most situations before receiving services from a specialist, the organization must either assign a primary care physician for purposes of making the needed referral or make other arrangements to ensure access to medically necessary specialty care. Medicaid policy in this area will be addressed in the next QISMC revision.

3.1.1.2　*Specialists. The organization provides or arranges for necessary specialty care, including women's health services.*

In the case of Medicare, the organization allows women enrollees the option of direct access to a women's health specialist within the network for women's routine and preventive health care services provided as basic benefits. When the organization permits women to choose an obstetrician, gynecologist or certified midwife as their primary care provider, this requirement will not cause any change in the organization's policies and procedures. However, organizations that do not allow such options must provide women with both a designated primary care provider or some other means for continuity of care and direct access to their women's health specialist. The organization arranges for specialty care outside of the plan provider network when network providers are unavailable or inadequate to meet an enrollee's medical needs.

In the case of Medicaid, the organization allows women direct access to a women's health specialist within the network for women's routine and preventive health care services while the organization maintains a primary care provider or some other means for continuity of care. Guidance on provision of specialty care outside of the plan provider network for Medicaid will be provided in the QISMC revision that follows publication of the Medicaid managed care final rule.

Both Medicare and Medicaid MCOs must also implement methodologies to project the amount and types of specialists necessary to serve their anticipated enrollees, clearly stating the approach for ensuring availability of pediatric specialists, among others (either within its network or as an infrequently utilized service under 3.1.1.). In addition, because many women use their gynecological provider (i.e., obstetrician, gynecologist, certified nurse midwife) for the delivery of primary care services such as annual breast exams, managed care organizations must provide women with direct access to a women's health specialist for routine and preventive health care services, which are defined as breast exams, mammograms, and pap smears. Provision of "direct access" requires that the organization may not require the woman to obtain any referral, or prior authorization as a precondition to seeking or receiving care from a women's health specialist.

If a Medicare organization requires its enrollees to obtain a referral in most situations before receiving services from a specialist, the organization must either assign a primary care physician for purposes of making the needed referral or make other arrangements to ensure access to medically necessary specialty care. Medicaid policy in this area will be addressed in the next QISMC revision.

Note that QISMC guideline 2.2.3.2 allows an organization to create formal subnetworks. In these cases, an organization can require an enrollee, at the time of initial selection of a primary care physician, to choose an entire subnetwork that may include women's health specialists. See 2.2.3.2 for further instructions on formal subnetworks.

3.1.1.3 *Complex needs. The organization has procedures approved by CMS (for Medicare) or the State Medicaid agency (for Medicaid) for: the identification of individuals with complex or serious medical conditions; an assessment of those conditions; the identification of medical procedures to address and/or monitor the conditions; and a treatment plan appropriate to those conditions that specifies an adequate number of direct access visits to specialists to accommodate implementation of the treatment plan, and that is time-specific, and updated periodically. The organization must also have procedures for ensuring adequate coordination of care among providers.*

To aid us in defining the concept of serious or complex medical condition, CMS contracted with the Institute of Medicine (IOM), which submitted in October 1999 a final report to CMS entitled "Definition of Serious and Complex Medical Conditions." This report can be purchased through the following web site: *www.nap.edu.*

The IOM report provides useful guidance to managed care organizations seeking to design a system for efficient identification and classification of enrollees with conditions which would benefit from careful and coordinated treatment planning, direct access to specialists and on-going coordination of services across the continuum of care. In the following sections, we have extracted material from the IOM's committee report with additional comments from CMS. Attached as an appendix to these standards is the Executive Summary of the IOM report.

Note that the committee chose to include only a subset of persons with serious or complex medical conditions, that is, they chose those with both serious and complex medical conditions. The committee determined that it was best to set this subgroup as a priority for consideration. CMS agrees with this recommendation.

MCOs should consider these recommendations, but retain the discretion to be creative in developing their own programs.

"Recommendation 1: The committee recommends the following language: A *serious and complex* condition is one that is persistent and substantially disabling or life-threatening that requires treatments and services across a variety of domains of care to ensure the best possible outcomes for each unique patient or member."

The committee reviewed a number of possible categories of conditions that might be considered serious and complex. These include, but are not limited to, life threatening conditions, conditions that cause serious disability without necessarily being life threatening, conditions associated with severe consequences, conditions affecting multiple organ systems, conditions requiring coordination of management by multiple specialties, and conditions requiring treatments that carry a risk of serious complications.

Organizations are expected to develop, in consultation with appropriate adult and pediatric clinicians, operational definitions that the organization will implement within its network of providers to identify such individuals. This standard does not require that an organization develop formal programs for every variety of complex condition, but that it establish a formal process for responding to any complex need as it arises in its enrollee population. The expectation is that the organization will establish a formal process that will identify the conditions for which more intensive care management is necessary and specify who in the organization will coordinate care for particular enrollees. Such a process should facilitate communication and information exchange among all treating health care professionals.

In its recommendations, the IOM committee indicates that it considered several alternative definitions prior to selecting its final definition, e.g., conditions affecting multiple organ systems. In the full report, the committee recommends that plans should use a combination of these different definitions, rather than just focusing on one definition. CMS agrees with this recommendation. A combination of measures is more likely to identify persons with serious and complex medical conditions. Therefore, CMS encourages M+C organizations to make use of several of the different definitions presented in the report.

"Recommendation 2: The committee recommends that MCOs design and implement strategies for routine screening and selection to identify those beneficiaries with serious and complex medical conditions. These strategies should be consistent with the guidance outlined in Recommendation 1 to determine which patients meet an organization's threshold for serious and complex medical conditions and would benefit from a coordinated care management strategy."

"The committee recommends that MCOs identify specific categories of patients or health conditions for which screening for the presence of serious and complex conditions should occur on a routine basis. The committee is of the opinion that screening an organization's entire population of enrollees is not a feasible, cost-effective, or efficient method of identifying subpopulations with serious and complex medical conditions. The committee feels strongly, however, that early efforts to develop screening methodologies should not be prescriptive; rather, innovation should be encouraged. Documentation of locally derived methods by MCOs will result in extensive nationwide experience that can be assessed and can lead to the identification of best practices and subsequent standardized methods for ongoing routine screening of patient populations."

"Recommendation 3: The committee recommends that MCOs develop a broad strategy for care management to enable patients and providers to achieve the best possible outcomes for each unique patient or member with a serious and complex medical condition."

"This care management strategy should include, but not necessarily be limited to, case finding, screening, and selection; problem assessment and identification of strengths; development of treatment or care plans; implementation of care plans with an emphasis on proactive interventions; and monitoring of care plan implementation and outcomes."

"Throughout the entire care management strategy for persons with serious and complex medical conditions, three principles should be evident. First, the care management strategy should reflect a commitment to continuity and coordination of care, as described among the requirements for National Committee for Quality Assurance accreditation. This entails monitoring continuity and coordination activities, analyzing data to identify opportunities for improvement, and taking actions to bring about improvements, as indicated. Second, the care process should include multidisciplinary perspectives and treatments, as appropriate. The care of persons with serious and complex medical conditions may require the assessment and treatment expertise of primary care providers; medical and surgical specialists; nurses and nurse specialists; social workers; pharmacists; occupational, speech, and physical therapists; rehabilitation specialists; behavioral and mental health professionals; and community-based services providers and resources. Access to expertise from these various disciplines should be available as needed. Third, and perhaps most important, patients and their family members should be involved at every step so that the care process incorporates the patient's expectations and preferences and documents the patient's role in achieving treatment goals."

The IOM Report further states:

"Recommendation 4: The committee recommends that MCOs develop a care management strategy that integrates the participation of all those involved in the care of the patient, including primary care physicians; medical and surgical specialists; nurses and nurse specialists; behavioral and mental health specialists; physical, occupational, and speech therapists; social workers; allied health professionals; and community-based service providers."

"Recommendation 5: The committee recommends that MCOs have programs in place to monitor care management plans for both process and outcomes for patients with serious and complex conditions at the level of population, patient, provider, and best practices of care."

The organization must also develop (in consultation with expert adult and pediatric clinicians), policies and procedures for assuring that all such individuals receive: (1) an assessment of all of their medical, psychological, and social conditions, and (2) the medical care needed to fully address and monitor those conditions. Where the assessment identifies needs for medical, psychological, or social services that are outside the scope of the organization's benefit package, the organization should have appropriate policies and procedures for making referrals to and coordinating care with appropriate external agencies and providers to be involved in the care of the enrollee.

The organization must also ensure that the implementation of the treatment plan (consistent with the enrollee's coverage) addresses the needs identified by the assessment. Effective treatment plans should establish individual goals for the patient, identify needed resources, and periodically evaluate outcomes and needs for further intervention. In the event the enrollee requires care from a specialist, the organization should provide direct access visits to the specialist(s) in sufficient quantity consistent with the patient's treatment plan. All treatment plans, therefore, should be: (1) developed by the primary care provider (or another designated member of the interdisciplinary team responsible for the patient) and the patient and his/her family (as specified in QISMC standard 2.2.4), (2) be established for a specific period of time, and (3) identify target dates for reassessment of progress toward and/or accomplishment of desired patient outcomes.

In addition to its general care coordination mechanism established under standard 3.2.1.1 and regulations under 422.112 (b)(3), the organization should have care coordination programs to facilitate communication and information exchange among professionals involved in the care of conditions requiring multiple sources of treatment or levels of care. This standard does not require that an organization develop formal programs for every variety of complex problem. Instead, the expectation is that the organization will identify conditions that are prevalent in its population and for which continuity and effectiveness of care would be improved through targeted programs. Effective programs (as described above) should set individual treatment goals for each participant, identify necessary resources, and periodically evaluate outcomes and the need for further intervention.

As previously indicated, the IOM committee did not define serious or complex, and only dealt with serious and complex medical conditions. Therefore, CMS does not expect MCOs to develop policies to deal with the broad spectrum encompassed by the phrase "serious or complex medical conditions" at this time. We will be reviewing how MCOs deal with different medical conditions to determine if revisions in this policy are warranted.

3.1.1.4   *The M+CO must make a good faith effort to provide written notice of a termination of a contracted provider within a reasonable time of receipt or issuance of a notice of termination to all enrollees who are patients seen on a regular basis by the provider whose contract is terminating, irrespective of whether the termination was for cause or without cause. When a contract termination involves a primary care professional, all enrollees who are patients of that primary care professional must also be notified.*

The M+C organization must make a good faith effort to provide written notice of a termination of a contracted provider, within 15 working days of receipt or issuance of a notice of termination as described in 42 CFR 422.204(c)(4), to all enrollees who are patients seen on a regular basis by the provider whose contract is terminating, irrespective of whether the termination was for cause or without cause. When a contract termination involves a primary care professional, all enrollees who are patients of that primary care professional must also be notified.

3.1.2   *The organization determines that all providers are qualified through the process established under standard 3.5.*

If the organization's subcontracts with providers allow those providers to enter into sub-subcontracts with other providers for services to Medicare or Medicaid enrollees, either the organization or its subcontractor must determine, pursuant to standard 3.5, that each sub-subcontractor is appropriately qualified and is not excluded from participation in Medicare or Medicaid.

3.1.3 *When medically necessary, the organization makes services available 24 hours a day, 7 days a week.*

This requirement is distinct from the requirement that the organization pay non-network providers for emergency services and urgent out-of-area services. These payment requirements are enforced in reviews of the organization's claims processing function and are not addressed in these standards. Instead, standard 3.1.3 restates a requirement of Medicare law and Medicaid regulations that the organization itself must make services available at all times.

This is not to suggest that the organization must maintain a separate facility around the clock, but rather to require availability of essential health care providers (physician, registered nurses, etc.) during normal business hours and, at a minimum, telephone contact/triage services by health care professionals outside of business hours. In the event that enrollees must be seen outside of normal business hours, there must be provisions for referring the patients in an expeditious fashion to a health care/emergency facility within reasonable distance from the enrollee.

3.1.4 *The organization ensures that the hours of operation of its providers are convenient to and do not discriminate against enrollees.*

Provision of "after hours" service, particularly for urgent care, is essential if inappropriate utilization of emergency room services is to be avoided. Therefore, this standard aims to ensure that:

(1) there is access to care after normal working hours (5 p.m. to 9 a.m.) for those urgent medical events that require attention after hours;

(2) the operating hours of provider sites allow for the provision of care to enrollees who are not able to take off from work to receive their care; and

(3) the hours of operation do not discriminate against Medicare or Medicaid enrollees relative to other enrollees.

3.1.5 *The organization ensures that services are provided in a culturally competent manner to all enrollees, including: those with limited English proficiency or reading skills, and those with diverse cultural and ethnic backgrounds.*

The delivery of culturally competent health care and services requires health care providers and/or employees to possess a set of attitudes, skills, behaviors, and policies which enable the organization and staff to work effectively in cross-cultural situations. It reflects an understanding of the importance of acquiring and using knowledge of the unique health-related beliefs, attitudes, practices, and communication patterns of beneficiaries and their families to improve services, strengthen programs, increase community participation, and eliminate disparities in health status among diverse population groups.

Activities to promote achievement of this objective fall under categories which include but are not limited to Organizational Readiness, Community Assessment,

Program Development, and Performance Improvement, for example. Under Organizational Readiness, MCOs should conduct educational programs to increase the knowledge of their staff about the unique health care beliefs, attitudes, practices, and communication patterns of the populations served by their plan. Title VI of the Civil Rights Act (see DOJ regulations 28 CFR Section 42.405 (d)(1)) specifically requires that MCOs provide assistance to persons with Limited-English Proficiency, where a significant number of the eligible population is affected. The organization may also be required to assess the language needs of beneficiaries in their service area, provide sufficient access to proficient interpreters, and disseminate written policies on the use of interpreters. In addition to the above, the provider network should be capable of meeting the cultural, linguistic, and informational needs of the beneficiaries residing in the service area. Ideally, the racial and ethnic diversity of the service area would be reflected in the provider network and staff of the organization. The literature has demonstrated that enrollees are more likely to seek and comply with health care services when delivered by one of their own racial or ethnic group. At a minimum, the organization must assure that all employees receive education regarding the importance of providing clinically competent and culturally appropriate services.

Community assessment consists of a market assessment to identify the specific health care needs of the beneficiary population as to enrollee groups health problems (e.g., some diseases are ethnically and genetically linked). Using existing and secondary data resources, organizations would collect data to the extent necessary to identify any special culturally-based health care needs among their beneficiaries. Program Development consists of implementation of formal programs and culturally sensitive patient education projects. The objective of such efforts would be to assure provision of comprehensive services which reduce and eventually eliminate cultural, linguistic, and informational barriers known to deter or discourage health-seeking behavior. And finally, Performance Improvement addresses an identified need or opportunity for improvement, either through a quality improvement project or other formal program which seeks to resolve undesirable differences in utilization of services and outcomes of care across all relevant racial, ethnic and cultural groups served by the managed care organization.

3.1.6 *An established organization seeking an expansion of its service area demonstrates that the numbers and types of providers available to enrollees are sufficient to meet the projected needs of the population and area to be served.*

It is expected that an established organization seeking an expanded service area will—

I. Identify the availability and accessibility standards that it will apply to the proposed service expansion area,

II. If different from the standards adopted for the existing service area, the organization will document the basis for these standards, and

III. Demonstrate that its has sufficient network capacity to meet the standards.

In addition, an organization that plans to furnish services through multiple formal subnetworks, as defined in the guidelines for standard 2.2.2, must ensure that each subnetwork has adequate capacity to meet anticipated needs of the population it is projected to serve.

3.1.7 *The organization establishes—*

3.1.7.1 *Standards for timeliness of access to care and member services that meet or exceed such standards as may be established by CMS (for Medicare) or the State Medicaid agency (for Medicaid), continuously monitors its provider network's compliance with these standards, and takes corrective action as necessary.*

An organization ensures access and availability of services by developing its own standards and continuously monitoring its own compliance with these standards. CMS or State Medicaid agencies may promulgate, or include in contracts, specific access standards to be met by the organization, in which case the organization's monitoring activities must be conducted in light of those standards. In an organization that serves both commercial and Medicare or Medicaid members, and whose commercial, Medicare, and Medicaid networks are not identical, assessment of compliance with availability and accessibility standards must be performed separately for the Medicare and Medicaid populations.

Access issues relating to particular services or population needs may be addressed as a part of the QAPI process. However, it is also expected that the organization will, as a routine administrative function, continuously assess access to all types of services and modify its network arrangements as necessary to correct any observed deficiency.

Standards

The organization must establish standards of timeliness of appointments and in-office waiting times for each type of service. The standards should consider the immediacy of member needs and common waiting times for comparable services in the community. An example of reasonable standards for primary care services might be:

I. Urgent but non-emergent—within 24 hours

II. Non-urgent but in need of attention—within one week

III. Routine and preventive—within 20 days

Standards should include criteria for classification of complaints by level of urgency.

The organization must ensure that affiliated providers are aware of the standards and have mechanisms in place for complying. For primary care providers, the organization should obtain documentation of backup arrangements for vacations and other absences, and ensure that backup providers are familiarized with plan procedures, such as approval requirements for referral services.

The organization must also have standards for responsiveness of member services telephone lines. The standards should specify maximum average waiting times to reach a non-recorded voice. In an organization with substantial low-income membership, these standards should take into account the likelihood that such members may not have access to touch-tone systems and may be using telephones outside their residences.

Monitoring

The organization must continuously monitor compliance with its own standards for timely access to services. Tools for monitoring might include:

I. Member surveys.

II. Analysis of member complaints and grievances.

III. Provider self-reports of appointment and in-office waiting times, supplemented by random calls or audits.

IV. For the organization's own services, test calls and ongoing monitoring of telephone abandonment rates (the percentage of callers who terminate a call before reaching an organization representative).

Note that the organization's work in this area must evaluate access and availability for all services, not merely primary care. Thus, the organization may not, for example, base its monitoring solely on general surveys of its enrolled population that do not yield information on availability of specialty or other services or do not provide a sufficient sample of enrollees requiring such services. (One possible source of this information would be reports by primary care providers of difficulties in arranging necessary referral services.)

Corrective Action

The organization must initiate corrective action when services are found to be inaccessible within the time frames specified by its accessibility standards. When the problem applies to an entire service type or specialty, this may involve expanding the organization's facilities or provider network. When the problem involves a specific provider, possible actions might include closing off the provider to new members or monitoring to ensure that the provider is treating the organization's members in the same way as non-members. The organization's procedures must include processes for assessing the effectiveness of corrective action.

3.1.7.2 *Policies and procedures, including coverage rules, practice guidelines, payment policies and utilization management, that allow for individual medical necessity determinations.*

Scheduling of utilization reviews, the presence of physician incentive plans and other policies may not interfere with or cause delay in services or otherwise preclude delivery of health care services which providers, through their education, experience and assessment of patient need, deem medically necessary for the individual patient.

3.1.7.3 *A policy encouraging provider consideration of beneficiary input in the provider's proposed treatment plan.*

The Consumer's Bill of Rights and Responsibilities states that, "Consumers have the right and responsibility to fully participate in all treatment decisions related to their health care. Consumers who are unable to fully participate in treatment decisions have the right to be represented by parents, guardians, family members, or other conservators." Further, it reports that patient participation in treatment decisions leads to improved satisfaction with care, enhanced outcomes and, subsequently, improved quality of life.

This respect for the right of the patient is essential given that consumers depend upon their health care providers to deliver expert consultation and advice which facilitates attainment of their health care goals and expectations. This responsibility is particularly great since patients must make critical decisions regarding their health care at a time when they are most vulnerable.

As enrollees are the ultimate health care consumer and partners with their providers, managed care organizations have a responsibility to ensure that enrollees are included in the planning and implementation of their care. As such, providers must: educate patients regarding their unique health care needs; share the findings of history and physical examinations; discuss potential treatment options (without regard to plan coverage), side effects of treatments, and management of symptoms; and, in general, recognize that the patient has the right to choose the final course of action among clinically acceptable choices. A choice of treatment must not be made without prior consultation with the patient as patient acceptance and understanding of the treatment plan will facilitate successful care outcomes.

3.2 *Continuity and Coordination of Care. The organization must ensure continuity of care and integration of services through arrangements that include, but are not limited to the following—*

3.2.1 *For Medicaid, MCOs should make use of a health care professional who is formally designated as having primary responsibility for coordinating the enrollee's overall health care; for Medicare, MCOs should develop policies that specify under what circumstances services are coordinated and the methods for coordination;*

For Medicare only, to meet this requirement, all organizations will need to develop written policies that specify the circumstances as to when services are coordinated and the methods for coordination.

Traditionally, many health maintenance organizations and similar entities have used a "gatekeeper" model, under which the enrollee's usual source of primary care served as the entry point for all other medical care services (often a distinct entry point was established for mental health and substance abuse services). While this model is still quite common, some organizations have systems under which either 1) a health professional other than the enrollee's usual source of primary care, such as a case manager, or 2) a case management team or interdisciplinary team coordinates services. In other organizations, enrollees may be free to obtain services from any network provider without authorization. The enrollee may have no usual source of primary care, and the organization may or may not have mechanisms in place for ensuring coordination and continuity. In these cases, it is acceptable for there to be plan-level case management for high-risk enrollees. Another approach is to use information systems to facilitate coordination of care.

These standards reflect the diversity of organizational structures by distinguishing among three different activities:

Delivery of primary care. Whether or not the organization uses a gatekeeper model, establishment of an ongoing relationship with a usual source of primary care plays an important role in promoting continuity and quality of care. The organization is therefore encouraged to make every effort to promote such a relationship, even in arrangements that allow direct access to providers other than the primary care provider.

Coordination of services. A health care professional, who may either be the primary care provider, a team of providers (for Medicare), or a plan employee who is a health care professional should have primary responsibility for evaluating the enrollee's needs, recommending and arranging the services required by the enrollee, and facilitating communication and information exchange among the different providers treating the enrollee.

Authorization of services. Many organizations have a two-step process for determining whether non-urgent, non-primary care services will be provided or paid for: (a) the service must be recommended by the primary care provider or service coordinator, and (b) the service must be approved through a utilization management system. However, Medicare and Medicaid enrollees have a right to request any covered service, whether or not the service has been recommended by the health professional responsible for coordinating their care. It is therefore important to distinguish between the coordination function described in this standard and the approval function described in standard 3.3, even if a single health professional may sometimes play a role in both functions.

3.2.1.1   *The organization's policies specify whether services are coordinated by the enrollee's primary care provider or through some other means;*

An organization may establish different mechanisms for different types of enrollees. For example, care of most enrollees might be coordinated by the primary care provider, while a case manager coordinates care of enrollees with complex needs, chronic illnesses, or functional disabilities.

An organization may provide for separate coordination of medical services and of mental health and substance abuse services, so long as the organization has procedures to ensure the exchange of necessary information between medical care providers and mental health and substance abuse providers, for example, with respect to prescribed medications. If the provider to whom an enrollee is referred for mental health or substance abuse services is not a physician, the organization must have procedures to ensure that the enrollee has timely access to a physician for medication evaluation and management, and for evaluation of comorbidity.

3.2.1.2   *Regardless of the mechanism adopted for coordination of services, the organization either ensures that each enrollee has an ongoing source of primary care; or offers to provide each enrollee with an ongoing source of primary care and provides a primary care source to each enrollee who accepts the offer.*

For Medicaid, the requirements are that each organization ensures that each enrollee has an ongoing source of primary care. For Medicare, the requirements are that organizations offer to provide each enrollee with an ongoing source of primary care and provide a primary care source to each enrollee who accepts the offer.

The organization's policies must specify who may serve as the primary care provider for an enrollee and the functions of this provider. The Medicare organization must also provide written notification to all enrollees that they have a right to choose a primary care provider.

Use of specialists. Although primary care is ordinarily furnished by general practitioners, family practitioners, pediatricians, internists, and sometimes obstetricians/gynecologists, it may be appropriate for some enrollees to obtain routine care from another specialist. There is some evidence that the overall care of patients with certain chronic medical conditions is most effectively managed by physicians outside the traditional primary care specialties (such as a geriatrician, an oncologist, an endocrinologist, or a general surgeon). Similarly, there may be enrollees for whom a psychiatrist coordinates medical as well as mental health or substance abuse services. The organization must have procedures for evaluating a request by an enrollee (or by a practitioner on the enrollee's behalf) to use a non-primary care specialist as his or her principal source of care.

Use of non-physician practitioners. An organization may permit licensed practitioners other than physicians to serve as primary care providers, consistent with requirements of applicable State laws. (Qualifications of such practitioners, and the degree of supervision required, are generally established under State law). If an organization designates non-physician practitioners as primary care providers, it must still ensure that each enrollee has a right to direct access to a physician for primary medical care. This right may be ensured in either of two ways: (a) the enrollee may choose between a physician and non-physician primary care provider, and may change this choice at any time; or (b) when the enrollee is not allowed such a choice, an enrollee with a non-physician primary care provider may have timely access to a physician upon request. For example, an organization might adopt a team approach, under which all enrollees seeking primary care are initially evaluated by a nurse practitioner or other qualified non-physician. However, the enrollee must always have an opportunity to request a follow-up appointment with a physician, and the enrollee's ability to do so may not be subject to the discretion of the non-physician practitioner.

Designation of an entity as primary care provider. An organization may allow an enrollee to select a physician group, clinic, federally qualified health center, or other facility with multiple practitioners as his or her primary source of care. To the extent feasible, the enrollee must be allowed to choose an individual primary care provider within the group or facility. In addition, the organization must confirm that the group or facility's medical recordkeeping practices are such as to ensure that necessary information is available to each provider furnishing primary care to the enrollee. (See standard 3.6.)

3.2.2   *Programs for coordination of care that include coordination of plan services with community and social services generally available through contracting or noncontracting providers in the area served by the organization.*

For Medicare organizations, such services include nursing home and community-based services. For Medicaid, these services are to be coordinated as specified by the State.

An organization should have a program or policies for assuring coordination among medical, mental health, and substance abuse services, and available social services or other community supports. For example, an organization with Medicaid enrollees must ensure coordination with the Special Supplemental Food Program for Women, Infants, and Children (WIC); this includes ensuring that the organization's providers refer potentially eligible enrollees to the program.

3.2.3 *Procedures for timely communication of clinical information among providers, as specified in standard 3.6;*

3.2.4 *Measures to ensure that enrollees: are informed of specific health care needs that require follow-up; receive, as appropriate, training in self-care and other measures they may take to promote their own health; and comply with prescribed treatments or regimens.*

The organization must ensure that enrollees receive the information they need to participate fully in their own care, including information on such subjects as: self-care, medication management, use of medical equipment, potential complications and when these should be reported to providers, and scheduling of follow-up services. For example, the organization's procedures should provide for patient education as part of its discharge planning process.

The organization must also make counseling and facilitating services available, on referral from providers or staff, for enrollees who are unable to, or are failing to, cooperate in their own treatment. Counseling services should include identification of social, financial, or other barriers that are preventing enrollees from following guidance or instructions from providers, with referral to appropriate social services as necessary.

3.3 *Service Authorization*

As was discussed under standard 2.4, the following standards apply to an organization's initial decision or determination in response to a request by an enrollee (or by a provider on behalf of the enrollee) for coverage of a service or continuation of a service previously approved. These standards do not apply when an enrollee requests a service directly from a provider and the provider is authorized by the organization to decide whether or not to furnish or arrange the service without referring the request to anyone else. Principles for determining when such a provider is making an initial decision or determination are discussed under standard 2.4. These standards do apply when an individual provider affiliated with a subcontractor of the organization must seek approval of services within the subcontractor's own internal review system.

For Medicare purposes, an organization's retrospective review of services is assessed as part of the claims processing function, rather than under these standards. For Medicaid, states may wish to use some parts of the following guidelines in assessing an organization's retrospective, as well as prospective or concurrent, reviews.

3.3.1   *The organization implements written policies and procedures, reflecting current standards of medical practice, for processing requests for initial authorization of services or requests for continuation of services.*

3.3.1.1   *The policies specify time frames for responding to requests for initial and continued determinations, specify information required for authorization decisions, provide for consultation with the requesting provider when appropriate, and provide for expedited response to requests for authorization of urgently needed services.*

Time frames and expedited responses: Medicare rules establish maximum time frames for an organization to notify an enrollee of an initial determination in response to a request for a service; States may establish their own time limits for Medicaid enrollees, or these may be established in state insurance law. This standard does not set a different maximum time frame for determinations, but requires each organization to establish its own time frames for responding to authorization requests and to monitor its own compliance with those time frames. The time frames may vary according to the urgency of the need for the requested service and the complexity of evaluating the request (so long as they do not exceed the applicable legal limits): The organization should be able to demonstrate that its time frames for different types of requests are reasonable in light of these factors.

Note that, under Medicare rules, an enrollee may request an expedited review when the enrollee believes that standard review time frames could jeopardize life, health, or ability to regain maximum functioning. These rules do not apply to Medicaid enrollees, and these guidelines do not specify expedited response requirements for Medicaid contractors. States should develop their own requirements in this area.

Information

The organization must notify affiliated providers of the information ordinarily required to process an authorization request, and of the circumstances under which additional information may be required. The organization's information standards must ensure that the authorization process is not unduly burdensome for provider staff or for enrollees. No information should be required that is not in fact used in the evaluation or recording of the request; in particular, submission of medical records may not be routinely required.

3.3.1.2   *Criteria for decisions on coverage and medical necessity are clearly documented, are based on reasonable medical evidence or a consensus of relevant health care professionals, and are regularly updated.*

An organization may develop its own clinical criteria for review of authorization requests or adopt criteria developed by outside resources. In either case, the organization's procedures must provide that criteria are reviewed before their adoption by affiliated providers, and must have mechanisms for periodic re-evaluation of the criteria in the light of scientific advances or changes in customary practice. If the organization has developed standard criteria for approval of a specific procedure or service, these criteria must be made available on request to any enrollee or affiliated provider.

3.3.1.3   *Mechanisms are in place to ensure consistent application of review criteria and compatible decisions.*

The organization must ensure that all employed or contracted reviewers understand coverage policies and review criteria. This may be accomplished through manuals, training programs, or other means. In addition, the organization must periodically assess the consistency of authorization decisions. Possible approaches include review of test cases by different utilization management staff or audits of samples of recent decisions.

3.3.1.4   *A clinical peer reviews all decisions to deny authorization on grounds of medical appropriateness.*

A clinical peer is, in the case of medical services, an appropriately trained and licensed physician (this does not require that the physician possess identical specialty training). Some state laws may require that the physician be licensed in the state served by the organization. For mental health and substance abuse services, a clinical peer is: (a) in the case of requests for inpatient hospitalization, a psychiatrist, a doctoral level clinical psychologist, or, in the case of substance abuse services, a certified addiction medicine specialist; (b) in the case of requests for other services, a licensed mental health or substance abuse professional. For other services, a clinical peer is an appropriately licensed practitioner (e.g., a dentist or nurse practitioner).

No denial of authorization on grounds of medical appropriateness may be issued before the request has been reviewed by the appropriate clinical peer. Other personnel (whether non-clinical, or clinical personnel not meeting the definition of a clinical peer) may approve requests, and may collect information for use by the clinical peer in evaluating a request. However they may issue a denial only on grounds clearly unrelated to medical considerations—for example, because the patient is no longer enrolled, or because the requested service is explicitly excluded from the enrollee's covered benefits. (Benefit determinations involving professional judgment, such as a determination that a given procedure was experimental, would require review by the clinical peer.)

This standard does not require (although some state laws may) that any authorization request submitted by a specialist be considered by a provider in the same specialty. However, the organization must have procedures under which the reviewing clinician may obtain specialty consultations; for example, in considering requests for complex, unusual, or highly specialized services.

3.3.1.5   *The requesting provider and the enrollee are promptly notified of any decision to deny, limit, or discontinue authorization of services. The notice specifies the criteria used in denying or limiting authorization and includes information on how to request reconsideration of the decision pursuant to the procedures established under standard 2.4.3. The notice to the enrollee must be in writing.*

Again, Medicare has maximum time frames for notice to enrollees. States may establish their own for Medicaid enrollees. Subject to these maximums, time frames for response are to be specified by the organization in its own procedures.

3.3.1.6   Compensation to persons or organizations conducting utilization management activities shall not be structured so as to provide inappropriate incentives for denial, limitation, or discontinuation of authorization of services.

Contracts with individual reviewers or with utilization review organizations may provide for compensation on the basis of time and/or of total numbers of authorization requests processed, but may not include any bonus or other incentive for denial of medically necessary services.

This standard does not apply to physician incentive plans, even though these may sometimes create indirect incentives to deny authorization of some services. For example, if an organization capitates a physician group to provide all ambulatory services for specified enrollees, the physician group may have an internal authorization system for specialty referrals. This is permissible, so long as the payment arrangement for the physician group meets Medicare and Medicaid standards for such arrangements (including standards prohibiting payment for denial of specific services to specific patients). It would not be permissible, however, for the physician group in turn to contract with an outside utilization review entity and then compensate the entity on the basis of service denials.

3.3.1.7   The organization does not prohibit providers from advocating on behalf of enrollees within the utilization management process.

No contract may implicitly or explicitly prohibit a provider from assisting enrollees in obtaining authorization for a service or pursuing reconsideration requests, for example by helping to document medical necessity or supplying scientific evidence of the appropriateness on the requested service. (Note that requesting practitioners are not necessarily parties in reconsiderations under the Medicare process; however, this does not prevent them from assisting the beneficiary in the process.)

3.3.1.8   Mechanisms are in effect to detect both underutilization and overutilization of services.

The organization has a medical affairs department that is responsible for regular review of claims, the payment system, encounter data and medical record review to assess the degree to which care is over- or underutilized. This includes processes such as utilization review and a MIS system with the capacity to generate comprehensive reports and data which is segmented by diagnosis, site of care delivery, provider identification, and other elements.

3.3.2   The organization furnishes information to all affiliated providers about enrollee benefits.

Provider manuals, supplemented as necessary by bulletins or other updates, must include clear explanations of covered services, including drug formularies and any general coverage decisions with respect to specific procedures or services.

3.4   Practice Guidelines and New Technology

3.4.1   The organization adopts and disseminates practice guidelines.

The aim of practice guidelines is to assist providers in clinical decision making, support consistency in treatment by an organization's affiliated providers, and promote improved health care. The organization should have an established mechanism for the adoption of guidelines. If administrative responsibility for adoption of guidelines is separate from administration of the QAPI program, there should be a system for interface between the two functions. For example, data on compliance with guidelines might be considered in the course of selecting topics for QAPI projects. (Note, however, that an improvement in compliance with guidelines, in the absence of evidence that improved health outcomes resulted, might not meet the requirements for successful QAPI projects as defined under standard 1.4.) A statement of clinical principles, rationales, and policies related to clinical performance measures used by the organization is a guideline.

This standard does not impose specific requirements for the number of different guidelines to be adopted or the range of conditions or services to be covered, although at least some guidelines should address areas other than preventive services. Each organization must develop its own priorities for adoption of new guidelines on the basis of population needs or identified variations in practice patterns within the organization.

3.4.1.1 *Guidelines are based on reasonable medical evidence or a consensus of health care professionals in the particular field, consider the needs of the enrolled population, are developed in consultation with contracting health care professionals, and are reviewed and updated periodically.*

An organization should adopt established evidence-based guidelines, such as those promulgated by the Agency for Health Care Policy and Research, expert consensus panels convened by the National Institutes of Health, or by medical specialty societies. If the organization does not utilize such guidelines, at a minimum they should have a process for developing new guidelines targeted to their own needs. (In regional or national organizations, this process may be centralized.) There should be a formal mechanism for consulting affiliated providers as guidelines are adopted and for reevaluating guidelines on a periodic basis.

3.4.1.2 *Guidelines, including any admission, continued stay, and discharge criteria used by the organization, are communicated to all providers and enrollees when appropriate, and to individual enrollees when requested.*

Guidelines must be disseminated through provider manuals, newsletters, or other communications. In addition, guidelines likely to be of interest to enrollees should be disseminated through enrollee newsletters and other educational materials. Possible examples might be guidelines that include recommendations relating to self-care or that relate to services the enrollee can initiate, such as immunizations or periodic screenings.

3.4.1.3 *Decisions with respect to utilization management, enrollee education, coverage of services, and other areas to which the guidelines are applicable are consistent with the guidelines.*

Practice guidelines are advisory documents, intended to assist providers without superseding independent clinical judgment, and are not identical to review criteria or coverage determinations. However, decision-making in these and other functional areas should not be inconsistent with the provider consensus on the basis of which guidelines are adopted. Enrollee education efforts should include information on guidelines for preventive care. Also, performance indicators selected for a QAPI project should, to the extent feasible, include measures of providers' compliance with guidelines that are relevant to the topic.

3.4.2 *The organization implements written policies and procedures for evaluating new medical technologies and new uses of existing technologies.*

For the purpose of this standard, new technologies include clinical interventions, procedures, pharmacological treatments, and devices. There must be an identifiable official or unit within the organization responsible for evaluation of such technologies. The organization's policies must specify criteria to be used in this evaluation and must establish procedures for: collection of scientific evidence; review of findings by the Food and Drug Administration and other regulatory bodies; consultation with affiliated practitioners and outside experts; and communication of coverage decisions to providers.

3.4.2.1 *The evaluations take into account coverage decisions by Medicare intermediaries and carriers, national Medicare coverage decisions, and federal and state Medicaid coverage decisions, as appropriate.*

Organizations with Medicare and/or Medicaid enrollees may not adopt policies that uniformly exclude from coverage services or items approved under national Medicare coverage determinations (although financial responsibility for newly approved services may be delayed under section 1876(d)(2)(B) of the Social Security Act), coverage policies of local Medicare intermediaries or carriers, or coverage decisions by the Medicaid agency, respectively. When more than one Medicare intermediary or carrier serves an organization's service area, the applicable coverage policy for any given enrollee is that of the intermediary or carrier serving the area in which that enrollee resides.

3.5 *Provider Qualification and Selection. The organization implements a documented process for selection and retention of affiliated providers.*

The organization must have written policies and procedures, approved by the policymaking body, for the selection and evaluation of providers. The policies should include criteria for credentialing of providers that are appropriate to the nature of the services they will be furnishing to enrollees. The process of provider selection should be integrated with the process, specified under standard 3.1, of establishing and maintaining an adequate network.

3.5.1 *For physicians and other licensed health care professionals, including members of physician groups, the process includes:*

3.5.1.1 *Procedures for initial credentialing, including: a written application, verification of licensure or certification and other information from primary sources, disciplinary status, eligibility for payment under Medicare and Medicaid, and site visits as appropriate. The ap-*

plication is signed, dated and includes an attestation by the applicant of the correctness and completeness of the application.

The Medicare organization must have written policies and procedures for the selection and evaluation of providers.

Credentialing is the review of qualifications and other relevant information pertaining to a health care professional who seeks appointment (in the case of an organization directly employing health care professionals) or who seeks a contract with the organization. Credentialing is required for all physicians and all other types of health care professionals who provide services to the organization's enrollees and who are permitted to practice independently under state law. Credentialing is *not* required for: health care professionals who are permitted to furnish services only under the direct supervision of another provider; hospital-based health care professionals who provide services to enrollees incident to hospital services, unless those providers are separately identified in enrollee literature as available to enrollees; or students, residents, or fellows.

The credentialing process begins with the completed application and attestation of correctness signed by the health care professional. The information collected must be no more than 6 months old on the date on which the provider is determined (for example, by a credentialing committee) to be eligible for appointment or contract. All items must be verified prior to the appointment of the health care provider, with the exception being in the case of a pending Drug Enforcement Agency (DEA) number.

Application

The applicant completes an application for appointment or affiliation. The application includes a work history covering at least five years and a statement by the applicant regarding: any limitations in ability to perform the functions of the position, with or without accommodation; history of loss of license and/or felony convictions; and history of loss or limitation of privileges or disciplinary activity.

Verification of Information

A "primary source" is an organization or entity with legal responsibility for originating a document and ensuring the accuracy of the information it conveys. Primary source verification may be achieved through the use of industry-recognized verification sources.

A managed care organization must verify the following from primary sources and include in the credentialing records:

1. a current valid license to practice—verification must show that the license was in effect at the time of the credentialing decision;

2. if applicable, clinical privileges in good standing at the hospital designated by the provider as the primary admitting facility;

3. if applicable, a valid DEA or Controlled Dangerous Substances certificate (CDS)—the certificate must be in effect at the time of the credentialing decision. However, if a practitioner's DEA certificate is pending, the managed care

organization may credential the practitioner provided the managed care organization has adopted and implemented a process under which other DEA-certified contracted practitioners write all prescriptions that require a DEA number. The process must also include verification of the newly issued DEA certificate.

4. education and training, including evidence of graduation from the appropriate professional school and completion of a residency or specialty training, if applicable;

5. board certification in each clinical specialty area for which the provider is being credentialed if the provider states that he/she is board certified on the application;

6. current, adequate malpractice insurance meeting the organization's requirements;

7. a history of professional liability claims that resulted in settlements or judgments paid by or on behalf of the provider; (This information can be obtained from the malpractice carrier or from the National Practitioner Data Bank.)

8. for physicians, information from the National Practitioner Data Bank;

9. information about sanctions or limitations on licensure from the applicable state licensing agency or board, or from a group such as the Federation of State Medical Boards;

10. information on previous sanction activity by Medicare and Medicaid—verification through the most recently issued report. (This may be obtained through the HHS Medicare and Medicaid Sanctions and Reinstatement Report or through direct contact with the Medicaid agency or the Medicare intermediary.)

Site Visit

The organization must establish a policy for conducting site visits. At a minimum, the organization should consider requiring site visits of high-volume specialists or other high-volume licensed providers, including high-volume non-physician providers. Its procedures should specify the criteria for determining that a provider is "high-volume."

Site visits should be conducted by clinical personnel (or teams including clinical personnel). They should include an evaluation of the site's accessibility, appearance, and adequacy of equipment, using standards developed by the organization. In addition, the visits should determine whether the site conforms to the organization's standards for medical record keeping practices (as required under standard 3.6.2) and confidentiality requirements (established pursuant to standard 2.2.1).

It is the responsibility of the organization to decide the frequency of site visits, as part of its site visit policy. Each organization's site visit policy will be reviewed per CMS's monitoring protocol (for Medicare) or per the State's monitoring protocol (for Medicaid). For example, any organization that adopts a time verification standard of 2 years will have an acceptable time verification standard for purposes of CMS Medicare monitoring. However, if within the two-year period the organization becomes aware of conditions at the site which suggest compromised safety or other concerns related to the care delivery setting, the organization will be expected to perform a site visit as soon as possible to assess the facility and identify corrective actions.

QISMC does not establish a methodology for conducting medical record reviews. However, QISMC does direct each organization to verify that its providers' enrollee health records meet its own standards.

Written Policies and Procedures

A Medicare organization must have written policies and procedures for the selection and evaluation of providers. These policies and procedures must conform with existing credentialing requirements and the antidiscrimination procedures contained under standard 3.5.5.

3.5.1.2 *Procedures for recredentialing, at least every two years, through a process that updates information obtained in initial credentialing and considers performance indicators such as those collected through the QAPI program, the utilization management system, the grievance system, enrollee satisfaction surveys, and other activities of the organization.*

The following must be re-verified from primary sources: licensure; clinical privileges, and malpractice coverage. Board certification must be verified only if the provider was due to be recertified or states that he or she has become board certified since the last time he or she was credentialed or recredentialed. In addition, the organization must re-query the National Practitioner Data Bank and obtain updated sanction or restriction information from licensing agencies, Medicare, and Medicaid. The organization should require that a provider who has been sanctioned or disciplined have a corrective action plan in place, and it should have procedures to ensure that the provider's plan is followed and is effective.

The organization must develop criteria for when it will conduct site visits as part of its recredentialing process. It should consider developing criteria that target high-volume providers, or those against whom complaints or grievances have been filed.

3.5.1.3 *A process for receiving advice from contracting health care professionals with respect to criteria for credentialing and recredentialing of individual health care professionals.*

Credentialing standards for types of providers and for specialists should be reviewed by clinical peers, through establishment of a credentialing committee or other mechanism. In addition, there should be a process for peer review when the organization is considering employing or contracting with a provider who does not meet its established credentialing standards.

3.5.1.4 *Written policies and procedures for suspending or terminating affiliation with a contracting health care professional (for Medicaid) or physician (for Medicare), including an appeals process.*

A formal process, including an opportunity for appeal, must be followed when an organization is suspending or terminating a provider's contract. The organization must notify all providers of its rules regarding affiliation with the organization, provide advance notice of adverse decisions, and provide for appeal including an opportunity for presentation of information and views of the providers.

Specific requirements for an M+CO that operates a coordinated care plan or network MSA plan providing benefits through contracting providers and that suspends or terminates a physician's contract are as follows:

1. The organization must give the affected physician written notice of the reasons for the action, including, if relevant, the standards and profiling data used to evaluate the physician and the numbers and mix of physicians needed by the M+C organization.

2. The organization must allow the physician to appeal the action, and give the physician written notice of his/her right to a hearing and the process and timing for requesting a hearing.

3. The organization must ensure that the majority of the hearing panel members are peers of the affected physician.

Specific requirements for Medicaid will be provided in the QISMC revision that follows publication of the Medicaid managed care final rule.

3.5.1.5 *Formal selection and retention criteria that do not discriminate against health care professionals who serve high-risk populations or who specialize in the treatment of costly conditions.*

Organizations may not discriminate against providers on the basis of factors such as license, certification, or nature of population served. For example, providers with a history of delivering services to inner city, rural patients, or those with chronic, long-term or complex care needs may not be prohibited from contracting and continuing service with the organization due to attendant costs and time involved in servicing such populations. This requirement is consistent with the Federal prohibition against organization practices that would reasonably be expected to have the effect of discouraging enrollment by eligible individuals whose medical condition or history indicates a need for substantial future medical services.

3.5.2 *For each institutional provider or supplier, the organization determines, and redetermines at specified intervals, that the provider or supplier:*

3.5.2.1 *Is licensed to operate in the state, and is in compliance with any other applicable state or federal requirements;*

3.5.2.2 *Is reviewed and approved by an appropriate accrediting body or is determined by the organization to meet standards established by the organization itself; and*

Accrediting bodies include the Joint Commission on Accreditation of Healthcare Organizations (JCAHO), the Accreditation Association for Ambulatory Health Care, the Commission on Accreditation of Rehabilitation Facilities, the Council on Accreditation, the Community Health Accreditation Program (CHAP), and the Continuing Care Accreditation Commission. This standard does not require that an organization accept the findings of an accrediting body in determining whether to contract with a provider, or that it reject providers that are not accredited.

However, an organization that does not rely on independent accreditation must develop its own standards for approval of institutional providers and determine that such providers meet those standards before including them in its network.

Primary source verification of accreditation and licensure are not required, unless otherwise provided in the organization's Medicare or Medicaid contract; that is, the organization may rely on documentation supplied by the institutional provider. Current documentation should be obtained at least every three years, and contracts should provide for notice from the provider of any change in its licensure or accreditation status.

3.5.2.3   *In the case of a provider or supplier providing services to Medicare enrollees is approved for participation in Medicare. (Note: This requirement does not apply to providers of additional or supplemental services for which Medicare has no approval standards.)*

Regardless of the organization's usual policies for determining that an institutional provider or supplier is qualified to serve its enrollees, an organization with a Medicare contract must ensure that its Medicare enrollees are served only by Medicare-approved providers/suppliers. Specific types of providers/suppliers for whom evidence of Medicare approval is required include:

1. Hospitals (JCAHO accreditation or Medicare certification)
2. Laboratories (Exemption from CLIA or a CMS-issued registration certificate, certificate, or certificate of waiver or accreditation)
3. Skilled nursing facilities
4. Comprehensive outpatient rehabilitation facilities
5. Outpatient physical therapy and speech pathology providers
6. Rural primary care hospitals
7. Home health agencies
8. Ambulatory surgery centers
9. Providers of end-stage renal disease services

For organizations with Medicaid enrollees, states may establish their own standards with respect to whether providers affiliated with the organization must meet standards for Medicaid fee-for-service participation.

3.5.3   *The organization notifies licensing and/or disciplinary bodies or other appropriate authorities when a health care professional's or institutional provider or supplier's affiliation is suspended or terminated because of quality deficiencies.*

Organizations contracting with Medicare and Medicaid must notify the appropriate State and Federal regulatory bodies and accrediting organizations upon suspending or terminating a provider because of quality deficiencies. This would include contacting entities such as State medical and nursing licensing boards and the National Practitioner Data Bank. In the case of a physician, the State medical boards that must be contacted include the Board of Medical Examiners, in accordance with the Health Care Quality Improvement Act of 1986. If the organization suspends or terminates its affiliation with a physician, or accepts the physician's surrender of his affiliation while he is faced with an investigation into possible incompetence or improper professional conduct, the organization must report to the Board of Medical Examiners the name of the physician, and a description of the acts or omissions or other reasons for the suspension or termination or surrender.

3.5.4 *The organization ensures compliance with Federal requirements prohibiting employment or contracts with individuals excluded from participation under either Medicare or Medicaid.*

This standard has relevance to several areas. First, if a provider opts out of Medicare, they may not accept Federal reimbursement for a period of two years. The other is related to the CMS Sanction List which identifies those individuals found guilty of fraudulent billing, misrepresentation of credentials, etc. The list is available on the Web and is published on a regular basis. Organizations employing health providers have a responsibility to check the Sanction list with each new issuance of the list, as they are prohibited from hiring or continuing to employ individuals named on that list.

3.5.5 *An organization may not discriminate against any health care professional, solely on the basis of the license or certification.*

An MCO may select the practitioners that participate in its plan provider networks. In selecting these practitioners, an MCO may not discriminate, in terms of participation, reimbursement, or indemnification, against any health care professional who is acting within the scope of his or her license or certification under State law, solely on the basis of the license or certification. If an MCO declines to include a given provider or group of providers in its network, it must furnish written notice to the effected provider(s) on the reason for the decision.

This prohibition does not preclude any of the following by the MCO:

(1) Refusal to grant participation to health care professionals in excess of the number necessary to meet the needs of the plan's enrollees (except for M+C private-fee-for-service plans, which may not refuse to contract on this basis).

(2) Use of different reimbursement amounts for different specialties or for different practitioners in the same specialty.

(3) Implementation of measures designed to maintain quality and control costs consistent with its responsibilities.

3.6 *Enrollee Health Records and Communication of Clinical Information. The organization implements appropriate policies and procedures to ensure that the organization and its providers have the information required for effective and continuous patient care and for quality review, and conducts an ongoing program to monitor compliance with those policies and procedures.*

3.6.1 *The organization makes a "best-effort" attempt to conduct an initial assessment of each enrollee's health care needs, including following up on unsuccessful attempts to contact an enrollee, within 90 days of the effective date of enrollment;*

To prevent gaps in service and facilitate identification of a primary care provider in a timely fashion, organizations must take every reasonable step to notify, schedule, and complete an initial, comprehensive assessment of enrollee's health care needs within 90 days of their enrollment. The assessment may take the form of a phone call, home visit, or questionnaire; it is not required to include a physical examination. Organizations will need to document when they have been unsuccessful in their attempts.

Any health risk assessment or approved instrument which accomplishes the following is acceptable:

(1) ensures that those with complex or serious medical or behavioral conditions are identified;

(2) identifies essential health care needs of enrollees which may require an expedited appointment with the appropriate provider;

(3) results in appropriate and timely care of the enrollee, such as an expedited appointment.

If the enrollee changes MCOs, but retains the same primary care physician who has already conducted an initial assessment, then the new organization does not need to conduct a new initial assessment. However, the new organization must receive information on the patient's current state of health from the provider/physician within 90 days. For example, the physician could provide to the new MCO information that he/she already had on file. This exception applies for enrollees who age in, are already under the care of the network providers, or who retain the same primary care provider when enrolling with a different organization. The organization may omit performing their own initial assessment on these enrollees, but must, nevertheless, have the kinds of information such as an assessment might produce.

3.6.2 *The organization ensures that each provider furnishing services to enrollees maintains an enrollee health record in accordance with standards established by the organization that takes into account professional standards.*

3.6.2.1 *The organization enforces standards for health record content and organization, including specifications of basic information to be included in each health record.*

At a minimum, each record should include:

1. Identifying information on the enrollee;

2. Identification of all providers participating in the enrollee's care and information on services furnished by these providers;

3. A problem list, including significant illnesses and medical and psychological conditions;

4. Presenting complaints, diagnoses, and treatment plans;

5. Prescribed medications, including dosages and dates of initial or refill prescriptions;

6. Information on allergies and adverse reactions (or a notation that the patient has no known allergies or history of adverse reactions);

7. Information on advance directives;

8. Past medical history, physical examinations, treatment necessary, and possible risk factors for the enrollee relevant to the particular treatment.

3.6.2.2 *The organization implements a process to assess and improve the content, legibility, organization, and completeness of enrollee health records.*

The organization should include a review of providers' record-keeping practices as part of any site visits it may conduct under standard 3.5. This review should also assess each provider's procedures for assuring confidentiality of medical and health information, as required under standard 2.2.1.1. The organization must have procedures for following up on deficiencies identified during site visits to providers, as well as deficiencies identified in records obtained from any affiliated provider in the course of QAPI or other record reviews.

3.6.2.3 *Enrollee health records are available and accessible to the organization and to appropriate state and federal authorities, or their delegates, involved in assessing the quality of care or investigating enrollee grievances or complaints.*

Contracts with providers must specify that records will be made available to government reviewers, peer review organizations, external quality review organizations, or other authorized entities.

3.6.3 *The organization ensures appropriate and confidential exchange of information among providers, such that:*

The requirements in this standard must be included in all provider agreements. Review of compliance should occur as part of reviews of recordkeeping practices under standard 3.6.2.2.

3.6.3.1 *A provider making a referral transmits necessary information to the provider receiving the referral;*

3.6.3.2 *A provider furnishing a referral service reports appropriate information to the referring provider;*

3.6.3.3 *Providers request information from other treating providers as necessary to provide care;*

Organizations that offer a point-of-service benefit, that allow enrollees to access in-network non-primary care services without authorization, or that serve dually eligible Medicare/Medicaid beneficiaries should emphasize in their educational materials the need for enrollees to inform their primary care providers about the services they obtain.

When a State's managed care program (e.g., by "carving out" certain services such as mental health care) or an enrollee's dual coverage by both Medicare and Medicaid creates a situation in which a Medicare or Medicaid beneficiary is enrolled in more than one managed care organization, each organization's providers may release, without the prior consent of the beneficiary (to the extent allowed under Federal and State law), individual, identifiable personal information pertaining to such a beneficiary to providers in any of the other Medicare and Medicaid managed care organizations in which the beneficiary is enrolled.

3.6.3.4   *If the organization offers a point-of-service benefit or other benefit providing coverage of services by non-network providers, the organization transmits information about services used by an enrollee under the benefit to the enrollee's primary care provider; and*

Information transmitted to the primary care provider must be sufficient to allow that provider to request additional information on the services in compliance with standard 3.6.3.3.

3.6.3.5   *When an enrollee chooses a new primary care provider within the network, the enrollee's records are transferred to the new provider in a timely manner that ensures continuity of care.*

Upon notification that an enrollee wishes to choose a new primary care provider, the organization must take steps to transfer the enrollee's complete medical record and allow the new provider access (immediately upon request) to all medical information necessary for the care of that patient. Transfer of records must not interfere or cause delay in the provision of services to the enrollee.

3.6.4   *The organization has policies and procedures for sharing enrollee information with any organization with which the enrollee may subsequently enroll.*

As the enrollee may have, depending on State law, the legal right to access his or her medical record, the organization must provide copies of all patient records to the new provider in order that they be available upon the enrollee's request. The organization must have in place authorization forms and policies which will safeguard the privacy of the patient record in transit. Further, it must assure that the information will be delivered in a timely fashion that does not impede continuity of care.

Appendix 11.D

QISMC Domain 4

DOMAIN 4: Delegation

STANDARD NUMBER	DESCRIPTION OF STANDARD

4.1   *The organization oversees and is accountable for any functions or responsibilities that are described in the standards of Domains 1 through 3 that are delegated to other entities. The following requirements apply to all delegated functions:*

With certain restrictions indicated below, an organization may, by written contract, delegate any activity required under or governed by these standards to another entity. However, an organization entering into a Medicare or Medicaid contract remains entirely accountable to CMS or the State for performance of any such delegated function. It is the sole responsibility of the organization to ensure that the function is performed in accordance with applicable standards. (Note that this standard is not meant to imply that the organization is legally liable for the actions of its subcontractors, for example in cases of malpractice; any such liability is established by State or local law.)

Special note must be made of "carve-out" arrangements, under which a managed care organization contracts with an entity to assume entire responsibility for a given type or category of service and delegates to that entity a broad range of basic management functions.

Such contracts are, perhaps, most common for mental health and substance abuse services, although some organizations use similar arrangements for prescription drugs, home health care, or other types of services. These arrangements are conceptually no different from those under which an organization capitates a single medical group to provide all physician and related ambulatory services and delegates management of those services to the group. Although the latter arrangements are never spoken of as "medical carve-outs," they are functionally comparable to "mental health/substance abuse carve-outs": the contractor assumes entire responsibility for management of a defined portion of the overall benefit package. Just as medical group contracts have never diminished the basic accountability of the organization directly contracting with Medicare or Medicaid, so with

---

mental health or other carve-outs. The prime contractor remains wholly account-able for the activities of its subcontractors.

In the Medicaid program, "carve outs" can also refer to the practice whereby a State Medicaid agency (as opposed to a managed care organization) enters into a separate contract with a managed care organization or other service delivery sys-tem, for a specific set of services, e.g., mental health and substance abuse, EPSDT, or dental services. In such instances, the managed care organization under con-tract to the State Medicaid agency to deliver the beneficiaries' primary medical care is not considered to have "delegated" the services "carved out" by the State Medicaid agency, and therefore is not expected to oversee or be accountable for such "carved out" services.

Because of the wide variety of organizational structures and contractual arrange-ments, it is difficult to develop simple guidelines for the review of delegated activi-ties. In any given situation, the review methodology to be adopted should be that which is least burdensome for reviewers and for the organization, yet which pro-vides positive assurance that the activity in question is being performed in compli-ance with these standards. For example, credentialing of providers might occur in several different ways:

1. The organization itself verifies the credentials of individual providers affiliated with its subcontractors. Review would focus directly on the organization's performance of this function.

2. An organization contracts with one or more independent physician groups, each of which is expected to verify the credentials of each affiliated provider. It would be impractical for a CMS or State reviewer to review compliance by the independent contractor(s). Instead, the organization itself must document that it has periodically reviewed the performance of each contractor, for ex-ample by verifying that all required credentialing information is present in a sample of each contractor's provider records.

3. An organization contracts with a single independent credentialing verification organization (CVO) to collect information about providers. The CVO, and not the organization, maintains documentation of verification of credentials from primary sources. If a single CVO provided services to multiple organizations in a state, a state Medicaid agency might review the CVO itself and deem in compliance all organizations that contracted with the CVO. Alternatively, the state might accept the findings of an independent body that accredits CVOs. For the purposes of Medicare, however, CMS does not at this time review CVOs or accept external accreditation of CVOs. It would therefore expect the organization to document that it has monitored the CVO's performance, again through a review of a sample of practitioner records. (Similarly, the or-ganization would be required to review the credentialing performance of any "carve-out" contractor, such as a national managed behavioral health care or-ganization.)

Again, as this single example illustrates, the variety and complexity of contracting arrangements makes it impractical to suggest a uniform method for review of delegated functions. As part of the advance preparation for on-site reviews, the reviewer and the organization should negotiate the most expeditious procedure. However, the burden of documenting a delegate's compliance with applicable standards ultimately rests with the organization.

4.1.1 *A written agreement specifies the delegated activities and reporting responsibilities of the entity and provides for revocation of the delegation or other remedies for inadequate performance.*

Contracts must indicate what functions have been delegated and must require the entity to comply with the requirements of these standards and of applicable law and regulations. When a function is only partially delegated, contract provisions must clearly delineate which responsibilities have been delegated and which remain with the organization. In the QAPI area, for example, the organization might develop topics for projects in consultation with an affiliated medical group but delegate the actual conduct of a specific project to the group. The agreement must specify how the delegate is to conduct QAPI activities, at what points in the process decisions by the delegate (for example, on data collection methodologies) are subject to the organization's review, and how the delegate's activities will be integrated into the organization's overall QAPI program (for example, through participation in an organization-wide committee).

It is especially important to identify instances in which a delegation has been made implicitly. For example, a contract with a medical group may hold the group responsible for providing or arranging for a wide range of ambulatory services in return for a fixed monthly capitation payment. The group is left to develop its own procedures for approving requests for referral services by its own primary care providers. If so, the utilization management function has been delegated, and the organization must ensure that the group complies with the standards for that function, including standards related to requests for expedited review.

4.1.2 *The organization evaluates the entity's ability to perform the delegated activities prior to delegation.*

The organization must document that it has approved the entity's policies and procedures with respect to the delegated function, and must verify that the contractor has devoted sufficient resources and appropriately qualified staff to performing the function.

4.1.3 *The performance of the entity is monitored on an ongoing basis and formally reviewed by the organization at least annually.*

The organization must have written procedures for monitoring and review of delegated activities. The nature of ongoing monitoring may vary according to the organization's past experience with the delegate and with the nature of the delegated activity. In the areas of grievance processing or utilization management, for example, monitoring may be more or less continuous, in as much as decisions by the delegate may be appealed to the organization. However, the organization must periodically verify that the delegate is in fact forwarding requests for reconsideration, and that its statistical or other reporting on these processes is accurate. In other areas, such as credentialing, annual review of the delegate's activities may be sufficient, particularly if the organization has ascertained in the past that the delegate is performing the activity properly.

The annual evaluation should be a comprehensive assessment of the delegate's performance, including both compliance with applicable standards and the extent to which the delegate's activities promote the organization's overall goals and objectives for the delegated function. If any problems or deficiencies are identified, the evaluation must specify any necessary corrective action and include procedures for assuring that the corrective action is implemented.

The organization must ensure that monitoring of delegates is carried out by staff of the organization who are qualified to assess the delegates' activities. For example, an organization that has delegated authorization of mental health and substance abuse services to an entity must use appropriately credentialed professionals to review the entity's authorization decisions.

4.2 *If the organization delegates selection of providers to another entity, the organization retains the right to approve, suspend, or terminate any provider selected by that entity.*

All contracts with medical groups or other entities serving Medicare or Medicaid enrollees must include this provision, so that the organization can assure that enrollees are not served by any provider excluded from program participation.

Chapter 12

The Future of Continuous Quality Improvement in Health Care

DONALD E. LIGHTER

◆ Introduction

Unquestionably, the application of quality improvement science to health care has just begun to produce results in the health care delivery system. Physicians frequently are distrustful of these efforts because of prior training and a general lack of information regarding the tenets of quality management. Payers are clamoring for inclusion of the quality improvement approach to provide value to the health services that they purchase. Patients—or consumers of health care, as they are more commonly labeled today—have tired of long waiting times for physicians, painful procedures, and impediments to receiving care. The system is not functioning optimally, and the cost-containment movement of the last 20 years will not provide the solution.

Payers have actively sought methods, such as managed care, to reduce the cost of care, and for a few years in the late 1990s, cost increases dropped to single digits annually; however, double-digit increases returned after only a short hiatus. These problems forced insurers, who were generally happy to process claims for administrative fees and a healthy profit, to initiate utilization management programs designed to ensure "appropriate" care according to guidelines established by panels of health professionals that often ignored exigencies caused by local variations in resources and access to care. Physicians have generally rebelled against these interventions, in spite of the best efforts of health plans to gain acceptance for their participation in patient care decisions. The net result of these changes has been an escalation in the enmity between insurers and providers, with increasing dissatisfaction among payers and consumers. This chapter addresses the need for a new approach to health care, incorporating a quality improvement focus rather than cost containment as a means of achieving true long-term cost reductions, while assuring consumers and payers that they are receiving valuable services. Pediatricians assess children in terms of benchmarks called developmental milestones, which are approximate ages at which certain developmental events should occur. This chapter will present some "quality milestones" as a means of measuring the health care industry's growth in quality improvement.

◆ Quality Milestone 1: Improved Information Management

Few in modern society have not felt the changes resulting from information technology during the last half of the 20th century. Computers and related systems have added a new dimension to life in highly industrialized countries, and the spread of this technology promises to revolutionize nearly every human endeavor throughout the world. Medicine has realized myriad benefits from this evolving technology, but in many ways, the health care industry still fails to exploit the advantages of the information revolution.

Electronic Medical Records

Computers and information systems have now become ubiquitous tools in the health care delivery system, but they are not being used optimally. Once physicians start using electronic medical records (EMRs), they find that the systems improve the quality of patient care (Marshall & Chin, 1998), and when the technology is offered at little or no cost, they adopt EMRs rather readily (Kouroubali, et al., 1998). As organizations become more integrated or as physicians become employees rather than independent practitioners, use of these systems tends to increase.

The advantage of an EMR resides in the ability to access clinical data inexpensively and expeditiously. Clinical studies using paper charts require substantial human time and effort to collect, record, and analyze data, whereas an EMR can make the process much faster and easier. In most cases, data sets from the EMR can be uploaded into a data repository and correlated with similar records from other providers, then evaluated with programs and tools as easy to use as a spreadsheet program. EMR systems are built from a database platform, allowing data to be selected and exported for analysis using relatively straightforward commands.

As more medical organizations automate patient care functions, a number of benefits will accrue. First, improved efficiency in the system will lead to lower administrative costs, freeing more financial resources for patient care. Studies of hospitals put the administrative costs of health care at over a quarter of the total cost of care (Woolhandler, et al., 1993) and more recent estimates have estimated administrative costs as consuming 31% of total health care expenditures (Woolhandler S, Campbell T, Himmelstein DU, 2003). Automated patient care can reduce a substantial portion of the costs of moving paper within and between organizations. From the standpoint of the health care delivery system, these overhead expenses add nothing to the quality of services produced by the organization, and the inability to easily find current patient care information serves as a serious barrier to providing care. The funds that are presently expended on this administrative overhead could be reallocated for patient care services or to reducing prices.

Second, patient care documentation will improve (Shiffman, et al., 1999; Spencer, et al., 1999, Kramer, et. al., 2003). The Shiffman study also demonstrated that compliance with clinical guidelines improved when the information was readily available at the site of care through the EMR system. Guidelines for documenting the clinical encounter are becoming more complex, and the ability of physicians to meet the criteria established by third-party payers and regulators will depend on their ability to document the care that was provided the patient (Taragin, et al., 1998). This and other studies indicate that the quality of documentation is improved because the computer can store large amounts of descriptive data that can be entered using a few keystrokes or mouse clicks. Improved documentation can be used more effectively in quality improvement (QI) studies, and the relatively standardized methods of entering and storing patient information incorporated into some medical record systems also provides better ability to analyze the information using computerized statistical analysis packages.

The information that is entered during the clinical encounter also can be analyzed in real time, and as systems become more capacious, concurrent processing can implement algorithms and decision-support systems to assist a practitioner's thought process at the time of the decision, rather than retrospectively after a quality breach has occurred. Prevention of errors produces substantially greater benefits than detecting and repairing errors after they have happened. Automated systems that use statistical methods like control charts and advanced heuristic algorithms can continually monitor the practice patterns of a practitioner and make recommendations at the time that a service is being rendered, rather than retrospectively dealing with an adverse outcome.

Finally, the EMR can improve the quality of care by providing information about contemporary practice recommendations and guidelines at the time of a patient encounter (Porcelli & Lobach, 1999; Nowalk, et al., 2003; Buller-Close, et al., 2003). Many providers face decisions at the bedside or in the office, armed with little more than an all-too-human memory and a prescription pad. Rapid access to reference materials will provide the knowledge necessary for good patient care, reducing the time necessary to find information and improving accuracy. Expediting the availability of pertinent information based on medical record input can prove invaluable in assisting practitioners in decision making.

Decision-Support Tools

Decision-support tools have evolved dramatically since they were first introduced in the 1960s. A number of decision-support systems currently exist for physicians (Bindel, et al., 2003), but some are now being adapted for patients as well (Berner & and Ball, 1998). Although these automated systems will not supplant physicians in the near future, the growth in knowledge bases available to individual patients will become more sophisticated with time, literally placing the world's medical knowledge at the disposal of everyone. These information resources can make the task of the provider much easier but also much more challenging. No longer will physicians be faced with patients who are largely uninformed about their conditions. Patients will become even more active participants in their care, resulting in increased commitment and adherence to treatment regimens. Physicians will no longer operate in a vacuum but will have more information than ever to make a decision (LaBresh, et al., 2003; Sausser, 2003), and computer systems will assist in synthesizing the information, forming hypotheses of potential diagnoses, and recommending diagnostic and treatment regimens. For many illnesses, computer systems will serve as "consultants" to advanced practice nurses (Caelli, et al., 2003), helping them make appropriate diagnoses and prescribe optimum treatment. Minor illnesses that presently require an expensive office encounter and testing will be handled using home telemedical systems, with decision-support programs that allow patients to self-diagnose and treat more of their minor maladies.

Using decision-support tools will become second nature to physicians. Many such tools now exist for nurses and other health professionals, e.g., for handling telephone calls in a call center (Hamill and Harris-Stevens, 1998; Campbell, 1998). As these computer support tools become more available to patients, many of the common causes for office visits can be eliminated and moved to home care or managed by midlevel practitioners. Physicians will be able to apply their more in-depth training to complicated cases that present a greater challenge to their skills and interests. In addition to their longer and more intense training, physicians will also have computerized tools that support their ability to care for more complex cases.

From better record keeping and reporting systems to automated knowledge bases that distill the best of the medical literature and professional consensus, these data management systems will serve physicians by presenting information in a usable form that includes preliminary analyses. Doctors often use resources such as toxicology databases for obtaining rapid information and treatment recommendations for toxic exposures and ingestions that are encountered infrequently. Similar databases will be available for other diagnostic dilemmas as well, allowing physicians to implement more appropriate diagnostic and therapeutic regimens and analyze more complex medical problems. As the sophistication of these information resources improves, physician intervention will become increasingly complex, justifying the immense investments in education and resources required to train a physician.

Knowledge-based systems will "learn" from experience. As physicians interact with these systems, the systems will store more experiences, and computer programs using statistical and heuristic techniques will translate the experiential data into useful information. This approach should be familiar to QI professionals because it emulates statistical process control. Statistical analysis of longitudinal data provides information on patterns of behavior of a system (disease state) that become part of the decision-making process for improving the system. These systems will have the ability to continually improve their recommendations by performing analyses of input data that add to the knowledge base.

These systems also will serve as repositories for QI data. Physicians must enter patient information in order to obtain recommendations from the system, so the system gradually accumulates more clinical data. This raw information can be used for other kinds of studies, producing assessments as simple as scatter plots to those that are exceedingly complex, like control charts and correlation analyses. These databases can be used to augment patient data in EMRs and lead to better definitions of disease states and even to identification of previously unknown syndromes and clinical disorders.

Some decision-support systems are presently designed to critique a practitioner's diagnosis and treatment (Harpole, et al., 1997; Leader, et al., 1996). Clinicians enter patient data (or the data is transferred from EMRs); the system analyzes the information and then either requests further information or produces a critique of the diagnosis and treatment plan. Although critiquing systems have had mixed acceptance with practitioners (Ridderikhoff and van Herk, 1999; van der Lei, et al., 1993), they show great promise in implementing QI systems, such as clinical practice guidelines (CPGs) (Shahar, et al., 1996; Sintchenko, et al., 2003; Jeannot, et al., 2003). Combining critiquing technology with CPGs would provide intervention at the site and time of care, thus reducing errors and leading to more appropriate care. A few studies indicate that such systems can reduce prescription errors (Bates, et al., 1998; Kuperman, et al., 1998; Hume, 1999; Peth, 2003).

Decision-support systems will become prominent over the next few years in health care for augmenting patient self-care and improving the quality of care rendered by health care professionals. The systems needed to provide this support are becoming more available, and the quality of the advice produced by the computerized tools will become increasingly useful, making their application for improving the quality of care much more practical.

Telecommunications and the Internet

The Internet has profoundly changed the nature of disseminating and acquiring information. This phenomenon is not limited to any one sector of society but has gradually infiltrated nearly every human venture. Once the realm of academics and computer geeks, the Internet now can be accessed from any number of telecommunication machines, including home television sets. The health care industry is just now beginning to capitalize on the ubiquity of the Internet and use the technology for something other than advertising. New programs and equipment, such as wireless access to information, will be applied to improving patient care at an accelerating pace, increasing access to care, and improving communications between providers and consumers of care.

For example, a care management program for individuals with congestive heart failure now usually entails a phone call from a nurse case manager with a reminder to perform daily weights and adjust doses of medications according to changes in those measurements. Each telephone call may take just a few minutes, but the time required providing this interaction for a large cohort of people can become expensive. Using Internet technology, consumers can access their medical records over a secure connection with the provider's office, enter a weight (or, better yet, stand on a scale connected to the host computer via a secure connection), and transmit the weight to the provider's record keeping system. A set of rules can then be invoked by the system to have the patient change the dose of medicine according to the change in weight. The consumer's interaction with the system can be at a comfortable pace, and the task of the case manager then becomes to track down those individuals who have not interacted with the system at the appointed time. Handling exceptions is a better use of a health professional's time, and involving consumers in managing their own care regimens often builds self-confidence and adherence.

The Internet is also being used to facilitate communications between providers and patients. From e-mail communications to educational Web sites, providers are finding that consumers appreciate the convenience of these new modes of interaction (Hammond, et al., 1998; Pergament, et al., 1999). E-mail provides a convenient mode of communicating routine information to patients, as well as a means for individual consumers to contact physicians directly without cutting into other patient care activities. Web sites can provide information rapidly and conveniently, eliminating the need for the 2:00 AM telephone call to ask about the dose of acetaminophen for a child. Routine medication refills, requests for information, and management of chronic, nonemergent conditions present other opportunities for using this new technology. In short, the Internet provides numerous prospects for improving patient care through better communications, and with the development of "Internet II," a high-speed, dedicated infrastructure for telecommunications, these promises will be realized in the near future (Quade, et al., 1999).

Telemedicine

With the growth of advanced telecommunication modalities and a broadband infrastructure, telemedical consultations are being conducted throughout the world, and the use of the technology is changing health care in ways that have been the subject of science fiction until now. A telemedicine system consists of a local video system, perhaps in a physician's home office, connected to a remote video system that is usually dozens of miles away, with all of the necessary instruments for a physician to perform an examination. The consulting physician sits at a console at the local site, and the patient examination is coordinated at the remote site by a health professional such as an advanced practice nurse trained to perform the physical examination under the consulting physician's direction. Special instruments transmit images and information such as electrocardiograms over the telecommunications link for the physician to evaluate. Using this information, the physician can make a diagnosis and initiate a treatment regimen. The obvious advantage of telemedicine is preclusion of the need for patients to travel long distances for consultation with specialists, but the promise of telemedicine reaches far beyond that obvious benefit.

Faster, more secure Internet connections speed video transmission over the Internet, making telemedicine applications much more common and available. Physicians and their peers communicate using these video links, just as between physicians and patients, quickly and clearly. Patients now can have some of the common examination tools in their homes, such as scales and stethoscope attachments, to facilitate an examination by the health professional at a central site (Louis, et al., 2003; Rialle, et al., 2002), eliminating the need to make an office visit for many common medical conditions. Not only will this type of encounter be more convenient for the consumer (an electronic house call, so to speak), but it will also help make more efficient use of the practitioner's time as well (Cornish, et al., 2003).

Physicians and consultants will be able to communicate face to face in order to better exchange information. Such consultations will be more effective because specific patient characteristics may be displayed for use in coming to a correct diagnosis. The extraordinary capabilities of this technology should not be underestimated. Patients with relatively rare diseases can benefit from intervention by the foremost experts on that condition anywhere in the world, without traveling long distances from family and the community support network. In addition to the obvious cost savings, quality of care will be improved by providing consumers with the most advanced and appropriate care for virtually any medical condition. Providers will no longer be left struggling with difficult cases but will be able to establish collegial relationships with fellow professionals from around the world and manage clinical disorders in a collaborative environment.

Although some of this section may sound a bit utopian, most of the technology is available now (Marsh, 1998; Rowberg and York, 1999). Equipment costs have become much more reasonable as more powerful computers continually decrease in price, and insurers have become more amenable to supporting these efforts financially (McCue, et al., 1998; Pavlopoulos, et al., 1998; Marta, 2003). Although issues of licensure for physicians providing consultation across state or country boundaries remain unresolved, even these issues are not thought to be sufficient to inhibit the growth of telemedicine technology (Siwicki, 1999). As telemedicine becomes more ubiquitous, the quality of care can be expected to improve; however, without the remainder of the information infrastructure described for quality milestone 1, these improvements will be difficult or impossible to document. Thus, this milestone depends on the field of medical informatics achieving its maximum potential in the next few years, a goal that is attainable with commitments from providers, payers, and consumers.

◆ Quality Milestone 2: Health Care System Integration

The monumental changes in the health care delivery and reimbursement system detailed in Chapter 1 have moved the industry from unlimited funding and open access to finite budgets and constrained access to care, creating tremendous upheavals and ripple effects. One of these effects is the drive of health care organizations to acquire greater negotiating leverage with payers by integrating services across the health care continuum. Health system integration seeks to establish a health care organization that can supply all of the health needs of a population, including assumption of financial risk. Financial risk may include establishment or acquisition of an insurance or health maintenance organization component, or it may involve accepting capitation payment from an insurer to care for a population within a fixed budget.

Integrated delivery systems (IDSs) have a number of advantages and disadvantages. First, the system is able to serve all of the needs of a population without outside referrals. Convenience for the consumer is an obvious consequence, but greater control over the use of resources improves the ability of providers to influence the care of patients under their care. The challenge for IDSs is to make sure that all of the providers who appeal to a target population are included in the medical group. For example, if an integrated system includes all of the providers necessary for meeting the needs of a payer's employees, but not the particular hospital that the chief executive officer's spouse prefers for inpatient care, then the group may not be selected to provide care. On the other hand, including providers in an integrated system who cannot adopt a collaborative style or the QI philosophy can make the system unmanageable. Thus, any system must be carefully constructed to have maximum marketability and find providers who are willing to perform as a team.

Another advantage of an IDS is the ability to have uniform medical record systems and increased connectivity for transfer of information. These organizations often can implement enterprise-wide electronic record keeping systems, as well as automated referral and appointment systems that add to consumer satisfaction (Davidson and Chismar, 1999) and reduce the chance for errors. The benefits of automated systems were detailed in the previous section, but using these tools, IDS quality professionals can analyze care and design interventions that have a much greater probability of success.

Many IDSs work out innovative reimbursement arrangements with providers that encourage participation in QI activities (Earnest, et al., 1998; Greene, 1998). These arrangements can vary from economic incentives to professional recognition, but the relationship between the provider and the organization is one of the keys to provider participation in QI efforts. When providers have allegiance to the organization, QI efforts are usually met with more enthusiasm than if these efforts are instituted by an insurer or government agency.

IDSs also can influence provider education. Continuing educational programs can focus on quality issues in the organization, and the IDS can promote QI through educational sessions within the organization, as well as by leveraging funding for better outside educational experiences consistent with organizational goals and objectives. Education has become the mainstay of QI efforts because it provides an acceptable way of informing providers of new techniques and procedures that will improve quality. Coupled with other incentives, educational programs can prove helpful in promoting quality concepts and applications in the organization.

Finally, IDSs can instill QI values throughout the system. Leaders in the IDS have the opportunity to directly influence large numbers of providers across traditional supply chain lines to promote QI, and the collegial relationships that can be built in integrated systems should be used to propagate the quality philosophy throughout the enterprise.

The road toward health care system integration has been bumpy, however (Burns and Pauly, 2002). Many attempts at mergers and acquisitions have failed for a number of reasons, including insurmountable cultural differences and persistent economic issues (Goldsmith, 2002). The selection process for medical schools tends to favor those who function autonomously, and the training programs and residencies ingrain the concept of individual decision making and accountability in young physicians. Changing that mindset will be difficult because these deep-seated character traits make physicians less familiar with team-based health care. In response to new guidelines from the Accreditation Council for Graduate Medical Education (ACGME), training programs are changing to include specific curricula designed to enhance young physicians' ability to function in teams (Frey, et al., 2003).

Many hospitals and other health systems went through a period when they acquired physician practices in order to integrate their systems, but many found that the culture of the physician practice was incompatible with the management structure in the hospital (Swisher, et al., 1999). Many of these practices were "returned" to their physician owners, sometimes with disastrous results (Cook, 2002). Although these failures seem not to bode well for integrated health care, many successes have also occurred, and the future of health care integration in the United States appears assured.

◆ Quality Milestone 3: Consumerism

Consumers are becoming more involved in their care. Over the past 30 years, sources of medical information have proliferated, and the population in the United States has become increasingly better educated about its health care options. Medical suppliers such as pharmaceutical companies are advertising directly to consumers, rather than to health professionals because consumers are making more choices regarding their care and exerting greater influence on payers (Elliott, 2003). The consumer movement in health care is still in its infancy, but the power that it will bring to bear on the system will be profound (Riccardi, 1998; Kertesz, 1996; Wyke, 1997; McGlynn, 2003).

Consumers have an effect throughout the system, from payers to suppliers and providers. Payers such as managed care organizations are particularly aware of consumer influence. Most companies that offer health plans will at least offer two or three choices to employees. Because employees have a choice of plan, the health plans compete for these consumers through a number of sales and promotional activities, but the final determinant for enrollees to continue with a health plan for several years is how effectively the plan meets health needs. Plans that have poor member service or a limited network of providers lose members very quickly, limiting the benefits of preventive care and QI activities. Thus, these plans often fail to focus on QI because members who stay with the plan are generally not interested in these attributes. Loss of the preventive care focus makes a managed care plan little different than a traditional indemnity plan with utilization management or cost containment. Although cost-containment techniques work well in the early stages of managed care, they soon lose effectiveness and must be replaced by preventive health strategies to improve population health status and decrease the long-term cost of care.

Consumers are becoming increasingly interested in improving quality of life, as well as the quality of health care, and health plans that can deliver services that prevent disease as well as treat the catastrophic effects of disease will become the most successful. In addition to providing feedback for health plans and providers through surveys, consumers are organizing community coalitions that promote greater consumer involvement in health care choices (Borland, et al., 1994; Cheadle, et al., 2003). Berwick noted in a 1997 article that consumers must be enlisted to a much greater degree by the health care industry to improve the quality of care and the efficiency of the system (Berwick, 1997). Using business strategies such as mass customization and stratification of need, the system can at once be streamlined and made more responsive to customer requirements. In the 1982 best-seller *In Search of Excellence*, Tom Peters and Robert Waterman (Peters and Waterman, 1982) noted that the most successful companies were also the most responsive to customers and the most efficient, a finding that was confirmed 19 years later by Jim Collins in his book *Good to Great: Why Some Companies Make the Leap...and Others Don't* (Collins, 2001). These companies thrive on the challenges of consumer satisfaction, and they recognize that consumer delight, not just consumer satisfaction, will bring customers back again and again.

The needs projected by consumerism require health care organizations to pursue a QI philosophy to meet the objectives of long-term profitability and organizational success. Companies that simply satisfy customers may survive, but those that seek to excel must work to delight consumers with the level of service that they provide. Health care industry leaders in the future will thus embrace consumerism and find new ways of raising health care encounters to new levels.

◆ Quality Milestone 4: Education

The utility of education for improving the health care system can be seen in the consumer movement. Better-informed consumers make greater demands for quality health care, and better-educated providers are able to offer services that delight consumers and lead to greater demands for even higher-quality services. This unending cycle produces the impetus for much of the research activity in health care, finding new ways of dealing with clinical conditions that will relieve suffering and improve quality of life. The linchpin for the cycle, however, is education for both providers and consumers.

Educational resources have mushroomed with the advent of worldwide telecommunications. Free sources on the Internet allow consumers to access the latest information in the medical literature through any of thousands of Web sites that have health information (Krempec, et al., 2003; Oermann, et al., 2003; Kershaw, 2003). Many of these sites have been listed in other chapters, and the wealth of information that is available continues to grow every day. Nearly every provider group of sufficient size has contributed to the information available, with input about virtually every conceivable disease. On the other hand, the Internet can also offer erroneous advice, making it imperative for providers to help consumers find correct information and avoid erroneous or detrimental sites. Health care providers are becoming "knowledge navigators" who will assist consumers in finding methods of diagnosis and treatment by sifting through all of the information that can be accessed on the Internet and from other reliable sources. No longer will physicians and other health professionals serve as a fountain of knowledge; rather, they will be more involved in assisting consumers in their care by formulating an effective education and information acquisition strategy for each individual circumstance.

This approach is consistent with that described above under quality milestone 3 on consumerism. As consumers gain more influence in the system, their needs for improved information sources will continue to grow. The most effective providers will be those who work to empower their customers to assume responsibility and control of their own care. Extensive educational resources will be necessary to achieve this transformation, but investment in the infrastructure to provide these resources will be repaid by a healthier society and a more cost-effective health care delivery system. Consumers also seem to appreciate the ability to apply health information to their own circumstances (Geller, et al., 1999). However, educational programs and provider efforts must be properly structured and coordinated to avoid negative repercussions (Sofaer, 1997). Programs that are designed poorly, contain erroneous information leading to adverse outcomes, and generate consumer demands that cannot be met because of insurance benefit design or lack of local resources can lead to frustration and consumer distrust of the health care delivery system. Some have even suggested a new subspecialty, consumer health informatics, that will study consumer needs and help structure information resources so that they meet, and even anticipate, those needs (Ferguson, 1997).

Providers also require education in new methods of delivering services. In their role as knowledge navigators, providers will need to become proficient at using new sources of information, as well as find ways of exploiting these new technologies for disseminating their own quality messages. Constricted funding sources are making traditional methods of continuing medical education untenable, and providers are actively pursuing more convenient and less expensive methods of learning. Internet-based educational programs are proving ideal for physicians to learn new medical approaches with a minimum investment of time and money. Just-in-time education supports practitioners at the time that they need information, and innovative methods of providing these tools are being developed (Carlton, 1997; Ong, 2003; Leach, et al., 2003). Even using simple Internet access methods, practitioners can find necessary information much more rapidly than in the past, but they must be trained to use the new technology and not be penalized for trying to improve care.

Several of Deming's 14 principles allude to the need to educate the workforce to improve quality. Health care presents a new variation on that theme because providers must not only educate workers but educate their customers as well. Achievement of that objective will continue to require careful study by health system leaders, emphasizing those aspects of research and education that will improve care and efficiency in the system.

◆ Quality Milestone 5: Federal and State Government Program Emphasis on Quality

Two trends dominated health care economics at the end of the 20th century: (1) a decline in health care costs relative to the gross domestic product and (2) an increase in the proportion of the health care bill paid by government (Iglehart, 1999). In spite of the failure of federally led health reform in the early 1990s, government influence in health care grew tremendously in the last decade of the 20th century. The monopoly power exerted by federal and state governments has been the cause of extraordinary changes in the system, from serious reductions in funding for health care services to imposition of quality goals that often exceed the capacity of the industry to comply. Government programs have now been established to improve the quality of care in addition to the efforts to reduce the cost of care.

Some of these initiatives, e.g., the Cooperative Cardiovascular Project (Marciniak, et al., 1998), have demonstrated true improvement. The Centers for Medicare and Medicaid Services (CMS; formerly known as the Health Care Financing Administration) sponsored the Cooperative Cardiovascular Project as a way of improving the quality of care for Medicare beneficiaries who sustained a myocardial infarction. The QI organizations (QIOs, formerly professional review organizations) in several states were enlisted to report seven performance measures related to myocardial infarction, followed by improvement interventions designed by the QIO in each participating state. Nearly all of the QIOs reported improvements in some or all of the measures, bolstering governmental confidence in the QI approach.

Another example of success was the effort of the Agency for Healthcare Research and Quality (AHRQ) in developing CPGs for 19 clinical conditions. Although the Agency lost substantial amounts of funding in government cutbacks, these 19 CPGs were exemplary in their creation and format and provided a pattern for efforts around the country. The AHRQ clinical guidelines are available for public use on the agency's Web site (Agency for Healthcare Research and Quality, 1999), and numerous reports of organizations using guidelines have been published in the medical literature (Miller, et al., 1999; Tacci, et al., 1999; Sugarman, et al., 2003). Although some of the guidelines provoked a reaction from some medical organizations, they were generally well accepted, and the procedure for creating the guidelines and the format of the final documents established the approach that other organizations have adopted.

Other federal initiatives have created QI systems for almost every entity in the health care system from managed care organizations to laboratories in physician offices. Regulations and standards have been set in an effort to establish better quality, but to date there is no published evidence of improved outcomes resulting from these regulations. The managed care program, called the Quality Improvement System for Managed Care (QISMC), is discussed in greater detail in Chapter 11. The Outcome and Assessment Indicator Set that CMS has designed for assessing home health services represents another attempt by the federal government to evaluate the care rendered Medicare beneficiaries by another segment of the industry (Shaughnessy, et al., 1998). On the other hand, Medicare reimbursement is being increasingly tied to performance on quality measures, rather than on submitted costs or charges (Traynor, 2003).

State efforts have been much more disparate. For example, under the aegis of federal–state partnerships for maternal–child health, regional perinatal programs have evolved over the past three decades to organize hospital neonatal programs into different levels of care, depending on the severity of an infant's clinical condition (Johnson and Little, 1999). Most states monitor hospital performance and make regular reports to state legislatures (Epstein and Kurtzig, 1994), and in some states the information is released to the public. The Michigan Hospital Association, for example, places extensive reports of hospital performance on the organization's Web site at *http://www .mha.org*. Such information will become increasingly available as public demand increases.

Federal and state governments have had a profound effect on the health care industry, and all indicators suggest that the trend will continue. Government is the largest purchaser of health care services, and ensuring that Medicare and Medicaid beneficiaries receive quality care has become a prime directive for the CMS and the state agencies responsible for oversight of health programs. These efforts push providers to create the infrastructure necessary for QI, although sometimes with too much emphasis on bureaucracy and not enough on performance.

◆ Quality Milestone 6: Adoption of the Quality Philosophy

Drs. Deming, Juran, and others in the QI field recommended that American industry adopt the "new philosophy" of QI back in the 1940s and 1950s. Deming stressed to American managers that the post-World War II world had entered a new economic era and that knowledgeable industrialists should recognize and adapt to the new order. World economies were not likely to conform to a global system in which the United States would be dominant indefinitely, and Deming urged American industrial leaders to structure their companies to compete on quality rather than price. Dr. Joseph Juran brought similar beliefs to industries around the world, leading to the total quality management paradigm that took QI from the realm of statistical charts to that of strategic management.

American health care finds itself at a similar crossroads. As the health care sector transforms from a system of unfettered growth in supply and demand to a rational system in which the price of services responds to market forces that include consumer demand and payer preeminence, the health care industry must demonstrate value in the services provided for customers. The system will no longer pay for services just because consumers or physicians want them; rather, the value of the services must be proven using the scientific methods developed in world industry over the past 50 years (Laupacis, et al., 2002; Maynard and Bloor, 2003). This level of accountability is new in health care, and a backlash has accompanied these changes, led by providers and consumers legitimately concerned that the new order in health care could cause harm to those who need the system most. These concerns do not negate the underlying issue, however—that the health care industry has become accountable and must take an increasingly aggressive role in improving the value of services provided to society.

The efforts of state and federal regulatory agencies to ensure quality for Medicare and Medicaid beneficiaries by implementing standards and enforcing rules generally run counter to Deming's principles to eliminate quotas and rules. Conformance to the standards to demonstrate value should be considered only a penultimate goal, however. The ultimate result must be the adoption of the quality philosophy throughout the industry. Establishment of QI departments or the conversion of old quality assurance programs to contemporary performance improvement systems will not suffice: Management and workers must incorporate quality principles and methods into their daily work so that the pursuit of quality becomes entrenched in the system.

Many state and federal regulations, as well as the standards of accreditation agencies such as the National Committee for Quality Assurance, the Joint Commission on Accreditation of Healthcare Organizations, and Utilization Review Accreditation Commission, have requirements for specific outcomes that make the establishment of a quality infrastructure inevitable. For example, the QISMC standards for Medicare+Choice managed care plans require studies, interventions, and remeasurements for particular projects on clinical quality that could be performed ad hoc but that achieve much better results within a QI infrastructure. Unfortunately, however, these standards and requirements cannot mandate QI values in the organization. Inculcation of the QI philosophy into corporate culture must occur if the organization hopes to optimize the return from improvement activities.

This task falls to management. Health care executives, providers, and administrators must first accept the reality that society demands accountability, not just financial accountability, but also responsibility for quality of services and outcomes produced by the system. No longer will society accept rationalizations that there isn't enough money or "the patient didn't follow orders." A QI philosophy must place these problems in proper perspective, i.e., "we must find ways of improving the process so that the money is adequate and we serve the patient's needs using the resources available." A QI approach will provide the proper perspective. Managing quality will produce the desired containment of costs much more effectively than managing utilization. Society challenges the industry with the goal of universal, affordable health care, and it is incumbent upon health care providers and managers to respond to the challenge.

Thus, achievement of the sixth quality milestone will happen when health care organizations adopt the new philosophy, recognize that change is not coming but is happening now, and that organizational survival depends not just on effective cost management but rather on optimizing the quality of the organization's products and services. When this milestone has been achieved, the health care industry will regain the respect that it deserves.

◆ QI Is the Answer

Achievement of all of these milestones may seem improbable or even impossible. On the other hand, the health care industry has a window of opportunity to regain a preeminent position in society by adopting the QI philosophy and gearing the culture to continuous improvement and accountability.

QI tools are simply the accoutrements that must be used to implement the changes. The key to success will be a willingness to change, explore, and grow using the philosophy of QI that has served the business world so well in the past century.

◆ Discussion Points

1. What barriers exist in the health care industry to incorporating the quality improvement philosophy? How did these barriers arise?
2. How can improved information management enhance quality improvement efforts?
3. What advantages do electronic medical records provide quality improvement professionals who are implementing quality improvement studies and interventions?
4. How do clinical decision-support systems assist in improving the quality of care? What measures can be taken to make them more acceptable to practitioners?
5. What effects have innovations such as the Internet had on health care? How can they be used to improve the quality of care?
6. Briefly describe a telemedicine system and discuss the benefits of this type of technology for a quality-oriented organization.
7. List the advantages of integrated delivery systems for implementing quality improvement activities. How will the growth of these organizations influence the incorporation of quality improvement into the industry? What challenges do these organizations face to achieving success?
8. Discuss the role of the consumer in health care today. What factors have led to the growth of consumerism in health care?
9. How can education change the roles of stakeholders in the health care system? What innovations in education will be necessary in the future to assure continuous improvement?
10. How has the influence of federal and state government changed in health care over the past 30 years? Has government intervention had any positive effects?
11. What is the "quality philosophy"? Why is the establishment of a quality improvement department in a hospital not sufficient to serve the quality philosophy?

◆ Notes

Agency for Healthcare Research and Quality. (1999). *Clinical practice guidelines*. Retrieved October 2003, from *http://www.ahcpr.gov/clinic/index.html#online*

Bates D. W., Leape L. L., Cullen D. J., Laird N., Petersen L. A., Teich J. M. (1998). Effect of computerized physician order entry and a team intervention on prevention of serious medication errors. *Journal of the American Medical Association, 280*(15), 1311–1316.

Berner E., and Ball M. (1998). *Clinical decision support systems: Theory and practice.* New York: Springer-Verlag.

Berwick D. (1997). The total customer relationship in health care: Broadening the bandwidth. *Joint Commission Journal of Quality Improvement, 23*(5), 245–250.

Bindels R., Hasman A., Kester A. D., Talmon J. L., De Clercq P. A., Winkens R. A. (2003). The efficacy of an automated feedback system for general practitioners. *Informatics in Primary Care, 11*(2), 69–74.

Borland M., Smith C., Nankivil N. (1994). A community quality initiative for health care reform. *Managed Care Quarterly, 2*(1), 6–16.

Buller-Close K., Schriger D. L., Baraff L. J. (2003, May). Heterogeneous effect of an Emergency Department Expert Charting System. *Annals of Emergency Medicine, 41*(5), 644–652.

Burns L., and Pauly V. (2002). Integrated delivery networks: A detour on the road to integrated health care? *Health Affairs, 21*(4), 128–143.

Caelli K., Downie J., Caelli T. (2003, July). Towards a decision support system for health promotion in nursing. *Journal of Advances in Nursing, 43*(2), 170–180.

Campbell D. M. (1998). Developing a successful call center: One hospital's story. *Healthcare Information Management, 12*(2), 97–105.

Carlton K. H. (1997). Redefining continuing education delivery. *Computers in Nursing, 15*(1), 17–22.

Cheadle A., Beery W. L., Greenwald H. P., Nelson G. D., Pearson D., Senter S. (2003, April). Evaluating the California Wellness Foundation's Health Improvement Initiative: a logic model approach. *Health Promotion Practices, 4*(2), 146–156.

Collins J. (2001). *Good to Great: Why Some Companies Make the Leap...and Others Don't.* Harper Collins, New York, NY.

Cook B. (2002, October 7). QuagMeyer: A cautionary tale of a failing medical practice. *American Medical News.*

Cornish P., Church E., Callanan T., Bethune C., Robbins C., Miller R. (2003). Rural interdisciplinary mental health team building via satellite: A demonstration project. *Telemed J E Health, 9*(1), 63–71.

Davidson E. J., and Chismar W. G. (1999). Planning and managing computerized order entry: A case study of IT-enabled organizational transformation. *Topics in Health Information Management, 19*(4), 47–61.

Earnest M. P., Grimm S. M., Malmgren M. A., Martin B. A., Meehan M., Potter M. B., Steele A. W., Zocholl J. R. (1998). Quality improvement in an integrated urban healthcare system: A necessary journey. *Clinical Performance and Quality Health Care, 6*(4), 193–200.

Elliott V. (2003, April 28). FDA chief pledges changes to direct-to-consumer advertising guidelines. *American Medical News.*

Epstein M., and Kurtzig B. (1994). Statewide health information: A tool for improving hospital accountability. *Joint Commission Journal of Quality Improvement, 20*(7), 370–375.

Ferguson T. (1997). Health online and the empowered medical consumer. *Joint Commission Journal of Quality Improvement, 23*(5), 258–264.

Frey K., Edwards F., Altman K., Spahr N., Gorman R. S. (2003, September). The 'Collaborative Care' curriculum: An educational model addressing key ACGME core competencies in primary care residency training. *Medical Education, 37*(9), 786–789.

Geller A. C., Halpern A. C., Sun T., Oliveria S. A., Miller D. R., Lew R. A., Koh H. K. (1999). Participant satisfaction and value in American Academy of Dermatology and American Cancer Society skin cancer screening programs in Massachusetts. *Journal of the American Academy of Dermatology, 40*(4), 563–566.

Goldsmith J. (2002). Integrating care: A talk with Kaiser Permanente's David Lawrence. *Health Affairs, 21*(1), 40–50.

Greene P. (1998). Improving clinical effectiveness in an integrated care delivery system. *Journal of Healthcare Quality, 20*(6), 4–8.

Hamill C. T., and Harris-Stevens L. (1998). 24-Hour call centers and home health care. *Home Care Provider, 3*(6), 324–325.

Hammond W. E., Pollard D. L., Straube M. J. (1998). Managing healthcare: A view of tomorrow. *Medinfo 9* (Pt. 1), 26–30.

Harpole L. H., Khorasani R., Fiskio J., Kuperman G. J., Bates D. W. (1997). Automated evidence-based critiquing of orders for abdominal radiographs: Impact on utilization and appropriateness. *Journal of the American Medical Informatics Association, 4*(6), 511–521.

Hume M. (1999). Computer-aided drug selection can sharply cut adverse events. *Quality Letter for Healthcare Leaders, 11*(3), 10–12.

Iglehart J. (1999). The American health care system—expenditures. *New England Journal of Medicine, 340*(1), 70–76.

Jeannot J. G., Scherer F., Pittet V., Burnand B., Vader J. P. (2003, April–June). Use of the World Wide Web to implement clinical practice guidelines: A feasibility study. *J Medical Internet Research, 5*(2), e12.

Johnson K. A., and Little G. A. (1999). State health agencies and quality improvement in perinatal care. *Pediatrics 103*(1), 233–247.

Kershaw A. (2003, September 9–15). Patient use of the Internet to obtain health information. *Nursing Times, 99*(36), 30–32.

Kertesz L. (1996). Patient is king: Studies define customers' satisfaction and the means to improve it. *Modern Healthcare, 26*(18), 107–120.

Kouroubali A., Starren J. B., Clayton P. D., (1998, November). Costs and benefits of connecting community physicians to a hospital WAN. In *Proceedings of the American Medical Informatics Association Symposium* (pp. 205–209).

Kramer T. L., Owen R. R., Cannon D., Sloan K. L., Thrush C. R., Williams D. K., Austen M.A. (2003, September). How well do automated performance measures assess guideline implementation for new-onset depression in the Veterans Health Administration? *Joint Commission Journal of Quality and Safety, 29*(9), 479–489.

Krempec J., Hall J., Biermann J. S. (2003). Internet use by patients in orthopaedic surgery. *Iowa Orthopedic Journal, 23*, 80–82.

Kuperman G. J., Cooley T., Tremblay J., Teich J. M., Churchill W. (1998). Decision support for medication use in an inpatient physician order entry application and a pharmacy application. *Medinfo, 9*(Pt. 1), 467–471.

LaBresh K. A., Gliklich R., Liljestrand J., Peto R., Ellrodt A. G. (2003, October). Using "get with the guidelines" to improve cardiovascular secondary prevention. *Joint Commission Journal of Quality and Safety, 29*(10), 539–550.

Laupacis A., Anderson G., O'Brien B. (2002). Drug policy: Making effective drugs available without bankrupting the healthcare system. *Healthcare Papers, 3*(1), 12–30.

Leach A., and Haun D. E. (2003, April). Just-in-time training: A Web-based tool for needlestick injury. *Joint Commission Journal of Quality and Safety, 29*(4), 201–204.

Leader W. G., Pestotnik S. L., Chandler M. H. (1996). Integrating pharmacokinetics into point-of-care information systems. *Clinical Pharmacokinetics, 31*(3), 165–173.

Louis A. A., Turner T., Gretton M., Baksh A., Cleland J. G. (2003, October). A systematic review of telemonitoring for the management of heart failure. *European Journal of Heart Failure, 5*(5), 583–590.

Marciniak T. A., Mosedale L., Ellerbeck E. F. (1998). Quality improvement at the national level: Lessons from the cooperative cardiovascular project. *Evaluation and the Health Professions, 21*(4), 525–536.

Marsh A. (1998). The creation of a global telemedical information society. *Medinfo, 9*(Pt. 1), 249–541.

Marshall P., and Chin H. (1998, November). The effects of an electronic medical record on patient care: Clinician attitudes in a large HMO. In *Proceedings of the American Medical Informatics Association Symposium* (pp. 150–154).

Marta M. R. (2003, July). Telemedicine payment: Then and now. *Healthcare Financial Management, 57*(7), 50–53.

Maynard A., and Bloor K. (2003, May–June). Dilemmas in regulation of the market for pharmaceuticals. *Health Affairs (Millwood), 22*(3), 31–41.

McCue M. J., Mazmanian P. E., Hampton C. L., Marks T. K., Fisher E. J., Parpart F., Malloy W. N., Fisk K. J. (1998). Cost-minimization analysis: A follow-up study of a telemedicine program. *Telemedicine Journal, 4*(4), 323–327.

McGlynn E. A. (2003, January). Selecting common measures of quality and system performance. *Medical Care, 41*(1 Suppl), I39–I47.

Miller E. H., Belgrade M. J., Cook, M., Portu J. B., Shepherd M., Sierzant T., Sallmen P., Fraki S. (1999). Institution-wide pain management improvement through the use of evidence-based content, strategies, resources, and outcomes. *Quality Management in Health Care, 7*(2), 28–40.

Nowalk M. P., Middleton B., Zimmerman R. K., Hess M. M., Skledar S. J., Jacobs M. A. (2003, July). Increasing pneumococcal vaccination rates among hospitalized patients. *Infection Control and Hospital Epidemiology, 24*(7), 526–531.

Oermann M. H., Lowery N. F., Thornley J. (2003, September). Evaluation of Web sites on management of pain in children. *Pain Management in Nursing, 4*(3), 99–105.

Ong K. R. (2003, July–September). Just-in-time database-driven Web applications. *Journal of Medical Internet Research, 5*(3), e18.

Pavlopoulos S., et al. (1998). Design and development of a multimedia database for emergency telemedicine. *Technology in Health Care, 6*(2–3), 101–110.

Pergament D., Pergament E., Wonderlick A., Fiddler M. (1999). At the crossroads: The intersection of the Internet and clinical oncology. *Oncology (Huntington), 13*(4), 577–583.

Peters T., and Waterman R. (1982). *In search of excellence.* New York: Warner Books.

Peth H. (2003). Medication errors in the emergency department: A systems approach to minimizing risk. *Emergency Medical Clinics of North America, 21*(1), 141–158.

Porcelli P. J., and Lobach D. F. (1999). Integration of clinical decision support with online encounter documentation for well child care at the point of care. *Proceedings of the American Medical Informatics Association Symposium,* 1999:599–603.

Quade G., Novotny J., Burde B., May F., Beck L. E., Goldschmidt A. (1999). Worldwide telemedicine services based on distributed multimedia electronic patient records by using the second generation Web server hyperwave. *Proceedings of the American Medical Informatics Association Symposium,* 916–920.

Rialle V., Duchene F., Noury N., Bajolle L., Demongeot J. (2002, Winter). Health "Smart" home: information technology for patients at home. *Telemedicine Journal and E-Health, 8*(4), 395–409.

Riccardi V. (1998). Modern medicine; modern consumerism. *Administrative Radiology Journal, 17*(11), 10–13.

Ridderikhoff J., and van Herk B. (1999). Who is afraid of the system? Doctors' attitude towards diagnostic systems. *International Journal of Medical Informatics, 53*(1), 91–100.

Rowberg A. H., and York W. B. (1999). Developing a framework for worldwide image communication. *Journal of Digital Imaging, 12*(2), 189–190.

Sausser G. D. (2003, July). Thin is in: web-based systems enhance security, clinical quality. *Healthcare Financial Management, 57*(7), 86–89.

Shahar Y., Miksch S., Johnson P. (1996, October). An intention-based language for representing clinical guidelines. In *Proceedings of the American Medical Informatics Association Annual Fall Symposium* (pp. 592–596).

Shaughnessy P. W., Crisler K. S., Schlenker R. E. (1998). Outcome-based quality improvement in home health care: The OASIS indicators. *Quality Management in Health Care, 7*(1), 58–67.

Shiffman R., Liaw Y., Brandt C. A., Corb G. J. (1999). Computer-based guideline implementation systems: A systematic review of functionality and effectiveness. *Journal of the American Medical Informatics Association, 6*(2), 104–114.

Sintchenko V., Coiera E., Iredell J. R., Gilbert G. L. (2003). Comparative impact of guidelines, clinical data and decision support on prescribing decisions: an interactive web experiment with simulated cases. Retrieved from *http://www.jamia.org/cgi/reprint/M1166v1,* November, 2003 (subscription required).

Siwicki B. (1999). Telemedicine providers' progress impeded at the border: The need for physicians to obtain a medical license in every state in which they practice slows the growth of telemedicine. *Health Data Management, 7*(5), 94–102.

Sofaer S. (1997). How will we know if we got it right? Aims, benefits, and risks of consumer information initiatives. *Joint Commission Journal of Quality Improvement, 23*(5), 258–264.

Spencer E., Swanson T., Hueston W. J., Edberg D. L. (1999). Tools to improve documentation of smoking status: Continuous quality improvement and electronic medical records. *Archives of Family Medicine, 8*(1), 18–22.

Sugarman J., Frederick P., Frankenfield D., Owen W., and McClellan W. (2003). Developing clinical performance measures based on the Dialysis Outcomes Quality Initiative Clinical Practice Guidelines: Process, outcomes, and implications. *American Journal of Kidney Disease, 42*(4), 806–812.

Swisher K. N., Begun J. W., Ulmer D. L. (1999, January–February). Hospital-physician relationships in the integrated delivery system: An ethical analysis. *Clinical Lab Management Reviews, 13*(1), 3–12.

Tacci J. A., Webster B. S., Hashemi L., Christiani D. C. (1999). Clinical practices in the management of new-onset, uncomplicated, low-back workers' compensation disability claims. *Journal of Occupational and Environmental Medicine, 41*(5), 397–404.

Taragin M., Lauer M., Savir M., Sivan E., Siesel D., Aufgang B. (1998, November). HCFA documentation guidelines and the need for discrete data: A golden opportunity for applied health informatics. In *Proceedings of the American Medical Informatics Association Symposium* (pp. 653–656).

Traynor K. (2003, September 1). Medicare demonstration project ties quality to reimbursement. *American Journal of Health System Pharmacies, 60*(17), 1728–1732.

van der Lei J., van der Does E., Man in 't Veld A. J., Musen M. A., van Bemmel J. H. (1993). Response of general practitioners to computer-generated critiques of hypertension therapy. *Methods in Information in Medicine, 32*(2), 146–153.

Woolhandler S., Himmelstein D. U., Lewontin J. P. (1993). Administrative costs in U.S. hospitals. *New England Journal of Medicine, 329*(6), 400–403.

Woolhandler S., Campbell T., Himmelstein D. U. (2003). Costs of health care administration in the United States and Canada. *New England Journal of Medicine, Aug 21;349*(8),768–775.

Wyke A. (1997). Can patients drive the future of health care? *Harvard Business Review, 75*(4), 146–150.

Glossary

accreditation an act of certification of competence, used in health care to describe the process of audit and review performed by organizations such as the **National Commission for Quality Assurance** (NCQA) and the **Joint Commission on Accreditation of Healthcare Organizations** (JCAHO) to certify **managed care organizations** and provider institutions.

activity-based costing (ABC) a method of cost accounting that allocates costs according to explicit and implicit activities involved in generating the cost rather than arbitrary percentages or amounts.

administrative services in the context of this text, activities that are required to record, transmit, evaluate, and pay health care providers.

affinity diagrams a method of organizing a large number of ideas into logical groups through group consensus.

Agency for Healthcare Research and Quality (AHRQ) formerly known as the Agency for Health Care Policy and Research (AHCPR). A federal agency within the Department of Health and Human Services that is involved in funding health services research.

ambulatory care groups a system for classifying illnesses using clusters of diagnosis (**ICD**) and procedure (**CPT**) codes that groups these codes according to a framework designed by researchers at Johns Hopkins University.

analysis of variance (ANOVA) a statistical method for determining the degree to which group means vary between each other.

arrow diagram *see* **program evaluation and review technique attributes** data. Data sets that are composed of **discrete variables.**

attributes of conformance a list of data requirements for **ORYX** measurements created by **JCAHO.**

autocorrelation results in one time period influence results in other time periods; observations are not independent.

average length of stay (ALOS) a measurement of the average amount of time that individuals admitted to a hospital stayed in the hospital.

balanced score card (BSC) a strategic planning tool designed by Kaplan and Norton in the early 1990s to help managers consider all factors of importance to the organization during a planning process.

barriers analysis a formal method of reviewing a **process** to identify barriers to implementation.

benefits and barriers exercise (BBE)   a group exercise that helps individuals in the group recognize the possible advantages and detriments of proposed changes.

brainstorming   a method for a group to generate ideas by spontaneously offering them in rapid succession, without discussion or criticism.

brainwriting   a variant of **brainstorming** in which the group writes ideas down, rather than voicing them aloud.

CAHPS   *see* **Consumer Assessment of Health Plans Survey.**

capitation   payment mechanism for reimbursing providers in which a single amount is paid to the provider during a specified time period (usually monthly), regardless of the volume or nature of services rendered to patients.

care management   an extension of the **disease management** approach that includes preventive services and well-person care as a means to decrease the disease burden of a population, improve health, and decrease costs.

carve-in program   a program that reduces risk to a provider by having a subcontractor educate and staff the organization's **disease management** function for a specific illness. For example, a **managed care organization** may carve in a program for congestive heart failure provided by a subcontractor specializing in managing that clinical condition.

carve-out program   a program that reduces risk to a provider by subcontracting for specific services on a risk-sharing basis with another entity. For example, a carve-out program may include all diabetics in a health plan who are managed by an outside **disease management** program for a **capitation** payment per member per month.

case management   oversight of the care of an individual patient by an experienced health professional using **care management** algorithms and **clinical practice guidelines** (CPGs).

case solutions technique   a method of team building in which a business case from another organization or the published literature is presented to the team for solution. Cases are usually chosen to be similar, but not identical, to the task to be managed by the team.

Centers for Medicare and Medicaid Services (CMS)   the organization within the federal government concerned with financing and maintaining federal programs for health care, i.e., Medicare and Medicaid.

claims data   data sent to insurance companies by providers to procure payment for services.

clinical practice guidelines (CPGs)   systematically developed statements to assist practitioner and patient decisions about appropriate health care for specific clinical circumstances.

clinical services   activities required for providing health care to individuals, usually delivered by health care professionals.

CMS *see* **Centers for Medicare and Medicaid services.**

common cause variation variability in a **process** that is inherent in the system.

comorbid conditions diseases or clinical conditions that exist in the same patient at the same time.

consultant, team *see* **team consultant.**

Consumer Assessment of Health Plans Survey (CAHPS) a standardized survey used to evaluate health plans for specific characteristics by surveying customers and determining levels of satisfaction.

consumerism a philosophy that emphasizes the role of the consumer in the health care system.

contact capitation a method of **capitation** in which a provider is paid a capitation payment only when a patient uses the services of the provider.

continuous quality improvement (CQI) a management philosophy that mandates continually pursuing efforts to improve the quality of the products and services produced by an organization.

continuous variables numeric values that have an infinite number of possible values between two numbers.

control chart a chart that includes a measure of central tendency, e.g., the mean, and a measure of variability, e.g., the standard deviation, that provides information about the performance of a **process** and the presence of **common cause** or **special cause** variability.

control limit a boundary set for a **control chart** that determines the presence of **common cause** or **special cause variation.**

control limit, lower *see* **lower control limit.**

control limit, upper *see* **upper control limit.**

cost of quality analysis evaluation of a flowchart to identify steps that lead to increasing costs or decreased quality.

CPGs *see* **clinical practice guidelines.**

CPT codes *see* **current procedural terminology codes.**

credentials documentation of a provider's qualifications to perform services.

critical path method (CPM) *see* **program evaluation and review technique.**

critical to quality analysis evaluation of a flowchart to identify steps that must be performed correctly to ensure quality in the final product or service.

critiquing system a **decision-support system** that evaluates problem issues and the plan constructed by the provider or manager, then provides an appraisal and recommendations based on a knowledge base and appropriate software.

cross-functional team   a group of individuals, drawn from several functional areas in an organization, that is charged with performing a specific task.

current procedural terminology (CPT) codes   a coding system that associates specific numeric codes to medical and surgical procedures. CPT codes are adopted and maintained by the American Medical Association.

data repository   a large capacity computer system that stores data from multiple sources in a format that allows access to the data for extensive analysis.

decision matrix   a 1 × (mult sym)2 matrix that specifically relates advantages and disadvantages of specific choices to the list of choices. Each choice can be weighted to provide a score that best reflects the value of the choice.

decision-support system   a computerized system that provides information and data to decision makers at the time and site where decisions are made and implemented.

delegation   subcontracting or assigning a task to another entity.

deployment flowchart   a specialized flowchart that identifies specific individuals or departments in the organization who must be involved in implementing a **process** at each step.

diagnosis-related groups (DRGs)   a system for classifying illnesses and clinical conditions using clusters of diagnosis (**ICD**) codes that group these codes according to a framework supported by the **Centers for Medicare and Medicaid Services** (CMS). DRGs are most commonly used to define and pay for hospital services.

disease management   an approach to caring for individuals with specific diseases based on the concept of complete understanding of the disease, the therapeutic regimens that are of value in treating the disease, and the effects on the individual of treatments.

discrete variables   variables that have distinct numeric values with no intervening values between each number.

DRGs   *see* **diagnosis-related groups.**

durable medical equipment   instruments and machines that can be reused to provide health care, e.g., dialysis machines, canes, and crutches.

effective-achievable matrix (EAM)   a 1 × (mult sym)1 matrix used by quality improvement teams to determine which potential interventions will achieve the greatest effectiveness and be most achievable.

episodes of care   discrete time- or event-limited periods during the course of an illness that have an identifiable beginning and endpoint, such as an inpatient hospitalization for asthma.

fish bone diagram   a method created by Ishikawa to identify cause and effect relationships leading to a specific outcome.

Foundation for Accountability (FACCT) an organization created by Paul Ellwood that promotes implementation of quality improvement and performance measurement in health care.

functional silos the tendency for organizations to establish isolated departments that communicate poorly with each other, leading to lapses in quality and increased costs.

group chart a method of analyzing data with multiple characteristics on the same chart by grouping the data logically for entry onto the chart.

HCFA 1500 form an insurance billing form for medical providers, created by HCFA, that includes information for payment of an insurance claim, including patient information, diagnosis and procedure information, and other salient information.

Health Care Financing Administration (HCFA) *see* **Centers for Medicare and Medicaid Services** (CMS).

health maintenance organizations (HMOs) companies created to provide health care services throughout the continuum of health care. With emphasis on maintaining a state of good health, HMOs are designed to manage an individual's health care to promote the best outcomes possible, given the current state of technology and access to care.

health risk assessment (HRA) a method of reviewing a patient's history and physical examination to determine the patient's level of risk for requiring health services.

Health Plan Employer Data and Information Set (HEDIS) a group of measures for assessing health plan quality designed by the **National Commission for Quality Assurance** (NCQA) that includes clinical and administrative metrics of health plan performance.

heuristic a problem-solving technique in which the most appropriate solution of several found by alternative methods is selected at successive stages of a program for use in the next step of the analysis.

HMOs *see* **health maintenance organizations.**

ICD codes *see* **international classification of diseases codes.**

international classification of diseases (ICD) **codes** a widely accepted disease coding system used by insurers as a means of identifying specific diseases and complications for billing purposes.

index of severity a numeric method of adjusting the illness burden of a patient or cohort of patients to reflect the seriousness of an illness or group of illnesses.

insurer any **payer** that subsidizes health care services and assumes financial risk for the services being provided.

integrated delivery system (IDS) a health care system that can provide all services across the continuum of health care, including the assumption of risk for services rendered.

Ishikawa diagram   *see* **fish bone diagram.**

is–is not matrix   *see* **Kepner-Tregoe matrix.**

JCAHO   *see* **Joint Commission on Accreditation of Healthcare Organizations.**

Joint Commission on Accreditation of Healthcare Organizations (JCAHO)   originally organized to ensure minimum quality standards in hospitals, this private organization has **accreditation** programs for health plans and hospitals, as well as a flexible performance measurement system (**ORYX**).

just-in-time (JIT) **manufacturing**   control of the manufacturing process that emphasizes availability of production resources at the correct site and precise time in the production process needed to complete the production process with minimum inventory of production resources and finished product.

Kepner-Tregoe matrix   also called an **is–is not matrix.** Relates specific problems to potential causes (who, where, what, when, why, how) as a means of identifying issues causing quality problems.

L-shaped matrix   a matrix that relates a single variable to another single variable.

LCL   *see* **lower control limit.**

lean manufacturing   a manufacturing approach that emphasizes minimization of resource utilization and inventories.

list reduction   a method of combining and eliminating ideas generated during a **brainstorming** (or equivalent) exercise that improves the quality of ideas and ensures that they are germane to the issue of interest.

lower control limit (LCL)   the lower boundary of process variability, usually defined as three standard deviations below the mean.

managed care organization   one of several types of health insurance companies that exert varying degrees of control over provider activities through medical management processes or quality improvement processes.

matrix   a table in two or more dimensions that relates two or more variables to each other.

medical informatics   a branch of information science that deals with applications of information science to health care delivery and management. The field of medical informatics has evolved into a specific area of study by clinicians, computer scientists, and Internet-based medical information systems.

medical review criteria   issues in a **clinical practice guideline,** usually identified by an expert body of providers, that are expected to produce problems in implementation of the CPG or that may be a source of quality lapses that must be monitored.

Medicare+Choice the federal government term for managed care programs for Medicare beneficiaries.

morbidity the degree of illness and disability associated with a disease.

mortality medical term for death.

multivoting a technique of reducing the number of ideas generated during a **brainstorming** (or equivalent) exercise through multiple episodes of group voting and concurrence on each idea.

National Committee for Quality Assurance (NCQA) a private **accreditation** organization for **HMOs.**

National Guideline Clearinghouse a site on the Internet, supported by the **Agency for Healthcare Research and Quality** (AHRQ), that catalogs all **clinical practice guidelines** submitted to the AHRQ.

nominal group technique a more structured method of **brainstorming** that encourages input from all members of a group. Ideas are generated and presented sequentially by each group member, rather than randomly as in brainstorming.

nonconforming unit an instance of failure of an outcome to occur as planned, e.g., a patient with a postoperative infection or a Caesarean section instead of a vaginal delivery.

nosocomial infection an infection occurring in an institution due to spread of an infectious agent by the institution's procedures or staff.

obstacles to quality exercise a group method of identifying problems that will inhibit improvement of quality in a process.

operational definitions precise definitions of data or **performance measures.**

ORYX a performance measurement system used by the **JCAHO** for health care institutions, which allows the institution to formulate **performance measures** relevant to the institution's needs for quality improvement.

Outcome and Assessment Indicator Set (OASIS) a set of **performance measures** designed by **CMS** for home health agencies.

oversight team a team consisting (usually) of senior managers that provides direction for other functional and operational teams in the organization.

payer any individual or institution that pays for health care services, e.g., insurance companies, consumers, employers, etc.

per member per month (PMPM) a means of expressing utilization and cost measures in a standardized manner. The measure is expressed as an amount for each member for each month of the study or membership in a health plan.

per member per year (PMPY) a measure similar to PMPM but with utilization or costs aggregated over a year rather than a month.

performance-importance (P–I) **matrix** 1 × (mult sym)1 matrix that relates performance on one axis to importance on the other axis; relates customer measures of importance of a product or service to the ability of the organization to produce the product or service.

performance measures metrics that assess the operation of a process.

Performance Measurement Coordinating Council a committee consisting of the **JCAHO,** American Medical Association representatives, and the **NCQA** designed to create **performance measures** that can be used by all accrediting organizations in an effort to improve the measurement process.

pharmacy benefits manager an organization that subcontracts the management of a health plan's pharmacy benefits, usually including prior authorization for drugs, drug claims management, and pharmaceutical analysis.

plan-do-study-act cycle a quality improvement cycle created by Walter Shewhart to describe the approach taken to a quality improvement project. A plan is created to correct a quality problem, the plan is implemented, results of the intervention are measured, and then the intervention is modified to continue the improvement process.

plan-results matrix (PRM) a 1 × (mult sym)1 matrix that relates operational plans on one axis with results of the operations on the other axis; determines if plans have produced desired outcomes.

population an entire group of interest for statistical analysis. For example, the population of the United States may be of interest to the federal government, but the population of a health plan will be a subset of the population of the United States.

preferred provider organization (PPO) a financing mechanism for health care, usually involving a broker who negotiates reduced rates of payment to providers in return for directing a stream of customers to the provider's business.

process any sequential set of actions, steps, or functions that lead to an outcome or goal.

process cycle effectiveness the ratio of the amount of time actual work is done in a process to the total time required for the process to complete a cycle; measures the relative amount of slack time in a process.

program evaluation and review technique (PERT) a method originally designed by the US Navy for construction of nuclear submarines that produces a flowchart to describe the process that includes information about resources required at each step. PERT charts can be used in both planning and monitoring phases of project management.

provider profile a listing of provider **performance measures,** usually in graphic format, that compares the provider with others in the same specialty and/or community.

quality assurance   a method of quality management that identifies quality issues, sets minimum standards to be met for the issue, and then ceases work on the issue once the minimum standards are met.

quality improvement (QI)   a system of process analysis and statistical techniques that are designed to better understand processes and create measures of process capability that are used collaboratively to improve the process.

Quality Improvement System for Managed Care (QISMC)   quality improvement standards promulgated by **CMS** for **managed care organizations** serving Medicare+Choice beneficiaries.

regression analysis   a statistical method of relating a dependent variable to one or more independent variables.

relations diagram   a graphic representation of cause and effect dependencies in a process.

relationship diagram   a set of procedures to produce graphic representation of interactions and dependencies among entities, e.g., steps in a process.

repository, data   *see* **data repository.**

requirements and measures tree (RMT)   a diagram that correlates customer prerequisites for a product or service with each step in a process to which the prerequisite is related.

requirements matrix   a table that lists internal and external customer requirements and the outputs of the process that address the requirements.

risk corridor   a range of potential losses from payments for medical services that provides for cost sharing between providers and **payers** if **payment per member per month** or **payment per member per year** cost targets are not met.

risk pool   a financial arrangement in which the withhold amounts for several providers are held in a special fund from which the costs related to over- or unexpected utilization can be paid by an insurer.

risk sharing   a method of spreading the risk of providing medical services among several health care providers, institutions, and **payers;** several models for risk sharing are applicable, e.g., **capitation** and **carve-out** programs.

root cause diagram   also called a **why–why not diagram.** This diagram is a specific application of a **relationship diagram** that identifies a problem, then works through a **decision tree** process to pinpoint a solution.

run chart   a chart of time-series data that includes a median. Analysis of groups of points provides assessment of the presence of **common cause** or **special cause variation.**

runs testing   the statistical basis for evaluating a **run chart.**

sample   a subset of a population.

services, administrative   *see* **administrative services.**

services, clinical   *see* **clinical services.**

silos, functional   *see* **functional silos.**

six sigma   pioneered by Motorola. A program goal to reduce **nonconforming units** to fewer than 3.4 per million.

SPC   *see* **statistical process control.**

special cause variation   variability in a **process** that is caused by factors outside the system.

standard of care   a level of medical care to which all providers must adhere. Standards can be construed as minima or maxima, depending on the circumstance.

statistical process control (SPC)   quantitative methods of evaluation and monitoring business and clinical processes for the purpose of determining if the process is "in control," i.e., if the process is producing outputs within 3 sigma limits.

statistical thinking   a process to incorporate the principles of statistical analysis into evaluation of quality problems in order to quantitate the problems as much as possible, as well as to avoid overreacting to issues that are within normal range for the capability of a process.

stop loss insurance   insurance coverage that begins when a certain level of medical costs has been reached. For example, a stop loss policy can be invoked when an individual patient's care costs more than $50,000 or when a care manager's total cost of patient care exceeds $1,000,000.

storyboard   a graphical display of team efforts, using pictures, graphs, and some text. Storyboards are often used for large displays that highlight a team's progress toward a goal.

systems approach   evaluating and intervening in clinical or administrative situations with a view toward the entire person or enterprise rather than just one or a few components. The ability to synthesize a clinical or managerial plan based on all factors in the environment, rather than just single factors.

T-shaped matrix   a matrix that relates a single variable in a column to two other variables in rows; sometimes termed a $1 \times$ (mult sym)2 matrix.

tampering   treating a **common cause variation** as a **special cause;** usually causes erroneous interventions and untoward effects.

target chart   a variant of **control charts** that plots the difference between observed values and a **target value** on a control chart to determine the capability of a **process** to meet target goals.

target value   a goal set by an external authority or by the management of an organization.

Taylorism   often termed "the one best way," this management philosophy emphasized the duty of the manager to continually monitor worker performance and implement corrective actions when a worker deviated from expected work patterns. Management's task was to design the process and ensure that workers followed the correct procedures.

team consultant   an individual with particular expertise, e.g., in quality management science, who serves as an advisor to a team, rather than as a team member.

telemedicine   a method of providing medical care through a video communications interface with the physician at one site and the patient at another site.

throughput time   the time required for a **process** to complete a cycle from beginning to finish.

top-down flowchart   arrangement of a flowchart to indicate the importance of each step in a **process.**

total quality management (TQM)   a philosophy of conducting business in a manner that increases value to customers, employees, and society. The TQM philosophy entails continuous improvement in quality and reduction in cost of production.

transaction data   data recorded during or after a patient–provider interaction; can include insurance billing data or clinical record data.

tree diagram   a **relationship diagram** that provides a hierarchical representation of dependencies among steps in a **process;** most frequently used to translate concepts for improvement into specific actions.

UB-92 form   a universal hospital billing form for insurance claim submission; contains information similar to that on a **HCFA 1500** form for medical providers.

UCL   *see* **upper control limit.**

unbundling   a practice in billing insurance companies in which a provider will use several codes to describe a procedure, rather than one all-inclusive procedure code.

upcoding   a practice of assigning a procedure code with a higher intensity and reimbursement level to a service provided to a customer.

upper control limit (UCL)   the upper bounds of expected process variation, usually three standard deviations above the mean.

Utilization Review Accreditation Committee (URAC)   a private **accreditation** organization for **preferred provider organisations** (PPOs), **health maintenance organizations** (HMOs), and other health care service organizations.

warehouse, data   *see* **data repository.**

What's in it for me? (WIIFM)   a worker perception that any new initiative to improve quality or reduce cost should include some incentive for the worker.

why–why diagram   *see* **root cause diagram.**

withhold an amount or percentage of a **capitation** or fee for service payment held in a special account by a health plan in reserve for inappropriate utilization by providers. The withhold amount can be applied to any discrepancies between actual and expected costs for health care services.

work flow diagram a **relationship diagram** that tracks process flow on a diagram of the work site to identify the presence of unnecessary redundancy and rework.

work mapping methods of identifying the flow of resources through a **process** or processes with a chart or map that locates everyone in the organization involved in the process; also can be used as a means of acquainting team members with one another.

X-shaped matrix a matrix forming the shape of an X that relates four variables in groupings of 1 × (mult sym)2, i.e., one variable related simultaneously to two others.

Y-shaped matrix a matrix forming the shape of a Y that relates three individual variables to one another.

Z-statistic a normalized version of a statistic created by subtracting the group mean and dividing by the standard deviation; the **Z-statistic** reflects the number of standard deviations that a statistic varies from the mean of that statistic.

zero defects a philosophy espoused by Phillip Crosby to encourage organizations and workers to strive for zero defects in production of services or products.

Index

CPSIA information can be obtained at www.ICGtesting.com
233731LV00003B/9/P